Studies in language disability and remediation 1a

General editors:

David Crystal
Professor of Linguistic Science, University of Reading

Jean Cooper
Principal of the National Hospitals College of Speech Sciences, London

Also published in this series:

Working with LARSP

David Crystal

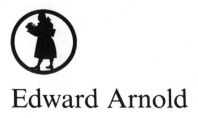

Edward Arnold

Introduction, sections 1.1–1.4 and part 4 © David Crystal 1979
sections 1.5, 1.6 and parts 2 and 3 © Edward Arnold (Publishers) Ltd 1979

First published 1979 by
Edward Arnold (Publishers) Ltd
41 Bedford Square, London WC1B 3DQ

Cloth edition ISBN: 0 7131 6117 5
Paper edition ISBN: 0 7131 6118 3

Working with LARSP.—(Studies in language disability
  and remediation; 1a).
  1. Communicative disorders
  2. Linguistic analysis (Linguistics)
  I. Crystal, David   II. Series
  616.8′55′0754

  ISBN 0–7131–6117–5
  ISBN 0–7131–6118–3

Printed in Great Britain by
Butler & Tanner Ltd, Frome and London

Contents

Contributors

Mary J. L. Auckland
  Clinical Chief Speech Therapist, Audiology Unit, Royal Berkshire Hospital
John M. Bamford
  Audiology Unit, Royal Berkshire Hospital
John Bench
  Audiology Unit, Royal Berkshire Hospital
Julie Brinton
  Chief Speech Therapist, Guy's Hospital, London
J. H. Connolly
  Lecturer in Linguistics, Leicester Polytechnic
D. B. Dennis
  Teacher in charge, Partially-Hearing Unit, Coleridge Secondary School, Cambridge
Paul Fletcher
  Department of Linguistic Science, University of Reading
Michael Garman
  Department of Linguistic Science, University of Reading
Corinne Haynes
  Chief Speech Therapist, Dawn House School, Rainworth, Nottinghamshire
Ella Hutt
  Remedial Teacher, John Horniman School, Worthing, Sussex
Elspeth Paul
  Formerly Chief Speech Therapist, Nuffield Hearing and Speech Centre, Royal National Throat Nose and Ear Hospital, London
J. E. Williams
  Peripatetic Teacher of Children with Impaired Hearing, Cambridgeshire Education Committee

General Preface

This series is the first to approach the problem of language disability as a single field. It attempts to bring together areas of study which have traditionally been treated under separate headings, and to focus on the common problems of analysis, assessment and treatment which characterize them. Its scope therefore includes the specifically linguistic aspects of the work of such areas as speech therapy, remedial teaching, teaching of the deaf and educational psychology, as well as those aspects of mother-tongue and foreign-language teaching which pose similar problems. The research findings and practical techniques from each of these fields can inform the others, and we hope one of the main functions of this series will be to put people from one profession into contact with the analogous situations found in others.

It is therefore not a series about specific syndromes or educationally narrow problems. While the orientation of a volume is naturally towards a single main area, and reflects an author's background, it is editorial policy to ask authors to consider the implications of what they say for the fields with which they have not been primarily concerned. Nor is this a series about disability in general. The medical, social, educational and other factors which enter into a comprehensive evaluation of any problems will not be studied as ends in themselves, but only in so far as they bear directly on the understanding of the nature of the language behaviour involved. The aim is to provide a much needed emphasis on the description and analysis of language as such, and on the provision of specific techniques of therapy or remediation. In this way, we hope to bridge the gap between the theoretical discussion of 'causes' and the practical tasks of treatment—two sides of language disability which it is uncommon to see systematically related.

Despite restricting the area of disability to specifically linguistic matters—and in particular emphasizing problems of the production and comprehension of spoken language—it should be clear that the series' scope goes considerably beyond this. For the first books, we have selected topics which have been particularly neglected in recent years, and which seem most able to benefit from contemporary research in linguistics and its related disciplines, English studies, psychology, sociology and education. Each volume will put its subject matter in perspective, and will provide an introductory slant to its presentation. In this way, we hope to provide specialized studies which can be used as texts for components of teaching courses, as well as material that is directly applicable to the needs of professional workers. It is also hoped that this orientation will place the series within the reach of the interested layman—in particular, the parents or family of the linguistically disabled.

David Crystal
Jean Cooper

Preface

This book has been written as a response to a demand for more detailed information concerning the application of the procedure described in *The grammatical analysis of language disability* (*GALD*: Crystal, Fletcher and Garman 1976). That book was primarily concerned to provide a theoretical perspective for work on language assessment and remediation, and thus a great deal of space was devoted to general issues. Since its appearance, LARSP has come to be used in a much wider range of clinical settings than we originally expected; also, the demand for in-service courses on the procedure has much increased, and it is being taught on diploma and degree training courses. As a result, we now know which aspects of the procedure give rise to the greatest problems of understanding, and we have accumulated much more experience in working routinely with LARSP in clinics and schools. The present book therefore tries to make good the deficiencies of *GALD*, by amplifying points of theory and practice which have led to misunderstanding, and by adding a large amount of illustration, some of which is re-analysed in workbook form (Part 4). Also, rather than attempting to summarize a wide range of LARSP's uses from assessment, remedial, research and teaching settings—and also to provide other points of view—I have asked some of the people who have been using the procedure in their work to contribute sections, and these are presented in Parts 2 and 3.

This book has one major limitation: it contains no example of the detailed application of the procedure to adults. Far fewer clinicians have begun to use LARSP routinely with adults than with children; and as a result of discussing why this is so, it seemed sensible to deal with the field of adult applications separately. We therefore anticipate a special publication on this topic. However, I am anxious that this decision should not foster the impression that LARSP is solely a child assessment procedure (as it has in fact been listed, in one bookseller's catalogue): the fact that it is more frequently used in this way seems simply to be a reflection of the clinical situation. The whole of Parts 1 and 4 can be applied directly to the analysis of adult clinical interaction, and indeed several of the insights discussed in Parts 2 and 3 are highly relevant to adult remediation. Nonetheless, we look forward to redressing the balance in due course.

For the present book, I have brought together a wide range of clinical examples to illustrate profile characteristics and grammatical structures, and I am most grateful to the many clinicians who have provided me with this material on the various LARSP courses, and who keep me informed of their progress in using the procedure. I owe particular thanks to the contributors to Parts 2 and 3, who have given this book an essential practical dimension. My colleagues Paul Fletcher and Michael Garman have not been co-authors this time, due to their individual writing and teaching commitments, but they have written sections of Part 2, and have provided advice and invaluable criticism at all stages of the compilation; and I am indebted to them for the way they have generously given their time to improve the book. My thanks, too, to Jill Tozer, for her speedy and accurate typing, and for her secretarial help with LARSP matters in general. As always, I have benefited from the editorial skills of Sarah Cohen and her colleagues at Edward Arnold, for transforming such an awkward typescript into something ready for printing; and I much appreciate the efficient handling of this complex setting by the staff of Butler and Tanner.

Above all, I thank my wife, Hilary, for the many ways she has helped the writing of this book: her work has affected every stage, from typing to proof-reading; and in her role as speech therapist, she has helped sharpen many of the clinical ideas expressed in this book. Without her support, *Working with LARSP* would have been much delayed, and much the poorer.

David Crystal
February 1978

Introduction

LARSP: Language Assessment, Remediation and Screening Procedure

A title of 16 syllables requires justification. Its purpose is to summarize the fundamental tenet of our investigations into pathological linguistic behaviour, that a *single* procedure can be developed which can integrate the three basic clinical operations of screening, assessment and remediation in the area of grammar. In the past, these tasks have usually been carried out separately. We may take an assessment tool, such as the Reynell or the ITPA, and establish levels of achievement accordingly; but having done this, there has been no systematic guidance about subsequent remediation. We may have learned a great deal about the child, in the process of carrying out the test, and some ideas for therapy may have sprung to mind, but there is no way in which these hints and impressions can provide the rationale for a therapeutic programme. The question 'What structure to teach next?' is still very much open. Conversely, if we take a remedial procedure such as one of the language-development kits or series, which list a definite sequence of teaching stages, then there will be plenty of guidelines concerning therapy, but in no way can these provide a principled basis for assessment or screening. The question 'What level of achievement has this child reached?' is still very much open. What is needed, it would seem, is a procedure which can relate these operations, showing how the skills of screening/assessment and remediation are functionally interdependent, and how information gained about any one can provide insights into the way in which the others may be implemented. The title, LARSP, reflects this general aim.

The term 'diagnostic', it should be noted, is noticeable by its absence. It would indeed be satisfying to contribute to the diagnosis of language pathologies, and to make predictions concerning the progress of a disorder and the efficacy of remedial measures; but at present insufficient empirical work has been done to enable us to provide a coherent linguistic account of the major clinical syndromes, or a set of criteria which would lead to more precise definitions of terms used in this field. We must begin with a detailed analysis of individual cases—to identify the linguistic characteristics of the disability of an *individual* patient or pupil (P), and to suggest guidelines for *individual* therapy. By looking in detail at samples of language behaviour, we can define immediate and long-term teaching goals, and then systematically explore the several different routes a therapist or teacher (T) may take in order to arrive at these goals. In due course we hope, by examining several cases of successful and unsuccessful therapy, to develop an explanatory account of the nature of linguistic intervention, and thus, ultimately, to contribute to a *theory* of language disability.

But a theoretical account of linguistic disability is a long-term and multi-disciplinary exercise, and in the meantime aims must be pragmatic—to make a useful contribution to ongoing therapy. What counts, however, as a 'useful contribution'? Evaluative criteria here must come, of course, from the professions involved (speech therapy, special education, etc.), and not from the linguist directly. Our interpretation of the clinical literature suggests that, to be justified, a linguistic procedure must be able to contribute to the main areas of clinical inquiry—as suggested above, to assessment and remediation, in the first instance. Its role must be judged, firstly, by the extent to which it provides T with *insight* into the character of P's disability, or of a disorder seen as a general type. By 'insight' here, two things are meant: (a) the observations made by the linguist were not being made by Ts working within traditional paradigms of inquiry (or which could not have been made thereby, due to their limited range); (b) the observations are productive, that is, they suggest patterns of assessment (by demonstrating the *systematic* nature of the data of disability, in given instances) and patterns of remediation (by making *predictions* concerning progress, motivating 'what to teach next?' and suggesting specific strategies of T–P interaction, e.g. the types of stimulus sentence to use).

Secondly, the role of linguistics must be judged by the extent to which it can introduce an element of conscious control into a clinical situation. This point, of course, applies to any technique of intervention, and indeed to the entire concept of speech therapy. The aim of the exercise is not solely to obtain progress in P, but to be sure that the progress obtained was due to the intervention of T, using T's professional expertise, and thus be able to explain the basis of any improvement or deterioration. It is a commonplace that many Ps can improve, given plenty of sympathy from relatives and a rich language environment. To what extent is improvement facilitated by therapeutic intervention? Sometimes it is possible to say with confidence that the therapy 'caused' the progress, especially when a rapid change in language ability is produced after a long period of stability or deterioration. It is even sometimes possible to arrange for comparative studies using control groups, though here the methodological and ethical problems are well known. But on the whole, verification of the efficacy of most therapeutic strategies is lacking, in scientifically convincing terms. If linguistic techniques are to be valuable, then, they should be able to introduce a greater measure of control over the nature of T–P interaction, thus helping to build up the professional confidence that clinical language work badly needs. There is no attempt here to suggest how far these techniques can help in achieving such a goal. By themselves they are not enough, as so many of the variables are non-linguistic in character. But it should be possible to show a *relative* gain in control, compared with most current practice; and it is just such an increased awareness of the linguistic variables involved affecting assessment and remediation that a linguistic procedure, such as LARSP, aims to provide, and by which it should be judged.

The notion of a profile

Dictionary definitions of *profile* indicate both the strengths and the weakness of the notion. 'An outline or concise sketch of an object,' runs one. It is plainly no more than a first approximation to an accurate description; but on the other hand it does imply that the salient, identifying features have been isolated. Notice, further, that a profile of an object becomes unrecognizable or confusing if *either* too few distinguishing features are given *or* too many. Nor is there any magical way in which the 'right' number and kind of features can be predicted in advance: they must be discovered empirically, and it is usually a lengthy process of trial and error. In this respect, language profiles are unlike, say, facial profiles: a detective's photofit kit works because of the limited range of variables involved in facial identification; the linguistic kit required is far more complex. But the principle is the same: every feature included in a profile kit—or chart—should be there because of its potential diagnostic value. There would be no point in having an item on a chart that was never used to discriminate individuals or groups. And thus it is with LARSP. The hundred or so linguistic features that occupy the bulk of the chart are there because they have been found to be useful, in the trial period when the procedure was being developed—that is, useful in the sense that contrasting assessments and remedial paths made use of such features. Naturally some features, or groups of features, turn out to be more regularly used than others— and in this the prospect of being able to make diagnostic judgements moves enticingly nearer—but all are demonstrably relevant to the task of coping with child and adult disability.

It is this principle which explains the varying amount of information at different points within the LARSP chart and the accompanying discussion in *GALD*. Some points in the language development process are pivotal, hence they need more attention if a profile is to 'catch' what is going on. This accounts for the main divisions of language into connectivity, clause, phrase and word levels, for instance; or the distinction between major and minor sentences, or between spontaneous and response utterances. At a more detailed level, the transitional information between Stages II/III, and III/IV is one area of particular significance (though frequently neglected in the clinical literature) (see below, p. 68); the clause-sequence complexity at Stage V is another (see p. 87), as is P's elliptical response patterns (see p. 45). From a remedial point of view, moreover, Stages I–V are especially relevant, hence the greater concentration. Stage VII in particular is very thinly characterized, so much so that some Ts have wondered why it is there at all. This Stage has largely mnemonic significance: it is included to remind people that several important grammatical features are still in the process of acquisition after age 5, and that a clinical disability could be grounded here. But the cases that arise are uncommon, and most Ts attend more routinely to the earlier Stages, which is where most of their caseload lies. As one T put it, 'If I have a child at Stage VII, I've more important things to do than profiles!' This attitude is not entirely valid. It is not an argument against profiles as such, but it *is* a limitation of this particular profile. The LARSP chart was not designed with Stage VII children primarily in mind.

The profile chart, in short, is an attempt to summarize the most frequently occurring indices of normal and abnormal grammatical development, and to provide a sufficient basis for plotting patterns of progress in this development. It might be possible to do this with fewer features on the chart, and omitting one or two features might make relatively little difference. But there is an enormous gap between the level of detail required by LARSP, or any similar procedure, and that found in the thumbnail-sketch assessments of grammatical disability common in the clinical literature, where the amount of information provided is insufficient to arrive at any coherent conclusion about the nature of the problem. It might be felt desirable, on the other hand, to *add* to the number of features on the chart— and individual clinicians have, we observe, often done this, e.g. expanding Stage VI errors to account for the more frequently occurring 'deafisms', subclassifying types of deviant sentences, or giving more information about types of verb at, say, Stage II (whether transitive, intransitive etc.). There are limits to the amount of complexity that a one-page chart can carry and a clinician assimilate, however, and rather than expand the chart in several directions simultaneously, more appropriate solutions are either (a) to redesign the chart, or a section of it, to meet one's personal needs (cf. the reports in 2.2 and 3.1 below) or (b) to develop the notion of 'micro-profiles'.

A micro-profile is a closer look at an area of the chart, using the same general procedure as was used to construct the chart as a whole. It is a necessary concomitant of any profile-oriented approach, which is—as already remarked—only a first approximation. It arises like this. We use the chart to obtain a more precise idea about which grammatical feature to focus upon, but having done this, we may still require more detailed information about the nature of the grammatical problem and its manner of acquisition. For instance, having identified Pronouns as a problem area (by an abnormally low figure at Stage III and a correspondingly high figure under 'Pronoun' at Stage VI Error), where does one go from there? It will be necessary to decide which pronouns to work on first, and in which grammatical and interactional contexts. To do this, one needs descriptive and developmental information of precisely the same kind as that required for the chart as a whole (see p. 11, ff below). A micro-profile for pronouns would then emerge, based on a synthesis of normal developmental findings, and this could be used as an assessment/remediation module, for that topic alone. *Any* label on the chart can be lifted out of the chart and given more detailed treatment, in this way. Whether it is worth doing depends solely on whether enough information has been accumulated in the language acquisition literature to make a Stages approach practicable. The point is discussed further below (p. 15), and micro-profiles of two areas are given in detail (1.7 and 1.8).

Is it possible to visualize the opposite of this process: the 'macro-profile'? This would be an attempt to construct profiles, encompassing not only grammar (which is the sole purpose of LARSP), but phonology and semantics—and perhaps even sociolinguistic and psycholinguistic development as well.[1] It is certainly possible, and desirable, to present data about disability in profile form for any of these areas;

[1] An example of a recent attempt to do this is Rieke *et al.* 1977.

but it is doubtful whether a single chart encompassing everything is more practicable or meaningful than the notion of a battery of profiles, implicit in the above.
The more variables one includes, the more difficult it becomes to see patterns
'across the board'. The various Stages one may wish to impose on the data are
not the same for the several areas. Nor in some cases is enough acquisitional information available for systematic profiles to be established—the dangers of over-
simplification and arbitrary selection are obvious. Rather than attempt to construct
a more grandiose profile of linguistic behaviour, therefore, we prefer to keep the
areas of investigation relatively small and compartmentalized—but never forgetting the arbitrary nature of the compartments so constructed, and the need to cross-
refer to other areas of language whenever problems are incapable of solution in
grammatical terms (cf. p. 16).

In principle, then, the notion of profile can be as large or as small as we care
to make it. In phonology, for example, we could construct a profile of the phonological system as a whole, or of the consonant system only, or of the plosive system,
or of initial plosives. . . . Underlying all such constructions, however, would be
the same concern to synthesize descriptive and developmental information, within
the context of assessment and remediation. There would also be the same belief
that profiles provide a constructive alternative to the limitations of working with
language scores. Single numerical scores for grammatical ability continue to be
widely used, and they can have utility; but with so many variables involved, such
scores are inevitably often ambiguous and indeterminate, and of negligible prog-
nostic value. We may, if we wish, reduce profiles to statistical configurations also—
and ultimately any normative or diagnostic procedure based upon this notion will
require adequate statistical support (cf. 3.1). But the essence of working with profiles is that the search for significant pattern is as much an intuitive as a mathemati-
cal skill, and is *always* multi-dimensional, involving repeated interpretive scans
of the chart in order to focus on sets of features which may suggest a significant
correlation. The process is illustrated throughout Parts 2 and 3.

Usage v. ability

A commonly-held fallacy about profiles is that they are a direct reflection of P's
ability. They are not: they reflect usage only. A profile is, in the first instance,
no more than a summary of the structures identified in a particular sample. We
may infer things about ability by interpreting the chart and the accompanying transcript, and this of course is the ultimate purpose of the exercise; but it must never
be forgotten that any such inferences constitute a separate process, made *after*
a profile has been compiled. In isolation, a profile tells us little about P's productive
control of a structure, nor about his comprehension of it. But this point is not
entirely negative.

Firstly, with reference to production. Given the occurrence of only one or two
instances of a structure in a sample, it might be premature to infer that P was
in control of that structure: the usages might have been produced by rote. On
the other hand, the fact that P did use those structures—as opposed to nothing

A	Unanalysed				Problematic		
	1 Unintelligible	2 Symbolic Noise	3 Deviant		1 Incomplete		2 Ambiguous

B	Responses				Normal Response									Abnormal		

						Elliptical Major				Full					
	Stimulus Type		Totals	Repet- itions	1	2	3	4	Full Major	Minor	Struc- tural	Ø	Prob- lems
		Questions											
		Others											

C	Spontaneous				Others	

		Minor			Social **10**	Stereotypes	Problems

Stage I (0;9–1;6) — Sentence Type

Major			Sentence Structure			
Excl.	Comm.	Quest.	Statement			
	·V·	·Q· **1**	·V· **7** ·N· **16**	Other **4**	Problems	

Stage II (1;6–2;0)

	Conn.	Clause		Phrase		Word
V X	Q X	SV **3**	V C/O **11**	DN **11**	VV	-ing
1		S C/O **6**	A X **8**	Adj N **4**	V part **7**	**3**
		Neg X **1**	Other	NN	Int X	pl
				PrN **9**	Other **2**	**1**
						-ed

Stage III (2;0–2;6)

		Clause		Phrase		
V X Y		X + S:NP	X + V:VP **1**	X + C/O:NP **4**	X + A:AP **2**	-en
	Q X Y	SVC/O	VC/OA	D Adj N	Cop	
let X Y	VS	SVA	VO_dO_i	Adj Adj N **2**	Aux	3s
do X Y		Neg X Y	Other	Pr DN	Pron	gen
				N Adj N	Other	

Stage IV (2;6–3;0)

		Clause		Phrase		
		X Y + S:NP	X Y + V:VP	X Y + C/O:NP	X Y + A:AP	n't
S	QVS	SVC/OA **1**	A A X Y	N Pr NP	Neg V	'cop
	Q X Y Z	SVO_iO_i	Other	Pr D Adj N	Neg X	'aux
				c X	2 Aux	
				X c X **1**	Other	

Stage V (3;0–3;6)

			Clause		Phrase		
		and	Coord. **1**	**1**	Postmod. **1** clause	**1** +	-est
how	tag	c	Subord. **1**	**1**			
		s	Clause: S		Postmod. **1** phrase		-er
what		Other	Clause: C/O				
			Comparative				-ly

(+)			(−)		
NP	VP	Clause	NP	VP	Clause

Stage VI (3;6–4;6)

NP		VP	Clause	NP		VP	Clause
Initiator		Complex	Passive	Pron	Adj seq	Modal	Concord
Coord			Complement	Det	N irreg	Tense	A position
						V irreg	W order
Other				Other			

Stage VII (4;6+)

Discourse		Syntactic Comprehension	
A Connectivity	it		
Comment Clause	there	Style	
Emphatic Order	Other		

Total No. Sentences **70**	Mean No. Sentences Per Turn **1·2**	Mean Sentence Length **2·6**

© D. Crystal, P. Fletcher, M. Garman, 1975 University of Reading

Fig. 1   John at 4;3

at all, for instance—is worth noting, as it at least provides T with a suggested line
of intervention, and whether there *is* a productive command of the structure can
be readily established, by eliciting (or failing to elicit) further structures of the same
type in a structured situation designed for that purpose. Similarly, a high figure
opposite a category needs to be carefully evaluated, in case it is the result of
repeated use of a reduced lexical range: Adj N 35 may count as a genuine instance
of productive control of that category, but this view would have to be modified
if it turned out that, say, 32 of the adjectives were colour adjectives. (The effect
of semantic considerations on the interpretation of profiles is discussed separately
on p. 18). A more complex example of the interpretive problem is given in Fig. 1,
which is part of the profile of a 4-year-old expressive language delayed child.
The profile is fairly typical, in that it shows a peak of usage (at Stage II, in this
case) and a thin scatter of smaller structures further down the chart. These
structures should not be ignored, as they may well provide the key to P's future
progress, but in the present profile we must interpret them judiciously. The sample
has brought to light an instance of XcX (/'Tom and Jèrry/), SVOA (/'me gòt 'one
'now/), and two instances of Adj Adj N (/'big 'black bòx/ and /'nice 'big bàlloon/).
Given the absence of any other structures at Stage IV, it would be premature
to attribute too much significance to the XcX and SVOA instances (there is evidently still some difficulty with earlier Stages). On the other hand, the fact that
big turns up on two separate occasions, in different lexical contexts, is more useful,
and suggests that perhaps there is some productive control here.

It is important to remember, also, that the profile chart is neutral about the
comprehension of the utterances located upon it (cf. *GALD*, 24). The fact that
a structure is used by P in an interpretable way is sufficient basis for it to be placed
on the chart. P may not fully comprehend what he has said, but—as in the case
of production above—the fact that a certain structure has been used at all is not
without significance. If it is suspected that comprehension is not present, then this
can be checked on in a structured situation. And the chart can then be used as
an index of comprehended v. uncomprehended structures (by marking the former
with one convention, the latter with another, as in Fig. 2). For example, if P says
'got pèncil/, when it is plain that he has not got one (and nor has anyone else),
this would still be analysed as VO; the inappropriateness of the remark would
be noted in the transcription margins. If there were a persistent mis-match between
expressive and receptive command of VO structures in this P, this would emerge
by the accumulation of marginal comments (or by the incidence of conventions
such as X and ? on the chart, as in Fig. 2). Likewise, if P says /bìg 'doggy/, choosing
the smaller of a pair, this would be analysed as Adj N, again with a marginal note
about the (semantic) error. The only cases where lack of comprehension is given
any direct reference on the chart is when it is possible to assign a clearly grammatical basis to the error. The above examples are not like this; but if P were to say,
for example, /'man 'bite dòg/ (when he means 'dog bite man'), or /I 'did gò/ (meaning 'I am going'), then apart from a marginal comment in the transcription, it
would be possible to incorporate the information within the Stage VI Error section
(see p. 96), which was explicitly designed to cope with incomplete command of

A

Unanalysed   **Problematic**

1 Unintelligible   2 Symbolic Noise   3 Deviant   1 Incomplete   2 Ambiguous

B

Responses

Stimulus Type		Totals	Repet-itions	Normal Response								Abnormal			
				Elliptical Major				Full Major	Minor	Struc-tural	Ø		Prob-lems
				1	2	3	4						
Questions													
Others													

C

Spontaneous   Others

		Minor			Social ✓6 ?2 Stereotypes			Problems			

Stage I (0;9–1;6) · Sentence Type

Major			Sentence Structure				
Excl.	Comm.	Quest.	Statement				
	·V·	·Q·	·V· ✓2 ·N· ✓6 ✗3 Other ✓1 Problems				

Stage II (1;6–2;0)

	Conn.	Clause			Phrase		Word
VX	QX	SV	VC/O ✓3	DN ✓4	VV ✓2		-ing 1
	✗3	S C/O	AX ✓2	Adj N ?6	V part		pl ✗3
		Neg X ✗4	Other	NN	Int X ✓1		-ed ✗2
				PrN ✓4 ?7	Other		

Stage III (2;0–2;6)

		X + S:NP	X + V:VP I	X + C/O:NP I	X + A:AP	-en
VXY	QXY	SVC/O ?4	VC/OA	D Adj N	Cop	
let XY	VS	SVA	VO$_d$O$_i$	Adj Adj N	Aux	3s
do XY		Neg XY	Other	Pr DN	Pron ✓3	gen
				N Adj N	Other	

Stage IV (2;6–3;0)

		XY S:NP	XY V:VP	XY + C/O:NP	XY + A:AP	n't
+ S	QVS	SVC/OA	AAXY	N Pr NP	Neg V	'cop
	QXYZ	SVO$_d$O$_i$	Other	Pr D Adj N	Neg X	'aux
				cX	2 Aux ✗1	
				XcX	Other	

Stage V (3;0–3;6)

how	tag	and	Coord. 1	1	Postmod. 1 clause	1 +	-est
		c	Subord. 1	1 ·			-er
		s	Clause: S		Postmod. 1 · phrase		
what	Other		Clause: C/O				-ly
			Comparative				

Stage VI (3;6–4;6)

(+)			(−)			
NP	VP	Clause	NP		VP	Clause
Initiator	Complex	Passive	Pron	Adj seq	Modal	Concord
Coord		Complement	Det	N irreg	Tense	A position
					V irreg	W order
Other			Other			

Stage VII (4;6+)

Discourse		Syntactic Comprehension
A Connectivity	it	
Comment Clause	there	Style
Emphatic Order	Other	

Total No. Sentences	Mean No. Sentences Per Turn	Mean Sentence Length

Fig. 2   One T's method of locating comprehension problems (X = structure used but not comprehended; √ = structure used and comprehended; ? = comprehension uncertain)

a grammatical pattern—in the former case, a Clause Word Order error (in addition to SVO at Stage III), in the latter case, a Tense error (in addition to the SV, Pron etc. further up the chart).

The above discussion relates primarily to T's assessment of expressive ability. It is of course also possible to use the chart as an index of comprehension. This would happen if T used the chart's organization to grade structures for presentation to P, as one would with any syntactic comprehension task. One aspect of Sarah's remediation (see p. 106), for example, involved T proceeding to elicit *VOA* (e.g. 'put dolly there'), then

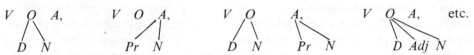

in general conformity to the chart's progression. A structured session based on *VOA* was profiled, and then compared with one based on *VOA* with *DN* expansion, and so on. The comparison indicated the extent for which the selected structures were facilitating responses, and provided a valuable clue to P's developing comprehension.

Finally, in all this, we must remember that a comprehension profile will not necessarily parallel a production profile for the same P. There is no neat relationship between comprehension and production, so that we can simply say the one always precedes the other (see Clark 1974, Clark *et al.* 1974, Rees forthcoming; and below on sampling procedures).

Three kinds of knowledge

Clinical competence requires three dimensions of linguistic knowledge. First, T must be able to *describe* P's linguistic behaviour; secondly, she must be able to *grade* the complexity of that behaviour; and thirdly, she must be able to analyse the *interaction* with P at an appropriate linguistic level. The LARSP profile extracts all three kinds of information from a sample: accordingly, it is worth devoting some space to a discussion of the significance of each dimension.

The descriptive issue facing T is simply summarized: how much grammatical apparatus is it necessary to master before patterns of disability can be described? In answering this, we would do well to remember the dictum 'Anything that *can* go wrong *will*, sooner or later.' There are no sacrosanct syntactic structures. Therefore the more grammatical knowledge we can acquire about the total linguistic system—i.e. an adult grammar of English—the more prepared we will be for coping with the unexpected syntactic eventuality. A selection of structures obviously has to be made in devising a practicable clinical procedure, but it is important to be aware of the principles on which the selection was made, and how to supplement the simplified description, as need arises. Chapter 3 of *GALD* outlines a set of structures which we have found to be an obligatory minimum in working with disability; but we do sometimes find it necessary to add to this description in analysing a given P, who may be subtly defective in precisely one of those areas on which chapter 3 has little or nothing to say. At this point, T ought to refer routinely to the appropriate sections of a reference grammar, such as the one we use (Quirk and Greenbaum 1973, or Quirk *et al*. 1972). Similarly, in the construction of micro-profiles (see 1.7), an essential step is the setting up of a framework in which the various structural alternatives in a grammatical area are described and interrelated. Working with pronouns, to take a clear case, we need to know how many there are, how they vary in form in different functions (e.g. *I* becoming *me*, *me* becoming *mine*), and what restrictions there are on their use in different parts of a sentence. This might take very little preparation. In more difficult cases, such as the modal verbs or complement structures, the amount of preparatory organizing will be much greater. But it is an essential step in developing a principled therapy. The alternative—to take the first examples of a structure that 'come to mind', without seeing how they relate to the rest of the grammatical area—can land T in diffi-culties. Witness the T who, wanting to work with Determiners, chose *some/any* to start with. They are very practicable forms to use, as they correlate easily with real situations, e.g. *Have you got some?* But their grammar is very tricky: *I have got some*, but not *I have got any*; *I haven't got any cake*, but not usually *I haven't got some cake*. P, of course, assumed the verb-negation system he knew from pre-vious language experience would apply in this case—with predictably confusing results.

The principle we advocate in describing P's linguistic behaviour is a deceptively simple one: *everything* P says in a sample must be explicitly accounted for on the profile chart. The more an analytic procedure leaves out, the less valuable it is as an objective tool. The information that has been omitted, due to the analyst feeling it (intuitively) to be less important, may well turn out to be significant, when comparing the sample with others, at a later date. The point is that, in the present state of the art, there is no way of guaranteeing in advance that a particular structural area will be of no value. The only safe procedure to follow, accordingly, is to ensure that everything linguistic is in. But how is this principle of comprehen-siveness compatible with that of selectivity, referred to above? The device used on the LARSP Chart which relates the two is the regular use of the 'Other' category. Any structure which is not given separate mention is placed anonymously under 'Other'. But this category is more than just sleight of hand. It has both pragmatic and diagnostic significance. Pragmatically, it permits the rapid categorization of several infrequent but syntactically awkward constructions (e.g. at Stage II, *in there* = Prep Adv, *another one* = Det Pron). Diagnostically, in 'normal' cases of lan-guage delay, the figure under 'Other' is always low—as would that of a normal child at that Stage. If the figure gets at all high, however, then this is immediately worth investigating further. In Fig. 3, we see such a profile, from a 4-year-old. The high Stage II and Stage III figures are striking. In this case, they reflect a frequent use of deictic words (*this, that, here, there, him, her*, etc.) as the heads of noun phrases. Examples from P's transcript are *put in there, give to him, give that one, want more that*. Vincent relied very much on such constructions, which is a strategy that works, of course, only when the context is sufficiently clear to provide referents for *there, him*, etc. His expressive language ability is therefore

A

	Unanalysed				Problematic	
	1 Unintelligible	2 Symbolic Noise	3 Deviant		1 Incomplete	2 Ambiguous

B

	Responses				Normal Response							Abnormal		
					Elliptical Major				Full			Struc-		Prob-
	Stimulus Type		Totals	Repet-itions	1	2	3	4	Major	Minor	tural	Ø		lems
		Questions												
		Others												

C

	Spontaneous				Others	

Stage I (0;9–1;6) — Sentence Type

Minor			Social **6**	Stereotypes		Problems

Major — Sentence Structure

Excl.	Comm.	Quest.		Statement	
	·V·	·Q·	·V· **6** ·N· **4**	Other **7**	Problems

			Conn.	Clause		Phrase		Word

Stage II (1;6–2;0)

	VX	QX		SV **4**	VC/O **9**	DN **7**	VV **2**	-ing
				SC/O **1**	AX **5**	Adj N **1**	V part **1**	
				Neg X	Other	NN	Int X	pl
						PrN **5**	Other **17**	

Stage III (2;0–2;6)

			X + S:NP	X + V:VP **4**	X + C/O:NP **21**	X + A:AP **7**	-ed
	VXY			SVC/O **5**	VC/OA	D Adj N **1**	Cop	-en
		QXY	VS	SVA **2**	VO$_d$O$_i$	Adj Adj N	Aux **2**	
	let XY		Neg XY	Other	Pr DN	Pron **24**	3s
	do XY				N Adj N	Other **14**	gen

Stage IV (2;6–3;0)

			XY + S:NP	XY V:VP	XY + C/O:NP	XY + A:AP	n't
		QVS	SVC/OA	AAXY	N Pr NP	Neg V	
	S	QXYZ	SVO$_d$O$_i$	Other	Pr D Adj N	Neg X	'cop
					cX	2 Aux	'aux
					XcX	Other **2**	

Stage V (3;0–3;6)

			and	Coord. **1**	1 ·	Postmod. **1** clause	1 +	-est
	how	tag	c	Subord. **1**	1 ·			-er
			s	Clause: S		Postmod. **1** · phrase		
	what		Other	Clause: C/O				-ly
				Comparative				

(+)			(−)		
NP	VP	Clause	NP	VP	Clause

Stage VI (3;6–4;6)

Initiator	Complex	Passive	Pron	Adj seq	Modal	Concord
Coord		Complement	Det	N irreg	Tense	A position
					V irreg	W order
Other			Other			

Stage VII (4;6 +)

Discourse		Syntactic Comprehension	
A Connectivity	it		
Comment Clause	there	Style	
Emphatic Order	Other		

Total No. Sentences	Mean No. Sentences Per Turn	Mean Sentence Length

© D. Crystal, P. Fletcher, M. Garman, 1975 University of Reading

Fig. 3 Vincent at 4;2

deceptively high, in this profile. As soon as Vincent was asked to talk about things and events *outside of* the immediate environment, his language markedly deteriorated (to Stage I–II levels).[2] The 'Other' category, in this instance, turned out to be the key to our understanding of Vincent's limitations, which had previously been overlooked: the everyday, familiar ring of deictic expression sometimes makes it difficult to see how limiting and ambiguous an area it is. (With normal children, parental tuition concerning the limitations of deictics comes very early, as the following dialogue illustrates:

> Parent (*downstairs, having heard a crash*) 'what's 'that nòise/
> Child (*upstairs*)   it 'fell òver/
> Parent   whàt fell 'over/
> Child   thàt did/
> Parent   whàt 'did/ (etc.))

The second main kind of linguistic knowledge required by T is how to grade the complexity of P's behaviour, and it is this which motivates the inclusion of the developmental dimension on the profile chart. The developmental dimension is essential, moreover, as only this can bridge the gap between assessment and remediation referred to on p. 3 above: the various stages recognized provide a ready-made framework for assessment, and motivate several possible remedial paths. The arguments for basing this dimension on the findings of studies of normal language acquisition were reviewed in *GALD* (25 ff): the argument is not that this provides the best possible basis, but the best available basis. If and when independent measures of cognitive/linguistic complexity come to be established, they may well perform better than acquisitional guidelines; but there is no likelihood of such measures becoming available in the near future, and the same applies to any of the other potential measures (e.g. difficulty of perception, memory, recall etc.). Language acquisition studies, however, while presenting some difficulties of their own (see below), are much less problematic. What must be emphasized, though, is that there is no necessary correlation between order of acquisition and the notion of complexity. The fact that there is a tendency for children to acquire structures and categories in a certain order is one thing. Whether a child finds any of these more or less complex than others is a quite different thing: too many other variables intervene (of which motivation to learn is perhaps the most relevant) to make any such correlation more than simply tentative.

As emphasized in *GALD* (60), the model of development in terms of discrete acquisitional stages derives from the empirical findings of the main grammatical studies of normal children. A synthesis has been made of the order of emergence of the various structures and categories along with the associated chronological range of the child samples. The fact that, to some degree, these stages display an apparent increase in complexity in terms of length (1 element, 2 elements, 3 elements, 4 or more elements) is not explicable in linguistic terms alone: any explana-

---

[2] This is the kind of reasoning lying behind the sampling procedure advocated in *GALD*, (87–8). The two samples of present and absent contexts make very different linguistic demands on P—see further below, p. 21. For a further example, see p. 202.

tion as to why these stages are as they are would have to refer in addition to developmental hypotheses concerning memory, attention, perception and cognition. The stages 'work', as a descriptive framework, and as a source of suggestions concerning the developmental relationships between structures, but the LARSP chart *per se* does not say *why* these particular patterns of relationship exist. Nor is any claim made about the typical strategies of learning used by children in arriving at these stages (see further p. 114).[3]

The Stages must, therefore, be seen as a reflection of the strengths and the limitations of the language acquisition literature. This is a literature whose data-base is almost exclusively middle-class, and this emphasis ought to be borne in mind when interpreting chronological ages. It is a literature, also, which is particularly strong on grammatical structures up to around age 4, and information about development becomes less well-grounded, accordingly, as we approach the later stages of the chart. But even within the early stages some topics and processes have been investigated much more thoroughly than others, and awareness of the relevant literature is essential if the fullest clinical use is to be made of any acquisition-based procedure. Both *SVO* and *SVA* are located at Stage III, for example; but far more analysis has been carried out of the uses of the former construction (and its transformational potential) than the latter. Likewise, Pronouns and Auxiliaries co-occur at Stage III, but the former has attracted more study than the latter, and we are therefore more confident about 'placing' the category at this Stage. Further comments on the accuracy and limitations of the various Stages will be made separately in Part 2. It is always in principle possible for fresh surveys of acquisition to broaden the data-base and suggest alternative orderings on the chart. The Stages are only as valid as the research on which they are based.

It must be remembered that the rationale for placing a grammatical category, such as Pronoun or Copula, on the chart is not the time at which instances of its use *first* appear, but the time period wherein the particular grammatical system seems to be undergoing its maximal rate of development, both in terms of increased frequency and—where relevant—membership of the category. Thus, for example, a pronoun may first be heard at Stage I, with errors still being made in their use at Stage VI; however, the most noticeable increase in the number of different pronouns used, and in the frequency of use of a given pronoun, takes place at Stage III, and this is why the item is lodged there. Placement in III also makes sense, in that the increased frequency can be related to other developments in syntax taking place during the same period (e.g. 3-element structures involving a relatively short *S* and long *O*, cf. Limber 1976).

The third kind of knowledge on the profile chart—the interactional dimension—is represented by Sections B and C (see also the putative Section D, p. 55 below). Two measures are involved: the ratio of P's spontaneous to response utterances, and the kind of response made by P to T's stimulus. The aim of this section is not to be exhaustive about interaction. It is simply to focus T's attention

[3] We also do not wish to underemphasize the potential importance of the *individual* strategy, in learning to use a structure (cf. e.g. Clark 1974, Limber 1973), though we feel this must be seen in the context of an invariant order hypothesis for most structures for most children.

on what may ultimately be the largest question which has to be faced: is P's failure to respond due to genuine inadequacy on P's part, or on T's inability to produce a stimulus within P's range? There is a common tendency to dismiss many patients as 'having reached their limit', 'ineducable' etc., and while this may sometimes be the only reasonable conclusion, it would be premature if the whole range of intervention procedures has not been tried. T can readily avoid this pitfall, but only if she is in principle aware of the levels of difficulty posed by different kinds of stimuli, can identify levels of response by P, and can react to these levels in appropriate ways. The LARSP procedure, as it stands, is only a partial answer in these respects. It focuses on P's responses, and spends little space on T. In later sections of this book, however, several further suggestions are made for ways of taking this area further.

In the meantime, it should be noted that Sections B and C are *not* developmentally oriented: they provide an analysis based on the response norms of adult interaction, and as such, sometimes make use of concepts which are inapplicable further down the chart (e.g. Abnormal responses, Repetition).

The remaining sections of the chart (Section A, and the bottom line) provide information of a mixed kind. Sentence length is partly descriptive, partly developmental; sentences per turn is interactional. The categories of Section A are partly there for methodological descriptive reasons (to simplify the analytic process, cf. p. 25), but they can be interpreted developmentally, and used as part of an assessment. Detailed comments on their role are provided below.

The focus on grammar

No procedure is a panacea. It selects certain features for attention and ignores others, and is therefore appropriate for a limited range of applications. Learning to use LARSP efficiently, then, is both a matter of understanding what is there on the chart, and also a matter of understanding what is *not* there. In this respect, the main consideration is to note that LARSP deals solely with grammar (syntax and morphology), not phonology, semantics, pragmatics, pre-linguistic vocalization, or the analysis of other aspects of communicative behaviour. The reasons for this focus are given in *GALD* chapter 1. Having chosen this focus, we have attempted to work with it consistently, drawing as sharp a dividing-line as possible between grammatical and other factors. Of course, ultimately any grammatical analysis must take into account its interconnections with these other factors, especially phonology and semantics. Sometimes, even, it is not possible to identify or analyse a grammatical construction without help from these directions. But while we accept the importance of using phonological and semantic criteria as part of the heuristic process (i.e. in arriving at our analysis), we do not describe phonological or semantic features as such on the LARSP chart.

In particular, this means that intonation patterns are excluded (and likewise gestures, facial expressions etc.), when these are used as substitutes for grammatical forms. The most widely-cited example here is the use of intonation as a means of expressing a questioning attitude—a rising pitch on a sentence in statement

form, as in *He's coming?* This is an important point, as before children learn to
question using conventional grammatical means, intonation may be used in a
similar way—and with many language-disordered Ps, this is the sole means they
have available in the early stages of language development. But the devices which
are adopted in order to anticipate or avoid grammar are not themselves grammatical. There is no neat one-to-one correlation between a language's intonation
patterns and its grammatical structures. Intonation is a notoriously ambiguous
marker, in isolation from semantic, contextual and other variables (see Crystal
1975, chapter 1). To take the present example, it is *not* the case that

(i)   rising pitches always signal a questioning attitude, or
(ii)   that grammatical questions always have rising pitches.

A low rising pitch on a statement (e.g. *that's ↓nice/*) may have a guarded, reserved,
or warning meaning (if the face is solemn), or a sympathetic, friendly meaning
(if the face is pleasant). A high rising pitch (e.g. *he's ↑cóming/*) may mean no more
than shocked surprise, there being no intention to ask for a response at all. In
P utterances, where there is often lack of a clear context, it is frequently totally
unclear whether a questioning or non-questioning intent is involved: e.g. P holds
up a bear and says, in a high rising squeak */téddy/*, T may take this to mean 'is
this a teddy?', or equally 'I've got a teddy (and am very excited about it)'. In short,
it would be misleading to put 'Intonation' onto the chart, at the top of the Question
column, as this would suggest a unique, unambiguous relationship between phonology and grammar which simply does not exist. It would also be inappropriately
placed, because the child's developing use of intonation is something which we
would expect to see on a phonology profile chart, not a grammatical one. We are
not, therefore, saying that no attention should be paid to uses of intonation such
as the above—solely that P's abilities here should not be confused with his
grammatical abilities. (A similar argument applies in relation to types of stimuli
in Section B, p. 40, and to other potential grammar/intonation correspondences
referred to later in this book.)

Other kinds of phonological information have also been excluded from the
chart, despite their developmental interest. In particular, we note the importance
of the various phonological stages which the child goes through as he approaches
the point where his utterances would for the first time be entered on the chart,
at Stage I. Such developments have been well described by Dore *et al.* (1976), who
point to the role of phonetically consistent forms in the stages we call transitional—
the second element of Stage II being 'anticipated', as it were, by a phonetic form
which is attached to the single-element utterance. Such patterns could be of considerable significance in assessment, and particularly in deciding when and how
far to intervene with work on a specific structure. But we have not incorporated
such interactions between phonetics and syntax into the chart.

Semantic information, likewise, is not directly represented on this profile chart,
e.g. information about the meanings of Stage I utterances, the semantic relationships between clause elements at Stage II (cf. Brown 1973), the patterns of lexical
over- and under-extension observed from the second year (cf. Clark & Clark 1977),

the interaction between the developing cognitive and linguistic systems, and so on. These would all be matter for a semantic profile chart. On the other hand, while the patterns displayed on the LARSP chart are not themselves semantic, it must not be forgotten that the *explanation* of the grammatical patterns which appear may indeed require reference to semantic factors. A good example is the deviance pattern found in Jannine (see p. 28), where an apparently grammatical problem (gross word-order errors) turned out to have a semantic/cognitive explanation—the only sentences which displayed such errors were those which were attempting to express a small set of semantic notions (in particular, to do with 'location'). A second example of the interplay between semantics and profile interpretation has already been mentioned (p. 9).

Developmental pragmatic (or sociolinguistic) information is also not represented categorically on the profile chart. By such a label we are referring to the different configurations and frequencies of structures used by a child in different social contexts, such as talking to parents, strangers, clinicians, other children etc. This point is taken up under Sampling, below: pragmatic information may not be present on the chart as such, but it is of course deducible from a comparison of profiles made in different social situations.

Part 1

The LARSP procedure

1.1

Sampling and transcription

Seven distinct stages are involved in making use of a procedure such as LARSP, each raising its own problems. These are:

1   sampling
2   transcription
3   grammatical analysis
4   profiling
5   interpretation
6, 7   remediation goals and procedures.

Part 1 reviews the difficulties most commonly cited in using LARSP with reference to these headings.

Sampling

The very first decision T has to make is the nature of the sample on which the profile will be based. In *GALD* chapter 5, we review several possibilities, and recommend a particular procedure—a 30-minute sample broken down into two 15-minute parts, one in which T talks to P about P's immediate environment, actions etc., and one in which the conversation is about absent situations. The reasons for choosing this particular sample-size are given on pp. 87–8 of *GALD*: we were primarily interested in devising a method which could be a viable foundation for research work using LARSP, with the ultimate aim of comparing groups of patients for diagnostic purposes. Hence we wanted a reasonably large sample, and one which would include a wide range of sentence patterns (this being the point of building in the contrast in subject-matter, as the present/absent distinction promotes the use of very different linguistic structures, e.g. deictic forms, tenses, sequences of clauses, cf. p. 14). It is also a sample size which corresponds well to a clinical session, and is thus easily introduced into the routine of clinical practice. On the other hand, it is evident that a full 30-minute sample will take some time to process. If T does all the work herself, it will take the best part of a morning to get from transcription to complete profile, and this is impracticable in several clinical settings. How may the problem of time be lessened, therefore? We have found four ways in common use, though we would commend only the first two:

(i) *T does not do all the work herself.* A considerable amount of time is taken up by the initial orthographic transcription of the tape, and if this can be given to an aide or other special helper, a considerable saving is obtained. (It is never to be seen as a secretarial task, however, cf. *GALD*, 91.) T should always check the transcription herself, of course, as – unless the transcriber is very experienced – there will be the occasional misinterpretation. A short training period in the main transcriptional conventions (especially on such points as putting sentences on separate lines, and leaving spaces where there are pauses) will always be needed. It is surprising how expert helpers can become at this task in a short time, especially if they know P.

(ii) *T reduces the size of the sample*. There is no magic in the '30 minute' rule: other sampling periods are possible and often more useful or practicable. With some (e.g. some severely subnormal) Ps, the sample size may have to be extended, to obtain enough data to provide a worthwhile analysis. But in most cases, the question is how *small* a sample it is possible to get away with. Everything, of course, depends on T's purpose. If the aim is a quick screening, to provide some general indications of immediate remedial goals, then a sample of 5 minutes may suffice, as a first step. Many Ts, we find, operate with a 10- or 15-minute sample. The LARSP approach works on such small samples, for two main reasons:

(a) A profile emerges fairly quickly, as the analysis of a single sentence can produce several marks on the chart, e.g. *The man is kicking the ball* will involve no less than nine marks (SVO, DN, Aux, DN, XY + S:NP, XY + V:VP, XY + O:NP, 3s, -ing);

(b) The vast majority of Ps have a *stable* linguistic pattern, in the short term: if we profile the first 5 minutes of an interaction, then the next 5, then the next etc., and compare the results, it will be noted that there are *far* more similarities than differences, and the differences become markedly less as the sampling proceeds. This is only what we would expect from such a sampling procedure, but it also means that any 5-minute sample is likely to contain the 'core' of P's structures, and thus be a reliable indication of P's system. This is *not* a deduction we can make for normal adults, or linguistically advanced children; but it does seem to be valid for the bulk of the language-disordered population. Ts, we find, can make confident judgements about the typicality or otherwise of a 5-minute sample, and it is this which we rely on in interpreting any profile results obtained in this way. However, to arrive at the profound level of understanding prerequisite for developing a full-scale assessment or remedial programme, larger samples will obviously be necessary.

(iii) *T does not do the prosodic analysis*. As might be imagined, we are not happy at such a short-cut. Too much of significance can be missed, and, at worst, one may end up with a misleading estimate of P's speech ability (T having read in 'complete' structures, or made different divisions from those suggested by the prosody). We cannot stress strongly enough the need for T to improve her skills in this area, if improvement is needed. Analysing speech without taking the prosody into account is a step in the direction of abdicating professional responsibility.

But having said this, we recognize that for some Ps a punctuation-based account may be better than no account at all. Hence if T is unable to proceed with prosody, whether for reasons of training or time, we would recognize the limited usefulness of a punctuated transcript in providing the input to the grammatical analysis.

(iv) *T does not use Sections B and C of the chart.* The developmental Section of the chart (below the thick black line) is certainly the Section whose purpose is most readily perceivable and immediately applicable. But in terms of arriving at a full assessment or any systematic remedial programme, focusing on Sections B and C is essential. The point is discussed further below (pp. 33 ff). A short-cut here can lead to quite erroneous conclusions being drawn about P's linguistic abilities (e.g. his spontaneity, creativity, or naturalness).

In relation to the problem of time, several pragmatic points should be borne in mind (cf. *GALD*, 24–5):

(a) T's first attempts to use the procedure will naturally be far more time-consuming than later work. In our in-service courses, for example, profiling time is reduced by over half, once the procedure has been gone through two or three times.

(b) The question of time must be seen within a long-term perspective: an extra outlay of time at certain points within a treatment programme may lead to great savings overall. But quantitative reasoning is very uncertain: what is more definite is the way in which any outlay of time on analysis of P's data leads to a more confident and systematic therapy. This is true for any linguistic procedure, on any language level; but it is particularly relevant for work in grammar, where there is a large number of simultaneously occurring variables that are impossible to assimilate and interpret in an impressionistic way.

(c) In practice, it is not necessary to sample and profile frequently. A single profile can, and usually does, provide T with enough indications of structural weakness to provide material for several therapeutic sessions. After an initial profile, a gap of 1–3 months is quite normal before T feels a further profile is needed to provide a systematic account of progress and fresh suggestions for remedial action. In particularly rapidly-moving and confusing patients, more frequent profiling may be warranted; but this is uncommon.

(d) Also, in practice, the analysis and profiling of many samples of delayed language is often less time-consuming than one might expect it to be, because the bulk of the utterances are at the early stages of development. The corollary is also worth noting: when first working with profiles, it is generally easier *not* to take samples of normal children. The profile chart becomes increasingly less useful, as the language of the subject matures. This is as it should be; but it therefore follows that using it on normal child samples after the age of about $3\frac{1}{2}$ is likely to be an experience that is atypical of routine caseloads, and therefore of limited value. Nor should one learn to use the profile on normal adult samples, because of the wide range of advanced problems encountered there (cf. *GALD* profile, 107).

Lastly, concerning speech sampling, the question arises of what one should do if a sample turns out to be largely unintelligible. If this is genuinely so—that is, no-one (including parents) can understand it—then this would be *prima facie* evidence for the need to work in the first instance on other aspects of communication than grammar. But if someone can understand some or all of it, it is perfectly in order for that person's 'translations' to be used as the primary data for analysis. A parent's helpful glosses may in the end be the only data T has to go on, and in such cases it is obviously desirable to use it (rather than consign the whole sample to the Unintelligible box, where it is is no use to anyone). We should always bear in mind the potential reading-in that parents do, but this is hardly likely to affect a profile in any serious way. Of course, if an intermediary is used in this manner, the point should be noted in P's profile records, for comparison with subsequent profiles where it would be hoped that P's language would become increasingly autonomous.

So far, the discussion of sampling has been wholly in terms of spontaneous speech; but the importance of two other kinds of sample, in some types of patient, should not be overlooked. Firstly, a profile may be made of some non-spontaneous speech sample, e.g. the set of responses to a fixed set of questions, or to a specific pictorial stimulus. An example of profile analysis based on a sample of imitation responses is given in Part 3.2. A further variable is whether the sample is of P talking to parent, clinician, or other children. Secondly, other media than speech may be sampled. Section 2.5, for instance, is based on samples of free writing provided in a given timespan. We might also want to use the procedure for the analysis of the signed patterns of contrived signing systems (i.e. those where the grammatical pattern of the language was being followed, e.g. the Paget Gorman Sign System), or any other language-based code.

Transcription

Practice in transcribing speech patterns, especially prosody, ideally needs to be carried out under the watchful eye of a phonetician, who can juxtapose the contrasts involved in ways that do not turn up in connected speech. A second method is to follow a transcription of speech while listening to the original tape. Several such recordings are now available in the foreign-language teaching context (e.g. Crystal and Davy 1976, O'Connor and Arnold 1973), and these are quite satisfactory for developing skills in this area.

The visual side of the transcription is also important, in particular:

(a) the sentence-per-line convention, helpful for smooth calculations of sentence-length, response patterns etc.;

(b) the use of the marginal convention—essential if such matters as zero response, inattention, incomprehension, etc. are to be correctly analysed. A good way of seeing if the margins are being sufficiently used is to get someone who has not heard the tape to read through the transcription: any inexplicitness will usually be quickly noted.

1.2

Analysis and profiling

In *GALD* chapters 3, 4 and 5, the various items listed on the profile chart are given some definition and discussion. Being an introductory volume, however, there was little detailed illustration of the different categories, and several questions of interpretation and methodology were pased over in silence. These questions fall into two types: (i) problems of grammatical analysis, i.e. deciding whether an utterance is to be analysed in grammatical terms, and, if so, which structures are involved; (ii) problems of profiling, i.e. ensuring that all the information recognized in the analysis is transferred onto the chart in a comprehensive and consistent way. These two aspects are complementary, in arriving at an understanding of why the chart has the form it has, and they are accordingly treated together in the following pages. The procedure will be to go systematically through the chart, from top to bottom, dealing with questions of analysis and profile procedure as they arise.

Section A

It is essential to appreciate the purpose of this section of the chart. It is basically a time-saving device, enabling T to avoid having to worry too much about utterances which are incapable of solution. Leaving out this information would be unsatisfactory, as the chart thereby would become a much less comprehensive record of P's utterances, and information of potential clinical interest would be missing (e.g. a decrease in the number of Unanalysed utterances over a period of time). On the other hand, we do not want too detailed a sub-classification of utterances in this section, as this would defeat its purpose. It would be possible to add to the categories recognized—for example, some LARSP users have added a category of Other to Section A—but we have rarely been motivated to doing so. A type of utterance which in some Ps does occur often enough to motivate a new category is illustrated in the following extract:

> T   what are you dòing/
> P   (*laughs*)
> T   tèll mé/ *etc.*

One can readily imagine instances where P's laughter is quite deliberate—a kind of response, therefore, but nonlinguistic in character. As the chart stands, the only place for (*laughs*) to go would be under Symbolic Noise, which makes this into a more heterogeneous category than its label suggests. Inserting an additional heading, such as Affect, to include all emotive nonlinguistic utterances (e.g. laughs, raspberries, whistles) may therefore be useful to some LARSP users.

Concerning the five categories currently recognized in Section A, a few remarks may be helpful, partly as caution, partly as amplification of the information given in *GALD*, 94 and 99–100. It should not be forgotten that all Section A information may need to be re-scrutinized at a later point, if the analysis of P's 'clear' sentences turns out to be less meaningful than was anticipated.

Unintelligible

(i) In clinical contexts, the usual reason for this is interference from the phonological system. Different kinds of intelligibility (e.g. whether dysarthric or dyspraxic) are not distinguished. What must be remembered is that the unintelligibility is interfering with our aim of *grammatical* analysis. If, therefore, an utterance is only partly unintelligible, whether it is to be analysed depends on whether the unintelligible portion affects our ability to make grammatical decisions. Take the following extracts, for example;

P   he gave me a 'big [flɔkuː]/ …
T   what have you got thère   *points to toy cars*
P   three ʔbàgs/

Neither of P's utterances is semantically intelligible, and one might even wonder about possible phonological problems—but the problems do not seem to affect the grammatical analyses. In other words, when the intelligibility difficulty is lexical, or located within a lexical item, it may be ignored, on the grounds that it is irrelevant to the chart's grammatical purpose. Similarly, a P who inserted irrelevant sounds predictably between words (e.g. 'the [suː] 'big [suː] 'man [ʃuː] …) could be analysed in the usual way, with the insertions discounted (cf. deviance below). The following examples, however, contrast clearly with the above:

(3 sylls) giving me/ = S? S + Aux?
'daddy '[iːtɛ] jùice/ = eated? eating? eat a? eat the?
[ɔlɪ]'red phòne/ = VO? D Adj N? Adj Adj N? etc.

Here it is impossible to assign any analysis with certainty,[4] and the utterances should therefore be logged under Unintelligible.

(ii) Unintelligible utterances, whether used as Responses or Spontaneous, are all placed in Section A, and no further reference is made to them under Sections B/C and on the bottom line of the chart. These Sections analyse *clear* sentences only.

(iii) Remember that, even with normal language samples, there may be utterances which are unintelligible, because of accompanying noise, speed of speaking etc.

---

[4] This contrasts with Ambiguous, where the alternative interpretations are quite specific: we know what we are choosing between, unlike the above.

Symbolic noise

Usually these occur in isolation, but we should note that sometimes they are integrated within a linguistic structure, e.g. *my ambulance go* [ni: na: ni: na:], [bi: p] *went the car*. The grammatical contexts are normally very restricted—the use of the verb *go* in these examples is typical—and as a result the sentences as wholes are unlikely to be representative of the rest of the sample. We suggest, then, that unless there is clear evidence of the 'noise' being institutionalized as a word (as in *he beeped at me*), the whole sentence is placed in Section A under this heading.

Deviant

By definition, deviant sentences are incapable of ready analysis using normal developmental and descriptive criteria (cf. *GALD*, 28–9). Their deviant form may be analysed in terms of morpheme order (e.g. *kicked man dog*), morpheme addition (e.g. *the cat a kicked*), morpheme omission (e.g. *the is in the garden*) or morpheme substitution (e.g. *he be speakly louding*). They may be totally uninterpretable (e.g. *chase there my is washing man*) or an interpretation may seem not to be too far away (e.g. *I saw was in a garden my daddy gone*). Many Ps produce an occasionally deviant sentence, but only a very few produce so many that it becomes a dominant characteristic of their output. In devising a clinical instrument for routine use, accordingly, it was felt that deviant sentences need be given only brief mention.

In using the Deviant category, however, we should note:

(i) T must be fairly convinced that the utterance is deviant before so assigning it, i.e. an impossible adult construction *and* an abnormal developmental pattern. If there is any doubt about this (e.g. if it may be a local dialect form, or if we think we have heard some normal children using it), we would give P the benefit of the doubt, and analyse it in the normal way. Obviously, the more that is discovered about language acquisition, the more precise this criterion can become.

(ii) The deviance may be trivial, e.g. due to a recurrent grammatical feature which pervades the whole of P's utterance. In certain psychopathological conditions, for example, a particular word or phrase may be interpolated between all other words in a sentence, e.g. *the yes man yes is yes coming yes*. Obscenities in particular may be used, and produce a similar, apparently deviant pattern. Likewise, P may regularly introduce a sentence with a specific phrase, or conclude it, e.g. *the trouble is* (*the man is coming the trouble is*). In all such cases, it is theoretically possible to class all such sentences as deviant, but little would be gained by so doing. Our inclination would be to disregard the interpolations, and analyse the grammatical residue in the normal way, to establish the extent of any genuine language problems. (The interpolations can of course be analysed separately elsewhere.)

(iii) Sometimes, the deviant sentences display no system—the word order looks random, or the errors are scattered across a wide range of constructions with no apparent pattern. Far more often than this, however, the deviant sentences contain useful information about P's difficulties—especially about those grammatical areas he is currently developing. This 'systematic deviance' may be immediately obvious. For example, one P, having reached Stage III, was receiving therapy aimed at expanding the *O* of *SVO* constructions. Contrasts of the sort *He's kicking a blue ball* v. *He's kicking a red ball* had been established in comprehension, but when it came to production tasks, P came out with sentences such as

> he blue kicking the ball
> he kicking the ball of a blue
> the ball is kicking is blue

despite the fact that he could still without difficulty produce *He's kicking a ball*, *A blue ball*, (in answer to *what's that?*) etc. The deviance in the above sentences is plainly related to the introduction of the adjective, and suggests that it was premature for T to take this remedial path so quickly (cf. p. 113). P was evidently being overloaded, and the whole of his carefully constructed grammatical system was in danger. The systematic deviance in this case acted as the warning signal.

Often the system in the deviance is by no means obvious at first sight. Careful detective work here is time-consuming, of course, and is worth doing only if P displays deviant utterances in sufficient quantity for these to pose a major assessment or remediation problem. An example of this is Jannine, a healthy child of above average intelligence, who at age 8 suffered a left hemisphere CVA of unknown aetiology, with a resulting temporary total aphasia. Data provided six months post-onset included the following sentences (see further, p. 110):

(1) mûmmy 'blow them 'up/
    'Margot and 'Mary and dáddy/ — 'brought sòmething/
    I like chícken/
    'how is a (=the) flỳing 'going 'on/
    I thìnk só/
    'put it 'up whère/
    because — a (=his) 'skin 'gets dàmp/
    that's a pòlar 'bear/
    'what's thát/

(2) (what did you do?) 'went to — bēd/ — 'on 'Christmas Ěve/
    and 'lots of 'toys to plây at/
    and 'Sharon — cámera/
    (did she take photos?) nó/ — Gûernsey/
    'Sindy's châir/
    twò 'Sindy's 'chair/
    a 'hat and a scârf/
    a 'cough and a còld/
    nòt 'initials 'on/ (referring to a new handkerchief)
    'seven — prèsents/ (=at seven o'clock there were presents)
    (what did you make?) cándlesticks/ — and — ángels/ and — kítchen roll/ — serviètte/
    (tell me about the horse) sòmetimes/ — a 'stripes 'down the tàil/
                       'step 'on your fòot/

(3) thìs 'horse/ is a 'mane—lòng/
    and 'went . a 'cut the nàil/
    'go to 'school—'every 'day—'when——'last wèek/
    màke óne/ a 'secret for dàddy/
    and I 'went 'my Sìndy 'set/

The puzzle is why a child who can produce such normal and advanced structures
as in (1) can, in the same sample, produce the highly confusing sentences of (2)
(requiring several T questions to clarify P's intent) and the different levels of
deviance in (3). Analysis of (2) shows that element omission is the main reason
for the confusions: subjects in particular are omitted, with the most frequently
omitted verbs being *be* and *have* (cf. <u>*I*</u> *went to bed*, <u>*we had*</u> *lots of toys*, <u>*she got*</u>
a Sindy chair, <u>*you've got a hat*</u> . . . .). Half the omissions in the total sample involved
'empty' subjects (*there is/are, that's a, it's a*); *I* was hardly ever used. As a result,
T is often not sure who P is referring to—whether an event is due to her or someone
else (e.g. P *a cough and a cold* T *who's got a cough* . . ., etc.). The items that are
kept, by contrast, are adverbials, especially of place and time, or NPs involving
the notion of possession, belonging, etc. The verbs of 'having' are a particular
problem (e.g. *Sharon camera*), but there is confusion when any kind of possessive
notion is involved (e.g. frequent omission of possessive pronouns). The deviant
sentences reflect these problems: *the horse* <u>*has*</u> . . ., *the nails* <u>*belong*</u> *to* . . ., *the secret
is* <u>*for daddy*</u>, *it does not* <u>*have*</u> *initials on*, <u>*there*</u> *were presents*, etc.
    There is an underlying pattern here, which can be indicated by the following
set of sentences:

> *there* is a cover *on the table*
> the table *has* a cover
> *that*'s the table *with a cover*
> the *table's cover* is . . .
> *its* cover is . . .
> *there* is the cover *for the table*

The basic notion of spatial location, with its extension to include attributes, personal possession etc., seems to be the main problem. P has spatial and temporal
concepts, but is having considerable difficulty in relating them to objects, actions
and (especially) agents. If we accept the hypothesis of the close cognitive relationship between space and time in early development (cf. H. Clark 1973), it is then not
surprising to find that sentences with temporal adverbials cause problems, and
that there are problems with tenses, etc. What the deviant sentences show is that
there is an 'overloading' kind of effect: P can cope with sentences if none of the
above notions is present (as in (1)); when she wants to express sentences with two
or three notions related to the above, then the Subject and Possessing Verb tend
to be omitted, leaving the spatial-temporal expression; and if she *does* introduce
Subject or Verb, and tries to get in the remaining notions, then the sentence 'col-
lapses under the strain', and we get deviance. The deviance, therefore, is an important indication of the limits of P's ability, in this case.

Incomplete

The point that must be emphasized immediately here is that this category includes only *grammatical* incompleteness. *He's coming*, for instance, said as a first utterance in a conversation, may be semantically incomplete, but it is a perfectly autonomous grammatical construction. The clearest cases of Incomplete are those where grammar and prosody coincide, e.g. *'he is—, the 'big—*. But what happens when there is a conflict between these criteria? We have found that prosody (sometimes accompanied by nonvocal activity, such as finger-snapping or gestures) is the only practicable identifying criterion, and this outranks all other characteristics. A sentence may 'look' grammatically complete, for instance, but not be so, e.g. *the 'man is 'coming* (no nuclear tone). Conversely, *the man wànts/* looks incomplete at the grammatical level, but prosodically is firmly finished (cf. the deliberate incompleteness of a T 'prompt', for example: 'this is á/). If the intonation was itself ambiguous, of course (e.g. a level tone), then the grammar would have to be followed. It is important to remember here that the simplified intonational transcription we use may not be an adequate guide to our decision about prosodic completion: an utterance with a nuclear tone may nonetheless be said in such an uncertain, wavering manner that we would not want to consider it finished in any sense (several of Mr J's utterances, in *GALD*, chapter 8, were like this, for instance). In such cases, a marginal note to that effect would be the appropriate way to draw attention to the point.

A second point concerning the identification of Incomplete sentences is to remember to discount obvious self-corrections, false starts, etc. If we did not do this, any sequence of stuttered syllables, or perseverated words, would have to be considered a sequence of incomplete sentences, and this would reduce the utility of the notion. A case of repeated opening was illustrated in *GALD*, 94, but not that of self-correction, which is a broader concept, including alterations in pronunciation and lexicon as well as grammar, e.g.

> he 'pound . 'found a pàcket/ (analysed as 'he found a packet')
> he 'saw his 'father . his mòther/ (analysed as 'he saw his mother')
> he 'said he'd go . they'd àll 'go to 'town/ (analysed as 'he said they'd all go to town')

In all such cases, there is an incomplete tone-unit, a brief pause, and usually an increase in prominence and tempo of the later part of the sentence. (There may also be articulatory indications, e.g. a glottal closure at the end of the corrected word.) In the following example, the tone-unit is complete, but the other prosodic features would remain:

> he 'saw his fàther/—his mòther I 'mean/ (analysed as 'he saw his mother', with the 'I mean' logged under Comment Clause at Stage VII)

But note two possible problems:

(i) If the first part of the utterance has a complete tone-unit, and the prosody is fairly even, it may be difficult to be sure that a correction was intentional, e.g.

> the people 'are hàppy/ — 'are smìling/

(ii) If a change in grammar becomes very radical, it may be necessary to take the second utterance as a fresh sentence, leaving the first as incomplete, e.g.

> the 'manager 'asked all the—thrèe cústomers/ 'wanted their mòney back/ and so the 'manager. ...

As with deviant sentences, it may be useful to refer back to the Incomplete category at a later stage of analysis. It might be, for example, that P fails to complete sentences if they begin with a certain construction (e.g. initiators, pronouns, an unstressed determiner)[5] or if the subject reaches more than a certain level of complexity (e.g. an extra adjective). As with Deviance, there may be systematic and unsystematic incompleteness, and, again as with Deviance, we need a good number of instances in a sample to make the detective-work worthwhile. Unlike Deviance, however, there may be a quite straightforward nonlinguistic reason for the incompleteness, such as a restricted auditory memory span (usually clearly distinguishable from any linguistic explanation by the greater randomness of grammatical structures found to be incomplete).

Lastly, can a sentence be incomplete anywhere other than at the end? Any cases where this might seem to be so are analysed in different ways on the profile chart, using the notion of ellipsis. The notion of incompleteness is inapplicable in cases such as 'on the cèiling/ (in response to 'where's the fly?'); and cases such as the 'boy a bàll/, which from an adult viewpoint might be considered to have a 'missing' middle section, are simply allocated to the appropriate place on the developmental section of the chart (in this example, S C/O at Stage II).

Ambiguous

In GALD, 94, an example is given of a common kind of ambiguity, where a single surface structure has two competing underlying interpretations (the man was killed by the tree). Most textbook examples are of this kind, and clinical samples often display them. There are however other kinds of Ambiguity, arising more out of what is not said, and these are also common, especially in the context of language delay. For example, Yesterday I lunch in the garden is unclear, in that it may be an attempt at Yesterday I lunched in the garden or Yesterday I had lunch in the garden. Because the analysis is in doubt (A S V A or A S V O A), the Ambiguous category should be used.

We should note, however, that all the available evidence should be taken into account before assigning a sentence to this category. If it is clear from T or P's accompanying activity or language what interpretation is relevant, the Ambiguous category should not be used. The passive/adverbial ambiguity cited above, for example, would in most circumstances raise no problem: it would be obvious from the context whether the tree had done the killing or not.

Prosody is a particularly crucial factor in deciding on ambiguity. For example, in moving from Stage I to Stage II, there is a stage where children bring two lexical

[5] Cf. the discussion of prosodic factors in Goodglass et al. 1967.

items into juxtaposition; but before a single intonation contour comes to be used, each lexical item retains its own contour, e.g.

> màn/———thère/
> màn/ thère/
> 'man thère/ *or* màn 'there/

This transitional stage passes quite quickly with normal children. In the case of language delayed children at this stage, however, it may take some time, and several potentially ambiguous situations arise.

> T   what's thàt/(*pointing to a picture of a man in a car*)
> P   màn/———drìving/

Here the problem is whether to analyse this as two Stage I sentences (*'N'*, *'V'*), or an (admittedly hesitant) *SV* at Stage II. The picture is no help, in such circumstances. Technically this is ambiguous, because of the prosody, as would be *màn/ drìving/*, where the prosody and grammar are even more obviously in conflict. If the tones rise, the ambiguity becomes even more complex (mán/drìving/), as a ´+` sequence is possible in adult English, and a decision over whether it is two tone-units or one is not always easy to make. In practice, Ts often resolve the ambiguity to their own satisfaction by observing P's accompanying actions, or seeing how much of the utterance P will repeat spontaneously, or paraphrasing P's utterance and seeing whether he is happy with the paraphrase. Relevant evidence may come from observing the extent to which there are clear cases of one or other of the alternative interpretations elsewhere in the sample: in the above example, if there were no Stage II structures elsewhere, it would be foolish to give a II analysis to this uncertain case; and vice versa. But there is always an element of risk in any such reasoning, and this should always be borne in mind.

The twofold relationship between prosody and syntax is in principle straightforward: prosody marks the boundaries between grammatical structures, and binds together the elements of grammatical structures. In practice, because of the vagaries of performance (e.g. stopping for breath mid-phrase) and the effect of attitude (e.g. more tone-units in angry speech), the correspondence between prosody and syntax is rarely simply stated. Thus for example, *pìg/jùmp/* could be analysed as Voc + V imp, with neutral intonation, or as SV with emphatic intonation. Sometimes it is simply not possible to decide, and Ambiguous must be used. Another common ambiguity, which occurs when P reaches Stage V, is whether two utterances linked by *and* constitute one sentence or two. For example, in the utterance

> the 'man's in a càr/—and a làdy's in a 'car/

it is initially unclear whether we are dealing with one sentence or two. The context may help: if there are two different pictures involved, and P turns from one to the other, an analysis of two sentences seems the better. If the man and the woman are in the same car, however, things are not so clear. With a longer pause, the two-sentence analysis is motivated; reduce the pause and one goes for a one-sentence analysis. Put a rising tone on *car*, and again, a one-sentence analysis is motivated, even with quite a long pause intervening. These are problems which affect the analysis of normal adult language too (see Crystal 1976, chapter 1), and they raise serious methodological and theoretical questions for linguistics. All T can do is adopt a consistent procedure when faced with such cases. It would be possible to put all such cases into the Ambiguous box, but this may mean dispensing with a considerable portion of the sample (especially if P is linking many clauses with *and*), and nothing would be gained. In order to progress, an arbitrary decision may have to be made, to take the least developed of the competing structures (to avoid overestimating P's ability): a Stage IV analysis, in this case, to be preferred to a Stage V.

Here is a final example of prosodic difficulty. The following sentences are clear:

it carries tanks and gùns/ v. it carries tànks/ — and gùns/
S   V   O   S   V   O   c   X
        X   c   X

The following utterance is not so clear:

it carries tànks/ and gùns/

In the present case, scrutiny of the rest of the sample helped the analyst by providing other utterances which could be placed in parallel to this one, e.g. *it carry torpedoes/ sometimes guns,* where the analysis SVO/AX is unavoidable, and this suggested a 2-sentence interpretation for the above. But often such extra clues do not exist, and there is no alternative but to use Ambiguous as the way out.

Sections B and C

Perhaps because of its complex appearance, or because of obscurities in our exposition in *GALD*, or perhaps solely because of lack of time, many Ts who routinely use the developmental sections of the chart fail to fill in Sections B and C. Obviously, the Stages analysis is methodologically autonomous, and may be completed without any reference to these sections. Sometimes, indeed, there is little point in referring to them, as when we are analysing a piece of spontaneous writing (cf. 2.5): as every sentence would be logged under Spontaneous, and as the distinction between one-element and more-than-one-element sentences would be obvious from the figures under the different Stages, the only 'new' information provided would be whether there was any element of repetition. But these cases are relatively rare, for most clinicians, and in most circumstances (certainly in all speech samples, but also in several non-speech contexts also) Sections B and C are highly relevant to an understanding of P's linguistic system.

The essential point to grasp is that while the developmental section of the chart can be *completed* without reference to B and C, it cannot be fully *interpreted* without such cross-reference. Whatever the range of figures found in the developmental section, their significance for assessment and remediation alters dramatically in the light of the different configurations of figures in B and C. For example, in

A	**Unanalysed**					**Problematic**		
	1 Unintelligible	2 Symbolic Noise		3 Deviant		1 Incomplete	2 Ambiguous	

B	**Responses**				Normal Response						Abnormal			
				Repet-	Elliptical Major				Full		Struc-		Prob-
	Stimulus Type		Totals	itions	1	2	3	4	Major	Minor	tural	∅	lems
		Questions											
		Others											

C	**Spontaneous**		Others	

		Minor			Social	Stereotypes	Problems

Sentence Type

Major — Social / Stereotypes / Problems

Sentence Structure

Stage I (0;9–1;6)

Excl.	Comm.	Quest.		Statement	
	·V·	·Q·	·V· **8** ·N· **11**	Other **9**	Problems

Stage II (1;6–2;0)

			Conn.	Clause		Phrase		Word
	VX	QX		SV **3**	V C/O **9**	DN **8**	VV **1**	-ing **7**
				S C/O	AX **2**	Adj N **5**	V part **7**	pl **2**
				Neg X **1**	Other **3**	NN	Int X	-ed **1**
						PrN **4**	Other **6**	

Stage III (2;0–2;6)

	VXY	QXY	X + S:NP	X + V:VP **4**	X + C/O:NP **2**	X + A:AP **2**	-en **1**
	let XY	VS	SVC/O	VC/OA **7**	D Adj N **6**	Cop **4**	3s **6**
	do XY		SVA	VO$_d$O$_i$ **1**	Adj Adj N	Aux **7**	gen
			Neg XY **1**	Other	Pr DN **11**	Pron **4**	
					N Adj N	Other	

Stage IV (2;6–3;0)

			XY + S:NP	XY + V:VP	XY + C/O:NP **2**	XY + A:AP **6**	n't
	· S	QVS	SVC/OA	AAXY	N Pr NP	Neg V	'cop
		QXYZ	SVO$_d$O$_i$	Other	Pr D Adj N	Neg X	'aux
					cX	2 Aux	
					XcX	Other	

Stage V (3;0–3;6)

			and	Coord. **1**	1 +	Postmod. **1** clause	1 +	-est
	how	tag	c	Subord. **1**	1 +			-er
			s	Clause: S		Postmod. **1** + phrase		
	what		Other	Clause: C/O				-ly
				Comparative				

Stage VI (3;6–4;6)

(+)				(−)			
NP	VP		Clause	NP		VP	Clause
Initiator	Complex		Passive	Pron	Adj seq	Modal	Concord
Coord			Complement	Det	N irreg	Tense	A position
						V irreg	W order
Other				Other			

Stage VII (4;6+)

Discourse			Syntactic Comprehension	
A Connectivity	it			
Comment Clause	there		Style	
Emphatic Order	Other			

Total No. Sentences	**55**	Mean No. Sentences Per Turn		Mean Sentence Length	

Fig. 4 'Neutral' developmental profile, lacking Sections B/C the developmental profile shown in Fig. 4, 55 sentences have produced a Stage II–III developing pattern (for the sake of simplicity of presentation, it is assumed that there are no Section A utterances to be taken into account). The interpretation of this profile changes markedly, however, when we correlate it with Figs. 5a and 5b. In Fig. 5a we see a 'pure' echolalic response pattern, of which the following are the distinctive characteristics:

(i) Most or all of the responses will be found under Structural Abnormality and Zero. There will always be a close correspondence between the figure under Repetition and that in the Totals column. For Question stimuli, the repeat of all or part of the question would automatically mean an analysis of structurally abnormal response.[6] For Other stimuli, this may not be the case (e.g. T 'that's a càt/ P a càt/).

(ii) For Other stimuli, responses which are not structurally abnormal or zero may be classified as full or elliptical, and here one would expect a spread of figures across the Elliptical range (the exact distribution will depend on the echolalic span): in Fig. 5a, the majority of utterances are two elements or less, and presumably the 3 full sentences used were fairly short ones.

(iii) No figures under Minor (Minor sentences would be unlikely unless T had ended her stimulus with a minor utterance (e.g. 'you put that thère/ yés/) or under Problems.

(iv) No spontaneous speech.

Note how the developmental section could be interpreted so as to reflect this: a preponderance of V C/O (A) structures, no developed subject structures, expansions towards the ends of sentences, and no minor sentences. On the other hand, the profile also (with one exception) resembles that which a language delayed child at this stage might produce with a phrase level bias. If this were the case, however, then Sections B and C would look more as in Fig. 5b:

(i) There are indications of spontaneous development.

(ii) The whole range of response categories is utilized, with a similar pattern for both Questions and Other stimuli. In particular, note the frequent use of minor sentences (this is the exception referred to above), and the use of the elliptical range.

(iii) Zero responses are much in evidence.

Other very different B/C configurations may be noted. Fig. 5c shows the language used by a P who has been taught a limited range of sentence patterns in structured situations:

(i) Full major sentences are the normal response pattern, evidently at the expense of elliptical constructions, i.e. the responses sound less natural and conversational (e.g. T 'where's the man gòing/ P the 'man is 'going to tòwn/).

(ii) Question stimuli, which promote clear structural responses, are well responded to; Other stimuli, where responses are often optional, and where P has to use more initiative, are responded to much less often (cf. high proportion of Zeros).

---

[6] One *may* repeat the question, as an echo-question (cf. *GCE*, 408 ff), but the intonation changes.

A

Unanalysed				Problematic	
1 Unintelligible	2 Symbolic Noise	3 Deviant		1 Incomplete	2 Ambiguous

B

Responses

Stimulus Type		Totals	Repetitions	Normal Response							Abnormal		Problems
				Elliptical Major				Full Major	Minor	Structural	∅	
				1	2	3	4					
50	Questions	40	40							40	10	
25	Others	15	15	5	3	1	1	3		2	10	

C

Spontaneous | Others

	Sentence Type	Minor				*Social*		*Stereotypes*		*Problems*	
Stage I (0;9–1;6)		**Major**					Sentence Structure				
		Excl.	*Comm.*	*Quest.*		*Statement*					
			·V·	·Q·	·V·	·N·	Other	Problems			

	Conn.	Clause			Phrase		Word
Stage II (1;6–2;0)		VX	QX	SV	VC/O	DN	VV	-ing
				S C/O	AX	Adj N	V part	
				Neg X	Other	NN	Int X	pl
						PrN	Other	
Stage III (2;0–2;6)		VXY		X + S:NP	X + V:VP	X + C/O:NP	X + A:AP	-ed
			QXY	SVC/O	VC/OA	D Adj N	Cop	-en
		let XY	VS	SVA	VOdOi	Adj Adj N	Aux	
				Neg XY	Other	Pr DN	Pron	3s
		do XY				N Adj N	Other	gen
Stage IV (2;6–3;0)		· S	QVS	XY + S:NP	XY + V:VP	XY + C/O:NP	XY + A:AP	n't
			QXYZ	SVC/OA	AAXY	N Pr NP	Neg V	'cop
				SVOdOi	Other	Pr D Adj N	Neg X	
						cX	2 Aux	'aux
						XcX	Other	
Stage V (3;0–3;6)	how		and	tag	c	Coord. 1	1 ·	Postmod. 1 clause	1 ·	-est
				s	Subord. 1	1 ·			-er
	what		Other		Clause: S		Postmod. 1 phrase		-ly
					Clause: C/O				
					Comparative				

	(+)			(−)		
	NP	VP	Clause	NP	VP	Clause
Stage VI (3;6–4;6)	Initiator	Complex	Passive	Pron	Adj seq	Modal	Concord
	Coord		Complement	Det	N irreg	Tense	A position
						V irreg	W order
	Other			Other			

	Discourse		Syntactic Comprehension	
Stage VII (4;6 +)	A Connectivity	it		
	Comment Clause	there	Style	
	Emphatic Order	Other		

Total No. Sentences	Mean No. Sentences Per Turn	Mean Sentence Length

© D. Crystal, P. Fletcher, M. Garman, 1975 University of Reading

Fig. 5   Four B/C configurations: Fig. 5a   Echolalic

A	Unanalysed			Problematic	
	1 Unintelligible	2 Symbolic Noise	3 Deviant	1 Incomplete	2 Ambiguous

B Responses

				Normal Response								Abnormal	
				Elliptical Major				Full		Struc-			Prob-
Stimulus Type		Totals	Repet-itions	1	2	3	4	Major	Minor	tural	Ø		lems
50	Questions	35	1	6	2	1			18	6	15		2
25	Others	18		4	2	1	1	1	8	1	7		1

C	Spontaneous	5	3	Others	2

Sentence Type

Minor		Social	Stereotypes	Problems

Stage I (0;9–1;6)

Major | Sentence Structure
Excl. | Comm. | Quest. | Statement
·V· | ·Q· | ·V· ·N· Other Problems

Stage II (1;6–2;0)

	Comm.	Quest.	Conn.	Clause		Phrase		Word
	VX	QX		SV	V C/O	DN	VV	-ing
				S C/O	AX	Adj N	V part	
				Neg X	Other	NN	Int X	pl
						PrN	Other	

Stage III (2;0–2;6)

	VXY / let XY / do XY	QXY / VS		X + S:NP	X + V:VP	X + C/O:NP	X + A:AP	-ed
				SVC/O	VC/OA	D Adj N	Cop	-en
				SVA	VO$_d$O$_i$	Adj Adj N	Aux	3s
				Neg XY	Other	Pr DN	Pron	gen
						N Adj N	Other	

Stage IV (2;6–3;0)

	+ S	QVS / QXYZ		XY + S:NP	XY + V:VP	XY + C/O:NP	XY + A:AP	n't
				SVC/OA	AAXY	N Pr NP	Neg V	'cop
				SVO$_d$O$_i$	Other	Pr D Adj N	Neg X	'aux
						cX	2 Aux	
						XcX	Other	

Stage V (3;0–3;6)

	how / what	tag	and / c / s / Other	Coord. 1 1+		Postmod. 1 clause 1+		-est
				Subord. 1 1+				-er
				Clause: S		Postmod. 1+ phrase		-ly
				Clause: C/O				
				Comparative				

Stage VI (3;6–4;6)

(+)				(−)			
NP	VP		Clause	NP		VP	Clause
Initiator	Complex		Passive	Pron	Adj seq	Modal	Concord
Coord			Complement	Det	N irreg	Tense	A position
						V irreg	W order
Other				Other			

Stage VII (4;6+)

Discourse		Syntactic Comprehension
A Connectivity	it	
Comment Clause	there	Style
Emphatic Order	Other	

Total No. Sentences	Mean No. Sentences Per Turn	Mean Sentence Length

Fig. 5b   Language delay

A	**Unanalysed**				**Problematic**		
	1 Unintelligible		2 Symbolic Noise	3 Deviant	1 Incomplete		2 Ambiguous

<table>
<tr><td rowspan="4">B</td><td colspan="2">Responses</td><td rowspan="2">Totals</td><td rowspan="2">Repet-itions</td><td colspan="4">Normal Response
Elliptical Major</td><td rowspan="3">Full
Major</td><td rowspan="3">Minor</td><td colspan="2">Abnormal</td><td rowspan="3">Prob-lems</td></tr>
<tr><td colspan="2"></td><td>1</td><td>2</td><td>3</td><td>4</td><td rowspan="2">Struc-tural</td><td rowspan="2">∅</td></tr>
<tr><td colspan="2">Stimulus Type</td></tr>
</table>

Stimulus Type	Totals	Repet-itions	1	2	3	4	Full Major	Minor	Struc-tural	∅	Prob-lems
46 Questions			**3**	**2**			**30**	**11**		**4**	
9 Others			**2**				**5**	**2**		**16**	

C	**Spontaneous**			Others		

		Minor				*Social*	*Stereotypes*	*Problems*	

<table>
<tr><th rowspan="18" style="writing-mode:vertical-lr">Sentence Type</th></tr>
</table>

Sentence Type

Minor

Major   Sentence Structure

Stage	Major					Sentence Structure				Word
	Excl.	*Comm.*	*Quest.*			*Statement*				
		·V·	·Q·	·V·	·N·	Other		Problems		

Stage I (0;9–1;6)

				Conn.	Clause		Phrase		Word
Stage II (1;6–2;0)		V X	Q X		SV	V C/O	DN	VV	-ing
					S C/O	A X	Adj N	V part	
					Neg X	Other	NN	Int X	pl
							PrN	Other	

					X + S:NP	X + V:VP	X + C/O:NP	X + A:AP	-ed
Stage III (2;0–2;6)		V X Y	Q X Y		SVC/O	VC/OA	D Adj N	Cop	-en
		let X Y	VS		SVA	VO_dO_i	Adj Adj N	Aux	3s
		do X Y			Neg X Y	Other	Pr DN	Pron	gen
							N Adj N	Other	

					X Y + S:NP	X Y + V:VP	X Y + C/O:NP	X Y + A:AP	n't
Stage IV (2;6–3;0)		S	QVS		SVC/OA	AA X Y	N Pr NP	Neg V	'cop
			Q X Y Z		SVO_dO_i	Other	Pr D Adj N	Neg X	'aux
							c X	2 Aux	
							X c X	Other	

				and	Coord. 1	1 ·	Postmod. 1 clause	1 ·	-est
Stage V (3;0–3;6)	*how*		tag	c	Subord. 1	1 ·			-er
				s	Clause: S		Postmod. 1 phrase		-ly
	what			Other	Clause · C/O				
					Comparative				

	(+)			(−)			
	NP	*VP*	*Clause*	*NP*		*VP*	*Clause*
Stage VI (3;6–4;6)	Initiator	Complex	Passive	Pron	Adj seq	Modal	Concord
	Coord		Complement	Det	N irreg	Tense	A position
						V irreg	W order
	Other			Other			

	Discourse		*Syntactic Comprehension*	
Stage VII (4;6+)	A Connectivity	*it*		
	Comment Clause	*there*	*Style*	
	Emphatic Order	Other		

Total No. Sentences	Mean No. Sentences Per Turn	Mean Sentence Length

© D. Crystal, P. Fletcher, M. Garman, 1975 University of Reading

Fig. 5c   Limited structural range

A	Unanalysed			Problematic	
	1 Unintelligible	2 Symbolic Noise	3 Deviant	1 Incomplete	2 Ambiguous

B   Responses

					Normal Response							Abnormal		
					Elliptical Major				Full		Struc-			Prob-
Stimulus Type			Totals	Repet-itions	1	2	3	4	Major	Minor	tural	Ø		lems
50	Questions		49	1	13	5	4		10	15	1	1		1
25	Others		22		3	1	2	1	8	7		3		

C	Spontaneous	36	1	2	Others 34

Stage	Sentence Type	Minor				Social		Stereotypes		Problems	
Stage I (0;9–1;6)		**Major**						Sentence Structure			
		Excl.	Comm.	Quest.				Statement			
			'V'	'Q'	'V'	'N'	Other		Problems		

Stage				Conn.	Clause		Phrase		Word
Stage II (1;6–2;0)		V X	Q X		SV	V C/O	DN	VV	-ing
					S C/O	A X	Adj N	V part	
					Neg X	Other	NN	Int X	pl
							PrN	Other	
Stage III (2;0–2;6)		V X Y	Q X Y		X + S:NP	X + V:VP	X + C/O:NP	X + A:AP	-ed
		let X Y	VS		SVC/O	VC/OA	D Adj N	Cop	-en
		do X Y			SVA	VOₐOᵢ	Adj Adj N	Aux	3s
					Neg X Y	Other	Pr DN	Pron	gen
							N Adj N	Other	
Stage IV (2;6–3;0)		S	QVS		XY + S:NP	XY + V:VP	XY + C/O:NP	XY + A:AP	n't
			QXYZ		SVC/OA	AAXY	N Pr NP	Neg V	'cop
					SVOₐOᵢ	Other	Pr D Adj N	Neg X	
							cX	2 Aux	'aux
							XcX	Other	
Stage V (3;0–3;6)		how	tag	and	Coord. 1 1+		Postmod. 1 1+ clause		-est
				c	Subord. 1 1+				-er
				s	Clause: S		Postmod. 1+ phrase		
		what		Other	Clause: C/O				-ly
					Comparative				

Stage	(+)			(−)			
	NP	VP	Clause	NP		VP	Clause
Stage VI (3;6–4;6)	Initiator	Complex	Passive	Pron	Adj seq	Modal	Concord
	Coord		Complement	Det	N irreg	Tense	A position
						V irreg	W order
	Other			Other			

Stage	Discourse		Syntactic Comprehension	
Stage VII (4;6+)	A Connectivity	it		
	Comment Clause	there	Style	
	Emphatic Order	Other		

Total No. Sentences	Mean No. Sentences Per Turn	Mean Sentence Length

© D. Crystal, P. Fletcher, M. Garman, 1975 University of Reading

Fig. 5d   Normal (3-year-old)

(iii) No spontaneous utterances—P has been taught to respond to specific situations and stimuli, and does not develop her reply in any way.

As a final example, Fig. 5d displays a normal 3-year-old pattern:

(i) A good balance of spontaneous to response utterances (about 1:2), unlike (b) above.

(ii) Both stimuli types responded to in similar proportions.

(iii) The whole range of categories utilized, with a good balance between full major, elliptical major, and minor sentences. There is less use of Zero than in (b) above, and a much better use of Full Major sentences.

These are some of the clear B/C patterns which emerge; there will obviously be many less clear patterns, which require special study. Figs. 5a–d should however be enough to illustrate the importance of these sections in reaching an assessment and planning remediation, and perhaps provide motivation to grapple with the technical problems which arise in working with structural distinctions of this kind. Several small but important methodological points must be borne in mind, if the procedure is to be used consistently, in addition to the general guidelines presented in *GALD*, 94–7, and these are now discussed.

Stimuli

The distinction between Questions and Others is made on *grammatical* grounds—in other words, phonological, semantic or 'speech act' factors are disregarded (though they would need to be taken into account in any attempt at linguistic assessment which went beyond grammar). This means that the only structures permitted under Question are those which are formally marked as such in the grammar of the language, viz. inversion, question-words or tag-questions (cf. *GALD*, 56). An utterance which has the grammatical form of a statement, command, exclamatory, or minor sentence is automatically placed under Others, *regardless of the intonation involved*. The status of intonation has already been discussed (p. 7): it would be impossible to classify stimuli consistently if an intonational criterion were allowed in, as the rising tone, whether high or low, is in no way a unique index of a questioning intent, but may express shock, surprise, warning and many other attitudes. But what if we encounter a T who clearly and regularly questions using a rising intonation on statements (or a P who asks questions using only this means)? Might it not give a misleading picture to assign all these stimuli to Others without further comment? If one feels this to be so, it would be perfectly possible to incorporate the intonational information onto the chart, by dividing the Others box (and the corresponding Response boxes) into two, or simply by adding a box for 'questioning intonation'; but we have not ourselves felt any need to do this.

The Stimulus boxes, as with any other category on the chart, can be given a more detailed subclassification, as detailed issues of assessment and remediation arise. The aim of this part of the chart, we must remember, is to focus the analyst's attention on what is probably the biggest remedial question of all: what kind of stimulus best promotes what kind of response. Bearing in mind that T is trying to exert some measure of *control* over P's language (cf. p. 4), the more known about stimulus–response interdependencies the better. As it stands, Section B contains very little stimulus information. Its aim, as already said, is more a mnemonic than a classification: T must not forget to pay systematic attention to this issue, in analysing her interaction with P. Having begun to look at this area, then, further subclassification may be necessary in order to make specific remedial suggestions.

What other categories might we recognize? The initial distinction, between Questions and Others, is well-motivated; the range of possible responses to a question is very restricted, compared with those which can be made to commands, statements, etc, e.g.

T   That's a cup
P   Yes   *or*
     It's a nice cup   *or*
     Is it?   *or*
     Give it to me *etc.*

Also, in clinical settings T uses questions in a much more frequent and systematic way than any other stimulus (there are usually at least twice as many Questions to Others in a sample).[7] For these reasons, a subclassification of Questions is likely to be more useful than of Others, and in *GALD*, 118 ff we present a wide range of possible stimulus types, c.g. forced alternative questions, *wh*-questions. It is evident that some questions pose more of a problem to a language deficient P than others: the 'open-ended' questions (cf. *GALD*, 124, e.g. *what's happening?*) seem more complex than those which give a specific structural clue as to how they should be answered, e.g. *where*-questions; and these in turn seem more complex than those where the world of possible answers has been tightly constrained (e.g. forced alternative questions: *Is it X or Y?*); and these in turn are more complex than those where a simple *yes/no* or non-verbal response would suffice (simple inversions, or questioning intonation utterances). Likewise, we could subclassify Others into the categories already mentioned (statement, command, exclamatory, minor), or add further categories typical of the clinical situation, e.g. prompts (*That's a—*).

Response v. Spontaneous

This distinction is based solely on a single grammatical criterion: the first *and only the first* sentence in P's utterance is classified as a Response. If other sentences follow, these are *all* classified as Spontaneous. There is a logical reason for this: for P to respond to T's stimulus, he must use at least one sentence, but he need not use more than one. Sentences other than the first are grammatically optional, not directly under the control of T's stimulus, and as a result may be legitimately called Spontaneous. Spontaneous also applies, of course, to the cases where no

[7] This is not the case with normal adult interaction, nor with normal child–child play situations (cf. *GALD*, 107), and as P's language becomes increasingly normal, so the Questions:Other ratio inverts.

T sentence immediately precedes, e.g. the utterances produced at the very beginning of a session (before T has said anything), or after a long silence or other major break in the session.

Once again, we must exclude semantic considerations. Take the following extract:

T   'what did you do yèsterday/
P   I 'went to tówn/—
        I got 'two càrs/
        my dâddy 'got them/ etc.

In a semantic sense, the whole of P's utterance is a response to the question; but in the LARSP procedure, only the first sentence is Response; the others are Spontaneous. (It is not difficult to see that the semantic criterion is a very weak and unsatisfactory one: almost anything can be a 'response', in a notional sense—a long monologue, a whole conversation, a book. . . .)

Response patterns

The first thing to note is the hierarchic way in which the range of possible response patterns is organized: initially, a response is seen as either Normal or Abnormal. If we cannot decide on the normality of a response (see below), we use the Problem box: this shows that at least responses have been made, even though their structural status is uncertain. If, *in addition to all this*, P's response is a repeat of some or all of T's stimulus, we also allocate the utterance to the Repetitions box (see further below).

Abnormal responses

As with stimuli, the basis of the distinction between normal and abnormal is grammatical. Under abnormal, we place all utterances which are totally unacceptable as syntactic responses to a given stimulus, or are extremely unlikely. The most obvious case of unacceptability is failure to produce any syntax at all, and as this is extremely common in clinical samples, with the varying figures here often aiding a differential diagnosis (cf. p. 35 above), a separate box is provided, headed 'Zero' (symbolized as $\emptyset$). Two problems arise in working with this category:

(i) Enough time must have been left by T for P to respond, before a decision about Zero is made. If T says

'where's the màn/ .
is he 'in the căr/

giving only a brief pause after the first question, it would obviously not be right to say there was a Zero response here. On the other hand, a transcription of

'where's the màn/———
is he 'in the căr/

would suggest Zero. Ultimately, only T can say whether she was waiting for P to respond, and whether the amount of time left was sufficient for P to do so. With many Ps, we can be fairly confident: if they do not respond immediately, they will not respond at all (e.g. due to problems of memory, or attention); hence T might produce another stimulus after only a brief delay, and yet be confident that there was a Zero response. But in principle, for all Ps, only T knows whether P should be credited with Zero or not: in the end it is a subjective decision, based on such indeterminate factors as T's patience, P's fatigue, and the like. Local circumstances may also intervene, e.g. if T asks a question, and before P responds something happens in the room which would count as a genuine distractor, there may be a long pause, and T may then need to re-phrase; but it would make sense not to count Zero in such a circumstance (to make the transcription unambiguous, a comment could be placed in the Marginal Column). Of course, we try to be as consistent as possible, in assigning Zero: our practice is to assign a Zero only to utterances followed by a triple dash in transcription (a pause equivalent to at least three pulses of T's rhythm, which is usually a minimum of 3 seconds), but we have noted that some Ts operate with a much shorter expectancy of zero, and some with a much longer one. Sometimes, the nature of the disorder is such that our norms of pausal expectancy have to be fundamentally altered: with SSN children, for instance, we may need to extend our normal pause time to perhaps 10 seconds or more, before we can be sure that no response was forthcoming. It is a familiar problem, and the cautionary point which has to be made is not to be over-rigid, and not to be afraid to extend the transcription system, if need be (e.g. introducing extra dashes, or inserting indications of absolute time).

(ii) It should also be emphasized that 'Zero Response' means 'no syntactic response when a syntactic response is possible', and not '... when a syntactic response is expected'. To illustrate the problem, let us take a T stimulus where a linguistic response is unnecessary, as in some comprehension exercises, e.g.

T   'show me the màn/——— *P points to man*
       'good bòy/. 'now 'show me ...

In such a case, do we mark Zero? The answer is yes, on the grounds that in *normal* adult–child interaction and in adult–adult situations comparable to this, some accompanying language is regularly used. It is not normal for adults or children to respond in total silence—*there, here it is, see, OK?* and many other utterances may be heard—and it is the degree of normality of P's interaction which we wish to capture in Section B. We therefore wish to indicate that P, when given the chance to use some language, did not do so, hence the use of Zero. Of course, we have to be sensible here: there is a clear difference between stimuli where a response is obligatory and those where it is optional, and in interpreting the figure in the Zero boxes, the fact that there has been a conflation should be born in mind. In theory, the only case where a Zero response would be disallowed would be one where no response of *any* kind was possible, but short of gagging P, it is difficult to think what this might be, as the following extract from an interaction with a language-delayed 5-year-old illustrates:

T   now 'don't sày ánything/
       'just 'point to the càr/
P   why̆/

In practice, situations of the comprehension exercise type illustrated above will be readily distinguished, if profiled, by a section B distribution of the following kind:

Stimulus Type

0	Questions
30	Others

The principle at stake is, once again, the chart's grammatical purpose. We want to know how far P is using grammar to respond. If he uses any other means of responding, *this is not taken into account on this chart*. Facial expressions, gestures, action responses (e.g. picking up the box in response to *where's the box?*), symbolic noises, indeterminate sounds, and so on, are not allowed to interfere with a decision that there has been a syntactic zero. (On a chart assessing communicative ability in general, of course, such aspects of behaviour would be very relevant.)

Under the heading of *Structural* abnormal responses, we include only those patterns which are syntactically deviant with reference to the structural stimulus used. Usually these responses follow Questions, as when a noun is given instead of an expected verb (e.g. T: 'what does the càr 'do/ P: màn/), or a *wh*-question is replied to by *yes*/.[8] But, although much less common, Other stimuli may be abnormally responded to, e.g.

T   'show me the càr/   T   'there's the màn/
P   wás a 'man/   P   she càme/

T   I can see a càt/
P   whèn

Such 'crazy' sequences may result from either specific failures of comprehension by P or expressive difficulties. In all cases, however, we are dealing with grammatical anomalies.

'Grammatical' is here primarily opposed to 'semantic'. Often P will produce an unacceptable response for semantic or extralinguistic reasons, e.g.

T   'where's the cár/   T.   'which one is grèen/
P   'in the bòx/   P   the càr/
T   nŏ/ it's 'in the gàrage/ ...   T   nŏ/ the 'car's blùe/ ...

It must be emphasized that these are *not* candidates for Structural Abnormality, as there is nothing wrong with the syntax of the response. Such anomalies provide interesting information about semantic development, which it is not the purpose of the chart to study. Conversely, a structurally abnormal response must not be missed if it happens to be semantically appropriate. Sequences such as

T   what's thàt 'car 'got/
P   dríving/

[8] As always, there are exceptions, as with the meditative adult *yes*, e.g. A *Where's that book I lent you?* B *Yes* (said slowly, and meaning 'hmm', 'I have a problem' etc.).

are anomalous on syntactic grounds; the fact that P has said something relevant to the topic must be ignored.

Sometimes, P produces an unacceptable response where it is difficult to be sure whether syntactic or semantic issues are involved. This is not surprising; there is no clearcut boundary between these two areas of linguistic inquiry. An example would be if a *when*-question were replied to by a *where*-phrase, as in:

T   when is he cóming/
P   in the gàrden/

The choice here is between allowing the sentence to stand as a normal one-element elliptical response, or not to analyse it at all, as structurally abnormal. If a decision cannot be made, then the appropriate place for the response is, of course, Problems.

Another problematic case, this time not involving semantics, would be one where the syntactic relationship of P's sentence to T's is unclear or ambiguous. Depending on how we see this relationship, we might accept the response or consider it abnormal, e.g.

T   It's a dòg/
P   rùnning/

Normal responses

Minor and Full Major responses seem not to cause many problems of analysis. We must remember that stereotyped sentences used as responses would go under the former heading, despite any surface similarity to Major sentences. Also, Major sentences are defined in terms of obligatory clause elements: Stage I sentences are still developing their major structure, and cannot be called 'Full'. Likewise, the 'immature' Stage II clause structures (SC/O, Neg X, and some QX, AX and Other) are analysed as elliptical in Section B (the analysis there being from the adult interactional point of view, and not from the viewpoint of the child's linguistic ability).

Elliptical Major sentences do require several comments. The motivation for counting ellipsis separately, it should be remembered, is to permit an estimate of the extent to which P is developing normal conversational patterns. Ellipsis promotes economy of utterance, avoids boredom, adds variety, and has several other purposes. It is important to know, then, how far P is able to take previous sentence structure for granted (an operation which requires cognitive as well as linguistic skills).

The unit of measurement which we have adopted for identifying the amount of ellipsis used is the *element of clause structure*. (We could use any other unit, such as number of words/morphemes/phrases, but all in our opinion would produce more complex procedures.) There are two possible ways of 'capturing' the notion of ellipsis: (a) to specify how much of the sentence has been left out; (b) to specify how much has been left in. We experimented with both approaches, before deciding on (b), on grounds of ease of working. The four columns (1,2,3,4), accordingly, represent the *number of elements of clause structure remaining* in P's response.

(1) Under 1 is included a single S,V,C,O, or A, as in:

T	'what's he dòing/		T	who's thàt/	
P	slèeping/ (=he's sleeping)		P	a màn/ (=that is a man)	
	V S V			C S V C	

Note: (i) the element may have quite an extensive phrase structure, yet still be only one clause element, e.g.

T   'where's he gòne/
P   'to his mùmmy's 'house/
        A

(ii) P may produce only a *part* of the element that would be expected in adult usage. This is still classed under the same heading, e.g.

T   'who 'gave you thàt/
P   màn/ (where *a man* would be normal)

(iii) As pointed out in *GALD*, 96, fn. 9, we do not know how far Ps using Stage I (and, to some extent, Stage II) sentences are in fact in control of the sentence structures they are apparently eliding. Presumably if P came out with the same 1-element response, regardless of the complexity of T's stimulus, this would be evidence to suggest that he was not operating with any clear notion of ellipsis. We have not researched this point, and therefore recommend that *all* elliptical responses (1,2,3,4) be interpreted simultaneously. Unlike Pattern (a), (b) shows that P is using 2- and 3-element sentences in addition to 1-element,

(a)

Elliptical Major			
1	2	3	4
20			

(b)

Elliptical Major			
1	2	3	4
20	11	2	

and is therefore likely to be in command of the range of structures used by T. (As already pointed out, the figure under 1 may also include the immature, apparently elliptical sentences of the Stage II child.)

(2) Under 2 is included any combination of two clause elements, as in:

T	what's he dòing/		T	'that's a 'nice mán/	
P	'kick bàll/ (=he's kicking the ball)	P	'man in gàrden/		
	V O			S A	

Notes (i) and (ii) above apply, e.g.

T	what's he dòing/		T	'who 'went to tòwn 'yesterday/	
P	'kicking 'big 'red bàll/		P	Ì did/	
	V O			S V	

(3)   Under 3 is included any combination of three clause elements, as in:

T   'what did he dò/
P   'kick a 'ball through that window/   P gave me a book/
       <u>V   O</u>   <u>A</u>   V   O   O

T   'how many visitors 'came to 'see you 'yesterday/
P   thrèe 'came from <u>Réading</u>/ (i.e. to see me yesterday)
       S   V   A

(4)   Under 4 is included any combination of four or more clause elements. These are much less likely to occur, but one fairly common pattern is that involving a subordinate clause, e.g.

T   'why did he còme/
P   because he 'wanted to 'give me a bòok/
       s   S   V O_i O_d

Problems

In this category is placed any utterance about whose status there is some doubt, e.g. whether Abnormal, whether Minor, whether Elliptical. We also include here any cases of doubt as to whether a sentence is spontaneous or not. As with all 'problem' boxes, the contents can be opened for re-inspection later in the investigation, should it prove necessary.

Repetitions

In addition to the analysis of responses in terms of Normal, Abnormal, and Problems, we indicate the number of P's utterances which are Repetitions of T's stimulus. Repetitions can be an important diagnostic feature: they may be a dominating characteristic, as in the echolalic pattern discussed above, or they may be an indication of a specific area of weakness (as when P repeats a stimulus-type he has failed to comprehend). We could find two very similar-looking profiles, but one might have a low Repetitions score, and the other a high one. Knowing this would lead us to interpret P's output in very different ways.

The idea of P 'repeating' T's utterance sounds simple, but certain methodological points need to be remembered, if the notion is to be used consistently.

(i) We are talking of grammatical repetition, not semantic, i.e. if P paraphrases T, this is not Repetition, e.g. T: *'it's your càt*/ P/ *Kàtie*/ (where Katie is the cat's name). Also, the notion has nothing to do with comprehension (which is why we do not use the term 'echolalia' here): whether P's repeated utterance is meaningful to him or not, it is nonetheless classed as Repetition.

(ii) To count as Repetition, it must be T's *immediately preceding* utterance which is involved, i.e. the sentence we take as the stimulus. This decision is not entirely arbitrary: it ties in with our expectations concerning echolalia, and it is reasonably easy to work with. If we did not restrict the notion in this way, there would be problems in deciding how far back in the discourse we would need to go before one of P's sentences would cease to be classed as a 'repetition'. For example, if T said *That's a boat*, and five minutes later, after several dozen sentences had intervened, P said *That's a boat*, we might be forced into calling this a repetition, which would be absurd. The same difficulty arises in principle, though, if only one sentence intervenes, e.g.

T   'that's a bòat/
     what ís it/
P   'that's a bòat/

Here we would definitely *not* want to talk of repetition. A little more problematic is the following example:

T   'that's a bòat/
     Ì'd like a 'boat like thát one/
     do yòu 'like bóats/
P   'that's a bòat/

Here there is some suggestion of an 'echo', but it is not entirely clear, and with cases of this kind, the analyst must simply be consistent. Any repetition span might be used—repeat of the previous one, two, three, ... *n* sentences: our approach restricts it to the immediately preceding sentence. Thus

T	'that's a bòat/	*or*	T	'that's a bòat/	*or*	'that's a bìg 'boat/
P	'that's a bòat/		P	bòat/		P	bìg/

are repetitions, but

T	that's a bòat/	*or*	T	'that's a bòat/
	go ón/		P	yès
P	'that's a bòat/			'that's a bòat/

are not.

(iii) As the examples just given illustrate, it is not the case that P must repeat *everything* in T's sentence—and in fact usually he does not. What is important is that the part of the sentence used be, formally, a repetition—and what this means in practice is that the intonation should be preserved. To change the intonation is no longer to echo, and we always credit P with a new utterance if he has done so. Thus, for example:

T	'that's a bòat/	*or*	T	that's a bòat/
P	a bóat/		P	thàt's a 'boat/

are not classed as repetitions.

These are examples of phonological changes—P's rising tone expresses query, his tonicity change alters emphasis. We must remember that if phonetically-based changes occur (i.e. there is no semantic contrast in evidence), there will be no cause to alter the classification of the sentence as repetition. This would be the case in sequences such as

T   'that's a bŏat/
P   thàt/   *or*   bòat/   *or*   bōat/

where P's utterance is weakly articulated, and where an impression of formal and semantic control is lacking—the classical echolalic effect. In such cases, a marginal note should be added to the transcription (e.g. 'echo') to remind T to discount the changed pitch contour.

In cases of uncertainty as to whether the pitch change is phonologically or phonetically conditioned, we avoid overestimating P's ability, and mark such sentences as Repetitions.

(iv) The forced alternative question has to be taken as an exceptional type of stimulus, in our view, in deciding on Repetitions. To ask 'Is it X or Y (or Z ...)' is a very different task from any other stimulus: to respond to such questions acceptably, a repetition is quite normal (often obligatory), and this places them in a rather different category:

T   is it a réd 'book or a blùe 'book/
P   a blùe 'book/   *or*   a réd 'book/

Such cases are therefore *not* logged as repetitions.

(v) Lastly, we must remember that sentences which are repetitions are placed on the chart twice: once for their response analysis, the second time to identify their status as Repetition. For example,

T   'that's a bòat/
P   a bòat/

is first of all classed as 1-element Elliptical Response, and then as Repetition. In this way we can distinguish readily (by the total under Repetitions) these Ps from those who use ellipsis in a more productive way, as in

T   what's thàt/ *etc.*
P   a boàt/

Totalling up

It is useful to have a quick indication of how many of T's stimuli were actually responded to by P in the sample. For instance,

B	Responses	
Stimulus Type		Totals
60	Questions	30
	Others	

means that of T's 60 stimulus questions, P provided 30 verbal responses. There seem to be no problems over counting stimuli, as long as we remember to count *only* stimuli (i.e. the utterance immediately preceding a P utterance). So, in the following extract, only the last sentence is counted as stimulus:

    T   'here's a càr/
         'put it on the táble/ —
         'a 'bit néarer/ —
         now 'put the 'man in the càr/

But how is the figure under Totals arrived at? Simply by adding all the figures along the line, *with the exclusion of* those under Zero (which by definition can hardly be counted as a verbal response!) and those under Repetitions (which have already been analysed as responses). This procedure may be checked in the following example:

B Responses				Normal Response						Abnormal		
				Elliptical Major				Full		Struc-		Prob-
Stimulus Type		Totals	Repet-itions	1	2	3	4	Major	Minor	tural	Ø	lems
71	Questions	60	7	14	7	1		13	20	1	11	4
36	Others	32	2	8	2			7	15		4	

The figure under Totals may be equal to the Stimuli totals, but obviously will never exceed it, and is usually much less, in clinical samples.

There is one complication, which may be seen from the following example:

    T   'what's thàt/
    P   (*2 sylls*) *or* 'it's a

Where P's response is either Incomplete, or one of the Unanalysed categories in Section A, how is this to be handled in Section B? As P's utterances are unanalysable, it is obviously not possible to be sure which is the relevant response category. We are left with two choices: to put these responses into Problems, or to ignore them completely. We chose the latter course, on the grounds that Section A utterances present problems that are so unlike any of the routine structural problems that to conflate them could be misleading. Is an attempt at a response (viz. an Incomplete) a response (albeit a 'problematic' one)? Is symbolic noise a response, in any comparable sense to the above? Unintelligible and deviant speech seemed more like genuine response Problems; but in the end we opted for consistency, and decided to exclude all Section A utterances from consideration. This means in practice that in the following sequence, we simply miss out lines 2 and 6 when completing Section B:

    1 T   'what's thàt/ —
       P   (2 sylls)
       T   a whát/ —
       P   tèddy/
    5 T   oh I sèe/ —
       P   it's a —
       T   go ón/

What are the results of this decision? It simplifies the Section B analysis somewhat, we feel, but a consequence of the decision will be that the total stimuli may appear to be greater than the available responses. For example, in the following array

B Responses				Normal Response						Abnormal		
				Elliptical Major				Full		Struc-		Prob-
Stimulus Type		Totals	Repetitions	1	2	3	4	Major	Minor	tural	Ø	lems
35	Questions	22	5	7	3	1		4	5	1	8	1
	Others											

a total of 22 responses is readily accounted for by all figures excluding Repetitions and Zero. If we now add the 8 Zero responses, we get 30. But there were 35 stimuli. The 'missing' responses will of course be examples of unanalysed Section A utterances, and we would accordingly expect to find in Section A a total of 5 (or more, if there were unanalysed utterances in Section C also). Here is a full Section A/B (it is in fact from Mr J's 2nd profile, taken from *GALD*, 175):

A Unanalysed	Problematic
1 Unintelligible 9 2 Symbolic Noise 3 Deviant	1 Incomplete 51 2 Ambiguous

B Responses				Normal Response						Abnormal		
				Elliptical Major				Full		Struc-		Prob-
Stimulus Type		Totals	Repetitions	1	2	3	4	Major	Minor	tural	Ø	lems
61	Questions	37	4	6	7			10	14		2	
122	Others	84	17	15	3			31	35			

37 responses to Questions +2 Zero = 39, i.e. 22 'missing'
84 responses to Other | no Zero = 84, i.e. 38 'missing'
60 utterances are 'missing' altogether, which is the sum of the utterances in Section A.

Spontaneous patterns

There is much less to be said under Section C, for obvious reasons: the only relevant subclassification is precisely that which is dealt with in the developmental section of the chart. It would be possible to develop a similar range of categories to those included in Section B, but we have not found this useful. The only information Section C provides, therefore, is what the developmental section does not contain, namely:

   (i) *Data concerning self-repetitions.* For similar reasons to those discussed under Responses, we need to keep a separate tally of any sentence which is a repetition of the immediately preceding sentence. The need for this may be seen by comparing the following two samples of data:

   (a)   my dàddy 'kick 'ball/—he kìck it/—my bròther 'kick it/—'me 'kick 'it tòo/
   (b)   my dàddy 'kick 'ball/—'me 'kick 'it tòo/ . 'me 'kick 'it tòo/ . 'me 'kick 'it tòo/

Both samples have 4 SVO(A) constructions, and identical analyses, but it would plainly be misleading to give a total to the hyperactive child who produced (b) which was identical to that given to the child who produced the range of novel patterns in (a). On the other hand, we cannot *not* analyse (b)'s sentences, as he did produce them, and needs to be credited with the appropriate number of SVO(A) constructions (as opposed to having used other sorts of structure, or said nothing at all). Repetitions are always analysed in terms of Stages. The way out of the problem is to analyse everything but to give a separate tally for immediate self-repetitions. Thus, in (b), the child has repeated *me kick it too* twice, hence 2 would go in the Repetitions box in Section C.

The same restrictions required for Section B also apply here, viz. formal identity and adjacency. If P changes his sentence even slightly (e.g. a singular noun becoming plural, or a falling tone becoming rising), there is no linguistic identity, and no self-repetition. And if he introduces a different sentence between two identical sentences, there is no self-repetition. For example:

he kìck it/ he kicked it/ he kìck it/

are not repetitions.

(ii) *1-element elliptical utterances.* We could have brought together all spontaneous sentences, giving them no subclassification at all; but there is one kind of sentence which P may use and which is not otherwise mentioned on the chart—a one-element sentence which is clearly elliptical, viz. S, V, C, O or A. This information is not available at Stage I (where one might think one-element sentences should go) for two reasons: firstly, not all of these sentences will go at Stage I (*bag, my bag, my nice bag*, etc. are all one-element (i.e. one-clause-element) sentences, but they would appear at different (phrase) Stages in the chart); and secondly, for those sentences which do consist of one word, we do not wish to attribute to the Stage I child who is using Spontaneous sentences such extensive knowledge of ellipsis. We are always very tentative about grammatical analysis at Stage I (cf. p. 119), and we think that to call the following P utterances clausal ellipses is misleading, from a developmental point of view:

T   what's thàt/
P   càr /— níce /—thère/—wánt/ *etc.*

Word-class	'N'	'Adj'	'Adv'	'V'
Clause	??C	??C	??A	??V

To say that *nice* is C is to say that the child has analysed it as deriving from an underlying structure of the type *The car is nice*. Some theoretical accounts of early child language dare to make this assumption, but we do not. Hence we do not analyse Stage I in terms of S, V, O, etc., but go for a much weaker characterization in terms of tentative word-classes.

But how do we handle such utterances in terms of Sections B and C, where we are dealing with interaction, not development? In Section B, we have already seen, an analysis in elliptical terms seems viable, in view of the potential prop of the immediately preceding utterance. But in Section C also, the utterances must be seen from T's viewpoint: how does T interpret them and reinforce them? If asked to gloss the spontaneous utterances above, T would undoubtedly treat them as ellipses, and expand them in some way, e.g. *It's nice, It's there, I want it*. This can be seen in the samples from the way T responds to a P who is using language of this kind, e.g.

P	càr/—níce/	P	càr/—wánt/
T	it is a 'nice 'car/	T	you 'want anòther one/

Under such circumstances, it would seem useful to add the 'missing' information to the chart, by counting separately any spontaneous utterances consistingly solely of a single clause element—hence the box under Elliptical Major 1. (If we wished, we could do the same for Elliptical 2, 3 and 4; but as already mentioned, there seems little point in this, as clausal information is dealt with routinely in the developmental section of the chart from Stage II on.) As P's language develops, the need for such a category becomes greater, and decisions about clausal status can be made with confidence, as would be the case in the following (adult) extract:

we had tèa in 'town yésterday/—at the 'new càfe/—the 'one in the
S   V   O   A   A   A   A

High 'Street/—it's 'not been òpen lóng/—a'bout a wèek/—and we 'saw
S   V   C   A   A   S   V

'Mrs Smith/. thè 'Mrs 'Smith/— 'in the 'entrance to the Dòrchester/—
O   O   A

'looking for àll the wórld as if . . .

There is one type of case where the figure under Spont. Ellipt. 1 is diagnostically very significant. Imagine a P who had learned or been taught only phrase and word-level structures. A possible developmental profile (if it had been allowed to develop unchecked) would be as in Fig. 6—no clause structure at all; no transitional information; and, therefore, each phrasal structure is a single-element sentence, e.g.

my dàddy/— — — in the gàrden/— — —'mummy and gràndad/— — — a 'big 'red bóx/
D   N   Pr D   N   X   c   X   D Adj Adj N

We have sometimes heard Ps who have developed a phrasal ability, with little or no clausal ability, not far short of that shown in Fig. 6. The rambling, uncoordinated, fluent and sometimes very confusing output of such children would be immediately reflected in the distinctive look of the Section B/C ratio: the 112 sentences of Fig. 6 might appear as:

B	**Responses**				Normal Response					Abnormal		
			Repet-	Elliptical Major				Full		Struc-		Prob-
	Stimulus Type	Totals	itions	1	2	3	4	Major	Minor	tural	Ø	lems
	10 Questions	10	0	7						3		
	4 Others	4	0	3						1		
C	**Spontaneous**	98	0	98	Others							

A   **Unanalysed**   **Problematic**

1 Unintelligible	2 Symbolic Noise	3 Deviant	1 Incomplete	2 Ambiguous

B   **Responses**

Stimulus Type	Totals	Repet-itions	Normal Response								Abnormal	
			Elliptical Major				Full Major	Minor	Struc-tural	Ø	Prob-lems	
			1	2	3	4						
Questions												
Others												

C   **Spontaneous**   Others

Stage I (0;9–1;6) — Sentence Type

Minor   Social **3**   Stereotypes **1**   Problems

Major   Sentence Structure

Excl.	Comm.	Quest.	Statement
	·V·	·Q·	·V· **2** ·N· **8** Other **4** Problems

Stage II (1;6–2;0)

			Conn.	Clause		Phrase		Word
	V X	Q X		SV	V C/O	DN **11**	VV	-ing
				S C/O	A X	Adj N **9**	V part **6**	**3**
				Neg X	Other	NN **2**	Int X	pl
						PrN **8**	Other **4**	**9**

Stage III (2;0–2;6)

-ed

			X · S:NP	X · V:VP	X · C/O:NP	X · A:AP
V X Y	Q X Y		SVC/O	VC/OA	D Adj N **7**	Cop
let X Y	VS		SVA	VOdOi	Adj Adj N	Aux
do X Y			Neg X Y	Other	Pr DN **8**	Pron **21**
					N Adj N	Other **7**

-en
1
3s
gen

Stage IV (2;6–3;0)

			XY · S:NP	XY · V:VP	XY · C/O:NP	XY · A:AP
· S	QVS		SVC/OA	AAXY	N Pr NP **1**	Neg V
	Q X YZ		SVOdOi	Other	Pr D Adj N	Neg X
					cX **2**	2 Aux
					XcX **4**	Other **3**

n't
·cop
·aux

Stage V (3;0–3;6)

how	tag	and	Coord. 1	1	Postmod. 1 clause	1 ·
		c	Subord. 1	1		
		s	Clause: S		Postmod. 1 phrase	**1**
what		Other	Clause: C/O			
			Comparative			

-est
2
-er
-ly

Stage VI (3;6–4;6)

(+)			(−)		
NP	VP	Clause	NP	VP	Clause
Initiator **2**	Complex	Passive	Pron	Adj seq	Modal	Concord
Coord **1**		Complement	Det	N irreg	Tense	A position
					V irreg	W order
Other			Other			

Stage VII (4;6+)

Discourse		Syntactic Comprehension
A Connectivity	it	
Comment Clause	there	Style
Emphatic Order	Other	

Total No. Sentences **112**	Mean No. Sentences (a) **8·0** (b) **0·9** Per Turn	Mean Sentence Length

© D. Crystal, P. Fletcher, M. Garman, 1975 University of Reading

Fig. 6   Profile of 'unchecked' phrasal development

Few stimuli are needed with such a child: one stimulus leads to an average of 8 sentences being produced (cf. Mean No. Sentences Per Turn, see p. 104). This is, accordingly, a very difficult and serious remedial situation. P has spontaneously begun to use her phrase structures all over the place. This carryover might have been a source of joy to parent or T at an earlier stage (where any increase in quantity is welcome, especially outside the clinical situation), but with increasing vocabulary and volubility, and no progress in clause structure to interrelate the highly developed phrases, increased ambiguity, incomprehension and frustration (by both T/parent and child) will result, e.g.

T   'what did you get for your birthday/
P   a 'lot of càrs/. 'from my dàddy/. a big 'racing 'car/
      'on my birthday/. 'all the children/. 'lots of càrs/

T might be forgiven for wondering what exactly daddy gave P, and what all the children were doing.

Contrast this with the following B/C profile, where the 112 sentences of Fig. 6 are distributed rather differently:

B **Responses**					Normal Response					Abnormal		
			Repet-		Elliptical Major			Full		Struc-		Prob-
Stimulus Type		Totals	itions	1	2	3	4	Major	Minor	tural	0	lems
100	Questions	62		59					3		2	
30	Others	23		22					1			
C **Spontaneous**		25		25	Others							

This is a much less serious remedial problem: the majority of P's sentences are still under the influence of T's stimuli, which suggests that T may be able to exercise a considerable measure of control over P's development.

All spontaneous sentences of at least two-clausal elements, and any one-element sentences that are *not* elliptical in character (e.g. a minor sentence) are classified under Others in Section C, e.g.

T   who was thère/
P   there was a 'big màn/—very 'big 'man/—
      Response (full Major) Spont.1

      he was 'walking a'round the ring/—a clòwn was 'following him/
            Spont. Other   Spont. Other

         nò/   two 'clowns 'were/—they 'got a búcket/ and 'put it òn him/—
    Spont. Other   Spont. Other   Spont. Other
      not nìce/—he 'got 'all wèt/
    Spont 1   Spont. Other

Section D?

Given that the purpose of Sections B/C is to focus T's attention on the interactional features of the sample, the question arises of how complete an account of grammatical interaction the Profile Chart provides. There is, indeed, a major omission which future revisions of the chart may well make good, but which we cannot at present remedy because the fundamental research needed has not been done. Some guidelines concerning the topic can however be introduced here.

Interaction in clinical contexts is not a two-step process of Stimulus and Response, as the above discussion appears to suggest. It is a three-step process: T Stimulus—P Response—T Reaction. Both the steps involving T are crucial in developing successful remedial procedures. What has often been commented on is the need for T to find a stimulus appropriate to P's language level, to avoid overestimating P's responses. What has been less noticed is the need for T also to react appropriately to P's output, and the various ways in which this can be done. Basically, two tasks are involved:

(i) if P's response is correct in all respects, T will need to provide the usual reinforcement, whether linguistic or otherwise;

(ii) but if P's response is incorrect, T must draw P's attention to the contrast between the incorrect and a correct response. In practice, there are a large number of reaction strategies, over which T should be in some degree in control. The most important distinctions in remedial situations are as follows:

(1) *General positive reinforcement*, unrelated to the structure of P's utterance, e.g.

    T   'what's thàt/
    P   a càr/
    T   yès/ ... 'that's rîght/ ... 'very gôod/ ... 'good bôy/ *etc.*

(2) *Explicit correction*, unrelated to the structure of P's utterance, e.g.

    T   'what's thàt/
    P   a càr/
    T   nó/ ... it's nǒt/ ... a cár (*with very wide rise, expressing disbelief*) ... I 'think its a bùs/ *etc.*

(3) *Repetition*, e.g.

    T   'what's thàt/
    P   a càr/
    T   a càr/   *turns page*
           now 'what's thìs/ ...

We permit necessary deictic changes (of pronouns, demonstratives etc.) under this heading, e.g. P *I see one*/ T *you see one*/

(4) *Check*, e.g.

    T   'what's thàt/
    P   a càr/
    T   a cǎr/ ... did you say cǎr/ ... a càr/ ís it/ ...

The marked 'echo-'intonation here (= 'have I got you right? is that what you meant to say') is often misunderstood by Ps, who think T is querying the correctness of the utterance (cf. (2) above). The facial expressions of (2) and (4) are of course very different, but if P is looking at a book, these will be of little help!

(5) *Structural expansion* of all or part of the grammar of P's utterance, e.g.

T   'what's thàt/
P   a càr/
T   that's a càr/ ... it's a càr/ ... it's a 'lovely càr/ *etc.*

(6) *Paraphrase* of all or part of the meaning of P's utterance, e.g.

T   'what's thàt/
P   a càr/
T   your dàddy 'drives one 'like thát/

(7) *Answer* to a P stimulus, e.g.

P   'what you gót/
T   a càr/

(8) *Comment* to P about the interaction, with no direct grammatical or semantic link with P's utterance, e.g.

T   'what's thàt/
P   a càr/
T   'sit stíll/ ... 'hold it cárefully/ ... I 'suppose you còuld 'call it thát/ *etc.*

(9) *Zero*, i.e. T proceeds to a new stimulus directly, giving no reaction to P's utterance, or (less commonly) stays silent, waiting for P to speak further, e.g.

T   'what's thàt/
P   a càr/
T   and 'what's thàt/
P   a bùs/
'T'   'what's thàt/
P   a càr/   *turns page to picture of bus*
     a bùs/   *turns page, etc.*

(10) *Other* reactions, as when T speaks to someone else in the room, speaks a commentary into the taperecorder, e.g.

P   a càr/
T   he's 'pointing at the bùs/

Four points should be noted:

(i) As with our treatment of responses above, we need to constrain the notion of Reaction to the immediately preceding P utterance.

(ii) These categories are not always mutually exclusive, and some in fact go regularly together, e.g.

(1)+(5)   yès/ it's a càr/
(2)+(5)   nǒ/ it's a bùs/
(3)+(1)+(5)   a càr/ thàt's 'right/ a 'big càr/

(iii) T may conflate reaction functions into a single sentence, e.g.

P   got càr/
T   you hàven't 'got a 'car/

which is (2)+(5) in one.

(iv) Similarly, T may use one sentence to act as both reaction and new stimulus, e.g.

P   I 'see the càr/
T   and 'who's in the 'car/

This, it will be appreciated, is a very adult and potentially complex interaction pattern for P to handle.

To illustrate this procedure more fully, here are two extracts from Hugh's transcripts (*GALD*, 150, 158), with T's reactions analysed along the above lines:

			Commentary
	T	'what's the làdy 'doing/—	*New stimulus*
	P	[kʌg]/ gìrl/—slèeping/	
	T	it's a lit/ it's a gìrl/ ìs it/—	*Ignore T's self-correction; Check, with (partial) structural expansion*
	P	slèeping/.	
	T	'what's she dòing/	*Zero*
	P	slèeping/.	
	T	slèeping/———	*Repetition*
		what are thòse/—	*New stimulus*
	P	'on a bìrd/	
10	T	yès/	*General positive reinforcement*
		they're 'on a bìrd/	*Structural expansion*
		it's 'what the 'bird flìes with/	*Paraphrase*
		'what do we càll them/	*New stimulus*
	P	fèather/	
	T	wìngs/.	*Check (P's poor articulation of 'feathers', which D glosses in l. 18)*
		yès/ (*said to herself*)	*Other*
	P	*wīng/	
	D	*fèathers/	
	T	fèathers/	*Other (T reacting to D's gloss)*

<table>
<tr><td>20</td><td></td><td>'what has your âeroplane 'got/
'not only the birds have gót them/ but
your âeroplane's 'got 'two of thóse/
hàsn't it/</td><td>New stimulus</td></tr>
<tr><td></td><td>P</td><td>yés/</td><td></td></tr>
<tr><td></td><td>T</td><td>'what áre they/</td><td>Zero</td></tr>
<tr><td></td><td>P</td><td>wìng/</td><td></td></tr>
<tr><td></td><td>T</td><td>yès/—</td><td>Zero</td></tr>
<tr><td></td><td></td><td>'makes it gò 'faster</td><td>Paraphrase</td></tr>
<tr><td></td><td></td><td>. . .</td><td></td></tr>
<tr><td>71</td><td>T</td><td>'what's thàt/—</td><td></td></tr>
<tr><td></td><td>P</td><td>gréen 'car/ ánd a/—'green . lòrry/</td><td></td></tr>
<tr><td></td><td>T</td><td>a gréen/cár/ and a gréen lòrry/</td><td>Structural
expansion</td></tr>
<tr><td></td><td></td><td>alríght/</td><td>General positive
reinforcement</td></tr>
<tr><td></td><td>P</td><td>'[ɔʒ] 'go hère/———
'put 'them 'like thàt/—</td><td>Zero</td></tr>
<tr><td></td><td>D</td><td>you 'put them like thàt/</td><td>Structural
expansion</td></tr>
<tr><td></td><td>T</td><td>'what còlour's 'that 'saw Húgh/</td><td>New stimulus</td></tr>
<tr><td></td><td>P</td><td>mè 'want/ a rèd/ 'red ràcing 'car/ . red—</td><td></td></tr>
<tr><td></td><td>T</td><td>you 'want a 'red ràcing 'car/—</td><td>Repetition
(? + Check)</td></tr>
<tr><td></td><td>P</td><td>m̀m/——</td><td></td></tr>
<tr><td>80</td><td>T</td><td>do you 'think I've gót a 'red *rácing 'car/</td><td>Zero</td></tr>
<tr><td></td><td>P</td><td>* yès/—
hère/
nò/—
yès/———</td><td></td></tr>
<tr><td></td><td>T</td><td>that rácing 'car/ is rèd/</td><td>Zero (i.e. this
is a new stimulus;
it would be
difficult to
decide what it is
reacting to,
earlier in the
dialogue—hence
Note (i) on p. 57)</td></tr>
<tr><td></td><td>P</td><td>yès/—
'got . tèn 'red 'racing 'car in hére/</td><td></td></tr>
<tr><td></td><td>T</td><td>tĕn 'red 'racing 'cars in 'there/</td><td>Repetition (deictic
change ignored)</td></tr>
<tr><td></td><td></td><td>I 'don't 'think I hăve/—
shall we 'see how 'many I hàve gót/——</td><td>Comment
New stimulus</td></tr>
</table>

If a Section D were incorporated onto the chart, accordingly, it would have to reflect the relative frequency and significance of the above categories in T/P interaction. For example, because of the importance of Structural expansion and paraphrase in developing children's language (cf. Brown and Bellugi 1965, Nelson *et al.* 1973, Bushnell and Aslin 1977), these categories should be tallied separately. Zero responses are worth noting separately, as they indicate the extent to which the interaction is more like an interview than a teaching session. Given the purpose of therapy, it might be useful to collapse the above ten categories into five types (plus the inevitable Problems box):

(1) Structurally unrelated, general responses—(1) and (2) above.
(2) Structurally related responses—(5), (6) and (7)
(3) Repetitions (3)
(4) Zero responses—(9)
(5) Others (irrelevant and T-orientated reactions)

giving a Section D as follows:

D Reactions	Repet-itions	General	Struc-tural	Ø	Others	Prob-lems

1.3

Developmental stages

Stage I

This stage is discussed at length in *GALD* (63–6), and seems to present few analytic problems in practice. It is also discussed in more detail below, in 1.7.

The distinction between Social and Stereotyped Minor sentences, however, is sometimes obscure. All Minor sentences, let us recall, are unproductive—that is, they have a sentence structure which has no potential for development using the normal grammatical rules of the language. We can 'do' nothing with *yes, mhm, ta, Jack and Jill went up the hill*, and so on. Some Minor sentence types have a very limited productivity (e.g. *Sorry > I'm sorry, How are you? > How am I?*), but compared with major sentences, the potential is highly restricted. If we were ever unclear as to whether a sentence is Major or Minor, the utterance would go in the Minor Problems box (to avoid overestimating P's language ability).

Similarly, if we were unclear about the distinction between Social and Stereotypes, the utterance would go into the Problems box. This rarely happens, in clinical situations, where only a limited use is made of either category; but in theory there are several possible points of confusion. The basic distinction we make is as follows. Social minor sentences are one clause element long (usually one word), and have a highly specific speech-act function, e.g. responding, greeting, thanking, apologizing. Stereotyped sentences, with more than one clause element involved, have more the appearance of a major sentence; they tend not to be restricted to a single social context, and may even be learned by heart (as in proverbs and nursery rhymes). Compare the Minor sentences of (a) with the stereotypes in (b):

(a)	yès/	(b)	'first cóme/'first sèrved/
	thànks/		'how do you dò/
	goodbўe/		'Christmas 'comes but 'once a yéar/
	párdon/		the 'grand old 'Duke of Yòrk/
	dàmn/		you're wèlcome/
	òh/		

Phrases such as the following, because of their single-clause-element structure and specific social function, would be classed as Social: *Good heavens, Merry Christmas, Happy birthday*. Occasionally, formal and functional criteria contradict: *I beg your pardon* is socially comparable to *pardon* (Social) but structurally like *I beg to differ* (Stereotyped). Any such uncertainty would be reflected in the Problems total.

These are some of the conventional (adult) Minor sentences. In the context of language development, of course, we can never be sure that the adult system is going to be shared by the child. He may use adult Minor sentences in a productive way, or develop his own minor sentences. This commonly happens with stereotyped sentences, in fact. Long before the child develops productive control over a grammatical pattern, he may use it in a stereotyped way, as a single unanalysable unit. This happens both with language-delayed children and adult dysphasics. The problem for T is that it is impossible to say in advance what P's personal stereotyped utterances will be—though this is usually obvious by the end of a session, because of their frequency of occurrence. A selection of stereotyped sentences, taken from different Ps at different times, shows the possible variety: *don't know, what do you think of that, I mean to say, me cuddle that, all gone now*.

Because of the cumulative impression of stereotyping that builds up throughout a sample, therefore, we recommend that a final decision about whether a sentence is stereotyped or not be made only in retrospect, once one has analysed the whole of P's language, and seen how frequent or productive the sentence pattern is. And of the two criteria, productivity is the more important. Both child A and child B may have the phrase *I can't* in their samples, but it may be stereotyped for A and not for B: the evidence would be the absence of any related structures in A, whereas these would be present in B, such as *I can, can I, can't I, can he, you can't*, etc.

A few other specific methodological points concerning Stage I are:

(i) The reason why sentences are not analysed in terms of single-clause elements (S, V, C, O or A) has already been discussed above (p. 52).

(ii) 'Q' can only be a question-word (*how, when, where, why; who/whom/whose, what which*; the compound Q *how much/many*). One-word sentences with questioning intonation are not to be placed under 'Q' (cf. p. 17), and if added to the chart would require a separate label. Note also that Q does not necessarily refer to the whole of the questioned clause element: with the nominal Qs (*what/which/who* etc.), the Q may be a Determiner, as in *Which books* (sc. *do you want*); this is also analysed as QX, as discussed further below, p. 64.

(iii) 'V' in the Command column can only be a verb in the 'unmarked' form (e.g. *go, sit*), used with imperative function; any other form (e.g. *going, sat*) is classed under Statement, whatever the co-occurring intonation. Context must always be checked to ensure that the verb's function is imperative and not statement. Uncertain cases are placed under Problems.

(iv) Vocatives (Nouns or Noun Phrases used to address or call someone, e.g. *John!, my dear Sir*) do not enter into clause structure, but stay outside it, e.g.

I've 'just 'bought a càr/
Jŏhn/I've 'just 'bought a càr/

They are therefore classed as Minor sentences (Social). If one is not sure that a noun has vocative function, this could be placed in the Minor Problems box.

Stage II

The following points should be emphasized, in the light of the discussion of two-element sentences in *GALD* (67–70):

(1) The 2-element labels listed under Clause and Phrase are not to be interpreted as having a fixed order: word order is still very fluid at 18 months, and is still inconsistent at 2 years, though the dominant patterns of the language are by then established. SV, then, usually applies to sentences where the subject comes first and the verb second, but the reverse order may be heard (and where it is obvious from the context that VO is not intended, e.g. the child who said '*tickle dàddy*/, and waited!). Similarly Neg X refers to 'Neg and X in either order' (e.g. *no pull, pull no*); and likewise for the other combinations, both at clause and phrase level. At phrase level, as it happens, we have never heard reversed word order for DN, V part, Int X and Pr N (*cat the, down sit, nice very, box in* etc. would seem to be deviant), but Adj N, NN and VV may be heard in either order (e.g. *red chair* v. *chair red, mummy bag* v. *bag mummy*, and *want go* v. *go want*).

(2) The distinctions between SC and SO, and between VC and VO, are unlikely to be needed at this Stage: both are included for the sake of completeness, but we recognize that it will often be impossible to be certain as to what verb, if any, has been omitted, if the C/O is a noun. Presumably *daddy ball*, said just after daddy has kicked the ball, is SO—that, at any rate, is how it will be interpreted—and *me David* is SC (for the present author, at least!) But it is not difficult to think of sentences where it is unclear which is involved, i.e. whether the post-verbal element is identical to or an attribute of the subject, e.g. P sees a picture of a man looking at another man painting a wall, and says *man painter* (= *is* or *sees* a painter). The distinction between C and O becomes far more important for remedial work once Copulas begin to be used, at Stage III.

(3) The label AX is a descriptive convenience, no more. We could have put Stage II AS, AV, AC, AO, AA (or SA etc.), but this would have been unnecessarily detailed. What we wish to note is P's use of an adverbial element: exactly which other element he uses it with could be the scope of a further mini-profile. Likewise, Neg X (or X Neg) is short for Neg S, Neg V, Neg C, Neg O or Neg A (again, with optional order), and the X in QX and VX has an identical range of application. (See p. 83 for the different sense of Neg X at Stage IV.)

(4) Neg (in Neg X, and Neg XY) is a separate clause element—albeit an immature and temporary one (cf. Note (7) below); therefore a sentence in which it occurs along with A will require two analyses: *there no*, for instance is A + Neg, and because *two* items of developmental information are involved in the one structure, the sentence is logged twice: Neg X and AX.

(5) 2-clause element Others are rare, there being so few patterns possible at this Stage, e.g. VO$_i$ *gave to him*. A common 'unclear' example is *allgone X*: it is difficult to know how best to analyse *allgone*. We have nothing to add to the para-

graph on Others in *GALD*, 69—apart, that is, from an apology for the inadvertent omission of a line of print in the book's first edition![9]

(6) A question of profiling method is raised by VX and QX, which recurs throughout the Question and Command columns at several stages—QXY, QXYZ etc. Do we give any additional analysis to the X, Y or Z? The answer is: No, at clause level; Yes, at phrase and word level, if relevant. The distinction between Statement, Question, Command and Exclamatory, it must be remembered, is made solely on the basis of the nature and ordering of elements of *clause* structure—hence, to have identified a Question, say, as having two clause-level elements (Q and X) makes it unnecessary to say this again elsewhere. If the profile chart were big enough, we could have printed QS, QV, QC etc., and thus made the contrast with the right-hand side of the chart explicit. But the chart is not big enough, nor is the explicitness really necessary, as questions, commands and exclamatory sentences tend to be so much less encountered in clinical language work that it would be a waste of effort.[10] Likewise, we do not provide a more detailed subclassification of the clausal function of Q in the cases of *what*, *which* and *who*. Take the two sentences *what came?* and *see what*: in the first, *what* is Subject; in the second, Object. There are different patterns of development here (cf. Tyack and Ingram 1977), but we do not devote space to them on the chart, for the same reason as given above.

On the other hand, phrase- and word-level structure, if used, is not affected by the Statement/Question distinction, nor is the existence of transitional information. Any information under these headings is, accordingly, inserted in the appropriate places on the right-hand side of the chart, as the following examples show:

'where dáddy/
Q   C   (Profiled as QX)

'where my dáddy/
Q   C   (Profiled as QX)[11]
D   N   (Profiled at phrase-level Stage II and at X+C: NP)

'what dóing/
Q   V   (Profiled as QX)
      -ing (Profiled at Word level)

'where 'my 'big cár/
Q   C   (Profiled as QX)
D Adj N (Profiled at phrase-level Stage III, and at X+C: NP)

---

[9] The omitted line reads: 'heading Other. Examples are *me sock* (?=put the sock on me), *mummy*.'

[10] The design of the chart would perhaps be clearer if the heading *Statement* were moved to be over the Clause column: at present, it looks as if Phrases and Words are statement only, which is not the intention.

[11] We need to know the clause element analysis (QC, in this example) in order to be able to mark the appropriate transitional information. If this were unclear (e.g. whether a sentence were QC or QS), the Ambiguous box would be used.

'where 'mummy and dáddy/

Q $\qquad$ C $\qquad$ (Profiled as QX)

X   c   X   (Profiled at phrase-level Stage IV, and at X+ C: NP)

The same principle applies for QXY, QXYZ, etc., as may be briefly illustrated:

'where 'daddy gò/

Q   S   V (Profiled as QXY)

'where my 'daddy is gòing/

Q $\qquad$ S $\qquad$ V   (Profiled as QXY)

D   N   Aux   (Profiled at DN Stage II, Aux Stage III; XY+S:NP, XY+V:VP; 3s and -ing at word level)[12]

Notes:

(a) Abbreviated questions (i.e. question-word plus preposition), such as *what for?, where to?, for when?, why not?* etc. are all analysed as QX.

(b) The distinction between Q-element and Q-word (see Quirk *et al.* 1972 (*GCE*), 394) causes a problem. In the adult language, the whole of *which book* (sc. *did you buy*), for example, is a Q clause-element (Q–S), but only the first item is a Q-word (which is functioning as Determiner in a noun phrase). This distinction has no parallel elsewhere in English grammar, and accordingly we have to adopt an ad hoc solution in profiling such usages. We could (a) ignore the distinction, and put the whole element under 'Q' at Stage I; (b) classify Q–Det usage separately at Stage II; or (c) subsume it under QX at Stage II. We do not follow solution (a), as this would be far too complex an assignment to the 1-element stage; nor do we follow (b), as it is often not easy to distinguish Q+Det from Q+Clause element in the usage of children at Stage II (e.g. *which book* might be 'which book did you buy' or 'which is the book'). We therefore follow solution (c), i.e. when the Q is a determiner in the NP (e.g. *what/which/how many/whose books*) the residual phrasal feature is still analysed as X, with a subsequent phrase structure analysis of D N. In *which red books* (*did you buy*), etc., the analysis is still QX, with a subsequent phrasal analysis of D Adj N. This is the *only* occasion where X is used in this column to refer to a phrasal element.

(7) A question of profile interpretation is raised by the categories of S O/C, Neg X and some instances of AX (and also QXY and Neg XY at Stage III, and QXYZ at Stage IV). These are the only 'immature' structures on the chart, i.e. structures which will not be found in the adult language, and which we would expect to drop out as P matures (SC→SVC, Neg X→Neg V, QXY→QVS, etc.). Gaps in the profile at these points are therefore a *desirable* feature to see emerging, as P reaches Stage III and beyond.

[12] In further examples below, profiling glosses are abbreviated as follows: Stage I=I, etc.; Clause level=C; Phrase level=P; Word level=W; Transitional=T; Other=O.

(8) Adj N. It must be remembered that Adj stands for *Adjectival*, not simply Adjective (cf. *GALD*, 53), i.e. it includes ordinals and quantifiers. As a descriptive category, it also includes nouns used as modifiers, either as possessives (e.g. *mummy's bag*) or as 'adnominal' (e.g. <u>railway</u> station); but developmentally and remedially, we feel these last constructions should be kept distinct from other Adjectivals, and they are in fact identified by a different label on the profile chart (NN). In *GALD* 53, we give examples of these constructions, by using the general category label Adj, and this, we now recognize, may mislead when it comes to the business of transferring analyses onto the chart. If, then, T finds it clearer to label the analysis of

the big railway station *and* the man's hat

as:

D Adj   N   N   D   N   N

instead of:

D Adj Adj   N   D Adj N

(as in *GALD*, 53), we recommend this should be done. All the following, then, would be NN at Stage II: *potato crisps, washing machine, doll's house, mummy bag, mummy's bag, mummies' bags*. Slightly more complex are examples like

mummy's red   bag
N   Adj   N

This, being a 3-element phrase, would be classified at Stage III.

(9) VV represents the earliest type of relationship between two 'main verbs'— the so-called 'catenative' construction. Most verbs govern nouns (as objects or complements), but some verbs govern verbs as well, and when they do they are said to be catenative verbs. Examples are: *want to go* (which would presumably first appear as *want go* or *wanna go*), *likes to stay, keep running, go walking*. The important point about these verbs is that they can build up into some quite complex sequences, e.g. *wants to keep going*, and these are discussed further below (cf. Hierarchic Organization, p. 72). For the VV structure containing an object (e.g. *want him to go*), see p. 94.

(10) *V part* is a construction which raises several analytic problems—primarily the confusion with the apparently similar V + Preposition + Noun Phrase. Resolving the ambiguity in the following sentence shows the contrast clearly:

He came across the road.

This can mean: (a) 'He moved across the road' (e.g. on a bicycle—i.e. a Prep Phrase functioning as A); (b) 'He discovered the road' (e.g. on a map)—a V Part. (a) and (b) are distinguished on both semantic and syntactic grounds. There are several criteria (cf. *GCE*, 811 ff), but the two most important are: (i) the V Part construction has a single meaning, with the component items constituting either an idiom or a very restricted interdependence, e.g. *bring up the children* has no opposite *bring down the children*—*bring down* has a quite different meaning; there is no such tight relationship between *come* and *across* in (a), cf. *he came across/ over/under/near ... the road*; (ii) the Part stays under the influence of the V, in various transformations, whereas in (b) the item stays with the NP, e.g. (a) transforms into (moving the A) *Across the road he came on a bicycle*; but (b) does not transform into **Across the road he came on a map*. The passive is also a useful transformational guide. Compare *he arrived after lunch* and *he arrived at the answer: *lunch was arrived after* is not possible, showing that *after* stays with the NP; *the answer was arrived at* is possible, showing the V Part construction. A third criterion is that V Parts take Nominal (*Who/What*) question forms, e.g.

When did he arrive? After lunch.
What did he arrive at? The answer.
(Cf. *When did he arrive after? *What did he arrive? At the answer.
?*What did he arrive after? *When did he arrive at? The answer.)

When there is no NP following, the problem of deciding whether it is V Part or VA is still there, and again a mixture of semantic and syntactic reasoning has to be used. Compare *look out* (the warning) and *look out* (=‘look outside’): the first is V Part, on the same grounds as (i) above; the second is VA, as *out* here can substitute for a wide range of other As (*look out/up/down/outside/out in the street...*)—putting it semantically, the *out* has a distinctly independent meaning from the verb *look*. On these grounds, *switch on, look at, find out*, and several hundred more are V Part; (*now I want you to*) *come down, run up, jump across* etc. are VA.

Note, finally, that there may be more than one Part in a multi-word verb, e.g. *put up with, check up on, look forward to*. These are classified as Stage III Phrases (Other). For a further subclassification of V Parts, see *GCE*, 815 ff.

(11) *Int X*. This is a very limited category, though its members are frequently used by some children, especially when their repetition value is discovered (e.g. I 'want a 'very 'very 'big 'kiss/). Examples other than *very* include: *pretty awful, really big, quite tired, all clean, terribly sorry*. Usually it is Int + Adj, but Int + Adv is possible (e.g. *very happily*), and there are a few others, e.g. *right in* (Int + Prep), and the Exclamatory patterns (*how nice, what charm*, cf. Stage V, p. 91). (Note in *that's the very book*, *very* is Adj; one cannot substitute other intensifiers— **the really book*, etc.)[13]

We also use this category to describe the periphrastic expression of comparison, which is distributionally very similar:

My box is more beautiful
S V   C
          _____
          Int   X

(When comparison is expressed clausally (*more beautiful than...*), the analysis is

---

[13] The example of *down there* in *GALD* (69) was a misprint: it should have appeared on the next line, under Other.

at Stage V.) Likewise, the comparative question form is best analysed as Int X at phrase level, e.g. *how big*?

(12) *Other*. This category is quite often required to handle Stage II sentences. Particularly common are Pr Adv—*in there, on here*; Adj Adj—*big three, three pink*; N Part—*coat off*; to v—*to kick, to go*, and any structures containing pronouns e.g. indefinite—*blue one, two each, very much*; interrogative—*red what?, in where?*; or personal—*to me, with them* (in all cases except interrogative, a mark would also have to be placed under Pron at Stage III phrase level).

Transitional Stages

Between Stages II and III, and III and IV, a different kind of information is provided on the profile chart, namely whether P has structurally expanded any of his clause elements. The ways of doing this are numerous in English, as may be seen from a single SVOA clause:

he	saw	her	then
the man	had seen	the lady	last week
some of the young men	had been seeing	every new American film	each week of the year
my two American friends who work at the office	had kept on trying to get to see	the new film that had been showing at the Odeon	every time they had had a day off work

The structural expansion of an element of clause structure—in other words, the development of noun phrases, verb phrases, and adverbial phases—is one of the most important syntactic developments in the early language acquisition period. Why might this be so? Consider what would happen if such expansion did not take place: sentences would increase in length, but stay totally 'telegrammatic', e.g.

'man 'kick 'ball gàrden/'me 'see báll/ — 'gone nów/ — 'why 'ball 'go thère/*etc*.

Also, as the motivation to express semantic attributes developed in P, there would be an increase in short, unvaried sentences of this type: in the absence of any other syntactic ability, a P who wanted to say *I see the big red ball* would have to say something like:

'I 'see bàll/it rèd/it bìg/

This is a not unfamiliar clinical problem, especially when compounded by increasing ability at Stage V, e.g.

'I 'see bàll/and it rèd/and it bìg/and ...

The 'effect' of such language as P matures is of never getting to the end of what he wants to say, and it is often a source of considerable parental frustration. In a similar manner, phrasal development which stayed isolated from clause structure would ultimately produce a confusing sequence of utterances, as already illustrated in the discussion of Spont. Ellipt. 1 (p. 52 above).

The use of phrases within clauses around age 2 also correlates with the development of the child's ability to make expressions cross-refer (especially backwards— *anaphora*): instead of spelling out a Noun or NP all over again, the child learns to use personal and demonstrative pronouns, and similar devices, e.g. *the man came in; he saw the cat* instead of *the man came in ... the man saw the cat.*

It should be noted, in passing, that 'pro-noun' really means 'pro-NP', as illustrated by

> *Man* coming. . . . *he*'s tall.
> *The big fat man* is coming. . . . *he*'s tall.

When we see such developments appearing simultaneously in children, it is evident that a considerable structural change is taking place in their grammar, one which has major implications for their subsequent language ability, and it is this which motivates us to give special prominence to it on the profile chart. In the Clause column, we tabulate clause structure; and in the Phrase column we tabulate phrase structure; but we need a separate space to handle the *interaction* between clause and phrase structure, and this is why the transitional line appears as it does.

In interpreting the formulae between Stages II and III, the variable function of X should be borne in mind: it stands for 'the other element of clause structure in the sentence being analysed'. Thus,

> X + S : NP reads: 'the sentence has two clause elements, one of which is Subject, and this Subject has been expanded into a Noun Phrase; the other element is not the focus of attention here.'
> X + V : VP reads: 'the sentence has two clause elements, one of which is Verb, and this Verb has been expanded into a Verb Phrase; the other element is not the focus of attention here.'
> X + C/O : NP reads: 'the sentence has two clause elements, one of which is Complement or Object, and this Complement/Object has been expanded into a Noun Phrase; the other element is not the focus of attention here'.
> X + A : AP reads: 'the sentence has two clause elements, one of which is Adverbial, and this Adverbial has been expanded into an Adverbial Phrase; the other element is not the focus of attention here.'

Examples of these are as follows (Word level analysis is ignored):

S expansions	Profiling
'my 'daddy gòne/	II C
$\underline{\quad S \qquad}$ V	II P
D N	II T (= Transitional)
X + S : NP	

S expansions	*Profiling*

the 'big 'man thère/

S A	II C (AX)
D Adj N	III P
X+S:NP	II T

the 'big 'fat 'men gòne/

S V	II C
D Adj Adj N	IV PO
X+S:NP	II T

V expansions

'daddy is gòing/

S V	II C
Aux v	III P
X+V:VP	II T

'boy 'want to còme/

S V	IIC
V V	IIP
X+V:VP	II T

O expansion

'kicking that 'big bàll/

V O	II C
D Adj N	III P
X+O:NP	II T

A expansion

'gone in the gàrden/

V A	II C
Pr D N	III P
X+A:AP	II T

If a 2-element clause has *both* elements expanded in this way, there is no change in the procedure: each element is taken in turn and its expansion noted, as in:

'my 'daddy is gòing/	II C
S V	II P
D N Aux v	III P
X+S:NP X+V:VP	II T (twice)

The process of developing transitional structure is not something which happens all at once between Stages II and III: progress is still being made between III and IV, and as the information is of potential diagnostic importance (see below), it needs to be made available. Hence we have a second transitional line at this point. The procedure for profiling is identical to that already explained: each clause element is examined in turn to see if it is expanded; if it is, a mark is placed on the chart at the appropriate place. As the sentences are now *three* clause elements long, we need two 'empty' letters to refer to the parts of the clause not being focused upon, X and Y. For example:

the 'man gòne nów/			
S	V	A	III C
D N			II P
XY + S : NP			III T

twò 'people	are 'going	in 'there/	
S	V	A	III C
Adj N	Aux v	Pr Adv	II P; III P; II P(O)
XY + S : NP	XY + V : VP	XY + A : AP	III T (× 3)

By the end of Stage IV, however, it would seem that the process of learning to use phrasal expansion is sufficiently complete for us not to need a further transitional line. It would have been possible to mark transitional information between Stages IV and V as follows:

the man	is kicking	the ball	in the garden
S	V	O	A
D N	Aux v	D N	Pr D N
XYZ + S : NP	XYZ + V : VP	XYZ + O : NP	XYZ + A : AP

but we do not feel that the extra effort involved brings any fresh insight into disability patterns. If P is not coping with these at the beginning of Stage IV, there is nothing within the new structure of Stage IV as such that will promote any improvement; and conversely, if he is expanding 3-element clauses well, his 4-element clauses will show a similar pattern. We therefore ignore any phrasal expansion in Stage IV or subsequently.

Notes
(a) All phrase structures except Cop and Pron can be used to expand clause elements, but of course there are restrictions. The likely patterns are:

S, O, C,	*A*	*V*
DN, Int X	Pr N	VV, Neg V
Adj N, NN	Pr DN	V Part
D Adj N, Adj Adj N	Pr D Adj N	Aux, 2 Aux

S, O, C,	*A*	*V*
N Adj N, N Pr NP	NN (e.g. *tomorrow*	Complex VP
Postmod clause	*morning*)	
Postmod phrase	Adj N, etc.	
I		
Coord		
Complementation		

(b) Subordinate clauses are also classed as element expansions (and logged, for convenience, under the same labels X + S : NP, etc.). The various types of subordinate clause are classified at Stage V. Thus, for example,

$$\begin{array}{ccc} \text{say} & \text{what} & \text{you did} \\ \text{V} & \text{O} & \\ \hline & \text{s} \quad \text{S} \quad \text{V} & \end{array}$$

is counted as X + O : NP, as well as Clause : C/O.

(c) In normal children, there is a considerable degree of correspondence between clause level and phrase level structural development. Profiles have a 'balanced' look about them. As a result of this, there is usually a match between the kind of phrasal expansion used and the general level of attainment. It would be an interesting P indeed who had a clause structure still at Stage II, say, and a well-developed phrase structure, and who used the phrase structure to expand the clause elements. This would produce sentences like:

$$\begin{array}{cc} \text{the 'man who be 'kicking the báll/} & \text{gòne/} \\ \underline{\text{S}} & \text{V} \\ \text{Postmod. clause at Stage V} & \end{array}$$

This would of course be a deviant pattern, in our terms.

(d) Clause elements in Questions, Commands and Exclamations, if expanded, are entered under transitional information, as this has nothing to do with the Statement/Question, etc. status of the clause, e.g.

$$\begin{array}{cccc} \text{put the book} & \text{in the corner} & & \\ \text{V} \quad \text{O} & \text{A} & (= \text{VXY}) \\ \text{XY} + \text{O:NP} & \text{XY} + \text{A:AP} & & \end{array}$$

Note the analysis of the following:

$$\begin{array}{cccc} \text{where} & \text{did} & \text{the book} & \text{go} \\ \text{Q} & \text{V--} & \text{S} & \text{--V} \\ \text{XY} + \text{S:NP} & & \text{XY} + \text{V:VP} & \end{array}$$

Hierarchic phrase structure

In the above illustrations, several examples have been given where 3-item phrases are used, e.g. D Adj N, Aux V Part. When it comes to profiling these structures, however, and the 4-item phrases which are a development of them, the question arises as to whether they display a hierarchic organization that should be represented on the profile chart. The question, in practical terms is: is D Adj N a single phrase structure containing 3 items, or is it a blend of D N and Adj N? Put in this way, both theoretical and methodological arguments would support the first of these analyses. If we opted for the second, we would have to be consistent with further expansions: D Adj Adj N would be what? D N + Adj Adj? or D Adj + Adj N? Plainly, some very arbitrary decisions would have to be made; and arbitrariness leads inevitably to inconsistency.

Most of the structures in the Noun Phrase are like D Adj N—Adj Adj N, N Pr NP, Pr D (Adj) N, N (Adj) N—and the one that might arguably be analysed as a separate process (Int X) we also treat in this way. Therefore

    very big engine
    Int Adj N

is profiled as a 3-element Other, not separately as Int X;

    very big red engine

would be a 4-element Other, and so on.

Coordinated words/phrases (XcX at Stage IV), however, are much more satisfactorily treated separately from the structures which enter into them, e.g.

            boy and girl
             X   c   X
    the big boy and the little girl
    ___X___   ____X____   IV P
    D Adj N   D Adj N   III P (x2)

The Verb Phrase, on the whole, is treated as the NP: the development of a syntactic process is tentatively handled in different stages as a continuity, though insufficient research has been done for us to be sure about the allocation to Stages in the following:

catenative

Stage II	V V	e.g.	*like walking, want to go*	Profiled as V V
Stage III	V V V	e.g.	*likes going walking, want to keep going*	Profiled as III PO
Stage IV	V V V V	e.g.	*likes to help go shopping*	Profiled as IV PO

particles

| Stage II | V Part | e.g. | *come in* | Profiled as V part |
| Stage III | V Part Part | e.g. | *put up with* | Profiled as III PO |

auxiliaries

Stage III	Aux V	e.g.	*is going*	Profiled as Aux
Stage IV	Aux Aux V	e.g.	*will be going*	Profiled as 2 Aux
	Aux Aux Aux V	e.g.	*may have been walking*	Profiled as IV PO

negatives

Stage IV	Neg V	e.g.	*is not going, isn't going*	Profiled as Neg V
	Neg Neg V	e.g.	*isn't not going*	Profiled as IV PO

But what happens when these processes are 'mixed'? Here it is important to keep track of two things: (a) the structural level of the processes involved, handled as above; (b) the overall complexity, arising out of the conflation of these processes—handled by putting a mark in the Complex VP box at Stage VI. For example,

He is hoping to go
I do want to go
S _____V_____   II C
   Aux V   V   III P (Aux)
                                              II P (VV)
                                              VI Complex VP

He has been wanting to go   II C
S _____V_____   IV P (2 Aux)
  Aux Aux V   V   II P (VV)
                                              VI Complex VP

He didn't want to go   II C
S _____V_____   III P (Aux)
  Aux Neg V V   IV P (Neg V)
                                              II P (VV)
                                              VI Complex VP

He did want to keep on trying to go
S _____V_____   II C
  Aux V   V   V   V   III P (Aux)
                                              IV P (Other)
                                              VI Complex VP

For other Stage VI complexities, see p. 94.

Stage III

The following notes should be read in relation to Stage III.

(1) At clause level, the direct-indirect object construction occurs, in two possible orders (*give me the book, give the book to me*). Of the two, the *to* construction seems to be developmentally prior (cf. Cromer 1975, Cook 1976). Notice that there are several similar structures, using other prepositions, e.g. *he took a book from you, he saw a man with you*, which are not O_d O_i, as they lack the transformational potential of the *to*-structure, i.e. one cannot say **he took you a book* meaning 'he took a book *from* you', **he saw you a man*. The only other preposition which is capable of being used in an O_d O_i relationship is *for* (cf. *I got a book for you→I got you a book*), and some grammars are doubtful even of this, preferring to analyse

all such sentences with prepositions other than *to* as SVOA. We include both *to* and *for* under O_d O_i.

(2) Also at clause level, Neg XY should be noted, as a development of Neg X, i.e. the negative item is still *outside of* the remaining sentence structure, i.e. it is not structurally dependent on any specific element of clause structure, but seems to modify the sentence as a whole. P may be intending *I don't want a drink* but he says, at this Stage, *no me want drink*, *want drink no*, or the like. The Neg is usually at the very beginning of the sentence, but it may occur at the end, or occasionally between the X and Y. For example in *me no car* (='I don't want to go in the car'), the *no* has no verb to attach itself to, nor does it negate *me* or *car*.

(3) Stage III phrase level is particularly important. At this Stage, we find major progress in the use of pronouns, auxiliaries and the copula, which are three central characteristics of a developed conversational style. The following points should be noted.

(a) *Auxiliaries*. This term includes *all* the primary and secondary auxiliaries of *GCE*, Palmer 1974, and others. e.g. *be*, *have*, *do* and the modal verbs (e.g. *may*, *can*).

(b) *Copula*. This term refers to the verb *be*, in its various forms, and then only when it is the *sole* verb in the clause. (When *be* is used along with another verb, it is then an auxiliary verb.) Thus,

I am cross			
He is Smith	are all	S V C	
You are happy		Pron Cop	

Note that there are various other linking verbs to be found in English (e.g. *he became/resembled a doctor, he looks well, it went wrong, it tastes/smells sweet*), and these might also be called copulas, though in a slightly different sense, because they have more intrinsic meaning than *be*. Because of their more complex meaning and uses, and their later acquisition, they are not included under Cop here, but under Complementation patterns at Stage VI.

Note also that, while *be* takes a Complement, not an Object, it is not the case that everything which follows *be must* be C. SVA constructions are also possible, e.g. *he is in the garden*, which answer such questions as *where?*, *when?*, or *how?*

(c) *Pronouns*. The important point to note here is that this term refers only to items used *in isolation* or as the *head* of a noun phrase. The main category (cf. *GALD*, 52) is personal pronoun (viz. *I/me, you, he*), but it also includes possessive pronouns (viz. *mine, yours*), demonstrative pronouns (viz. *this, that, these, those*), reflexive pronouns (*myself* etc.) and indefinite pronouns (e.g. *someone, one, none*). When these items are used in other constructions, however, they have a different status: *this car, mine book, her cat* are D N. The types of pronouns which are *not* listed under Pron on the chart are *relative* pronouns (s at Conn. Stage V) and *interrogative* pronouns (labelled as Q).

(d) As with Stage II, there are several structures that need to be placed under the heading of Other. At clause level, we might have, for example, *gone home now* (VAA), or *Johnny the letter to Mary* (= 'Johnny gave the letter to Mary', i.e. SO$_d$ O$_i$), as well as indeterminate constructions. At phrase level, all the following would be under Other: *in nice book* (Pr Adj N), *what a car* (Int D N), *to that one* (Pr D Pron), *my mummy's car* (D N N), *get on with* (V Part Part).

(4) The two developments in Question structures at Stage III were not explained in sufficient detail in *GALD*, 71–2, and consequently some amplification is in order.

QXY. As elsewhere in the Question/Command columns, the X and the Y refer to different, unspecified elements of *clause* structure. Thus, all the following are profiled under QXY:

<table>
<tr><td>what you doing</td><td>where you gone</td><td>who saw daddy</td></tr>
<tr><td>Q   S   V</td><td>Q   S   V</td><td>Q   V   O</td></tr>
<tr><td>why kick that ball</td><td colspan="2">who is going in the garden</td></tr>
<tr><td>Q   V   O</td><td colspan="2">Q   V   A</td></tr>
</table>

The phrase and word structure involved is profiled separately, in the appropriate columns, as with QX at Stage II. If we had left it like that in *GALD*, there would have been no problem. But we added a comment, which in retrospect has turned out to be highly misleading, intended to cover sentences such as the following: 'where 'my mùmmy/, 'what 'be gòing/. The stress pattern (omitted in *GALD*, 71) is different from the normal blend pattern, which would be 'where my mùmmy/, 'what be gòing/. It seemed to us that the '`/ pattern is what we would associate with a series of *clause* elements (cf. *GALD*, 68 (d)), and suggests that the blend structure is not yet well established. Only in such circumstances did we think it possible to say that 'the two phrase elements of a blend' as in 'where 'my mùmmy/ were to be analysed as QXY. However, this phenomenon has turned out to be not as systematic or frequent as was thought; it is difficult to work with consistently, and as a result the comment at issue will be deleted from future editions of *GALD*. The similarly misleading example under VXY (*GALD* 72), *kick big ball*, will likewise be replaced. *Where my mummy*, then, regardless of stress pattern, will be analysed as

$$\frac{\text{Q} \qquad \text{X}}{\text{D} \quad \text{N}};$$

kick big ball, regardless of stress, as

$$\frac{\text{V} \qquad \text{O}}{\text{Adj} \quad \text{N}}.$$

The only exception to this principle, as already noted (p. 65) is when the Q-word acts as Determiner or Intensifier as part of a phrase, e.g.

'What 'books búy/
Q–   –O   V =QXY

'How big thát/
Q– –C   S   =QXY

VS. This refers to the use of inversion of Subject and Auxiliary Verb in the expression of questions. Aux is always marked in the phrase column. At Stage III, VS appears as the only marker of question in a clause (e.g. *is he going*); at Stage IV, it appears along with a question-word (e.g. *where is he going*, QVS). What was left unillustrated in *GALD*, 71 was the range of sentences which would be profiled under this heading. In fact our practice is to allocate two types of sentence here:

(a) VS alone, e.g. *is he?*, *are they?*; *is he going?*, *have they gone?*;
(b) VS + one other element, to conform to the general pattern of Stage III being for 3-element clauses, e.g.

'is he 'kicking the báll/
V S   O   (or V S V O, if one wishes to note discontinuous
                          elements)

'have they 'gone to tówn/
    V   S   A

We left this second type implicit: if it had been spelt out on the chart, some such notation as VS(X) would have to have been devised. More complex clausal developments using VS would then be left to Stage IV, e.g.

is he 'kicking the 'ball nów/
V S   O   A

'will he be 'visiting us to'morrow at hòme/
V   S   O   A   A

all of which might be grouped under the additional label VS(X+).

These patterns are uncommon, in P samples, but they are important remedial goals, hence it may be useful for Ts wishing to work in this area to have guidelines such as the above in order to develop this part of the chart.

(5) Likewise, if it were felt desirable to develop *let* or *do* constructions at Stage IV, an additional notation would have to be devised, viz. *let* XYZ, *do* XYZ, for sentences such as:

'let 'mummy go 'shopping nów/
let   S   V   A

dò 'give 'me the bát/
do V O_i O_d

(Note that two-element *let*/*do* constructions, e.g. *let go*, *do that*, are analysed as VX at Stage II.)

(6) And further, if the XYZ specification were felt to be too gross, it would be possible to develop a mini-profile, to distinguish the various possibilities—QSV, QVO, QVA, etc. In this way, the Question and Command columns would

approximate more in size to the statement clause column, and the Chart would have to be redesigned to a much broader format.

Stage IV

The following clarifications should be noted, mainly to do with profiling method:

(1) The Stage refers to four *or more* elements of clause or phrase structure, hence the Other boxes will be more heterogeneous, as P moves nearer the adult language. All the following are Other:

he 'saw the 'man at 'home 'yesterday in Wòking/
S   V   O   A   A   A

he 'gave me a lètter this mórning/
S   V   O$_i$ O$_d$ A

in the 'big 'red càr/
Pr D Adj Adj N

It is likely that with further child language research, something systematic might be said about the development of structures of 5 or 6 items or more.

(2) AAXY means: AASV, AAVO, AASC, etc. The point to be made here concerns the function of adverbials in clauses. In a clause, there may be one S, one V, one C and one O (occasionally two—O$_d$ O$_i$)—but there may be an indefinite number of As, e.g. *he saw me yesterday, on a bus, with Mary, in the rain.* . . . It is the first sign of this in P's language (i.e. his using two As) which we give special mention to on the chart. The sequence AAXY is of course only mnemonic: the As may occur in any order at any position in the clause, e.g.

he 'soon gòt 'there/
S   A   V   A

'quíckly/ I 'went to tòwn/
  A   S   V   A

(3) *N Pr NP*. This was originally intended to cover solely cases such as the following: *boy on a dolphin, man in a warm coat, seat on the bus*. NP meant: one of the NP structures *so far* developed (Stages II–IV); N meant a single N. In the light of subsequent use of the chart in several centres, it has emerged that phrases such as the following are rather more common: *the boy on a dolphin, a big man in a warm coat*. By amending N to NP, these structures could be handled under the same heading (otherwise they would have to go under Other), and this does seem to make intuitive sense. The aim of this category, after all, is to emphasize the developmental point at which children put two noun phrases together, using the second as a means of postmodifying (i.e. specifying further the meaning of) the first. The preposition is the commonest way of doing this (the other ways all involve subordinate clauses—see Stage V). For example,

(Which man?) *the man in a raincoat*
on a bus
of steel
      NP   Pr NP

The two NPs are then analysed each in their own terms, as D N, Pr D N, etc. More complex postmodification than a single Pr NP is dealt with in Stage V.

A problem sometimes arises in differentiating a NP which is postmodifying, and one which is a separate Adverbial (cf. the V Part/VA distinction above, p. 67). Compare:

I saw the street from my bedroom
S V   O   A

I saw the man from the gasboard
S V   O

The transformational potential of A (mobility) is usually enough to show which we are dealing with (*From my bedroom I saw the street, *From the gasboard I saw the man*). This criterion should be borne in mind, then, whenever one encounters a sentence which has a temporal or locative Pr NP, and which could therefore receive either interpretation, the context being unclear. For example, *I saw the man in a coat* could mean either 'the man was in a coat' (−SVO, with postmodification) or 'I was in a coat when I saw him' (=SVOA). Intonation sometimes helps here, the A construction receiving a separate tone-unit, but it is not an infallible guide. The written language, likewise, sometimes uses commas: cf.

(a) I saw the man near the bar
(b) I saw the man, near the bar

The meaning of (a) is clear: 'the man near the bar' as opposed to 'another further away from the bar' (hence NP Pr NP). The (b) analysis is trickier. The (b) construction is SVOA if it means 'I was near the bar when I saw the man'; it is NP Pr NP if it means 'There was only one man in the room, and he was near the bar'. The contrast between *the man near the bar* and *the man, near the bar* is that of restrictive and non-restrictive modification (*GCE*, p. 858), and is not analysed separately in LARSP, as developmental norms are quite unclear. The important point is to be clear about the difference between either form of postmodification and the adverbial. A clear criterion is whether an expansion into a relative clause applies—*the man who was near the bar*. Only the NP Pr NP construction permits this.

(4) *X c X*. Quite a wide range of patterns is found under this heading, and some methodological guidelines are therefore needed. It is the occurrence of overt phrasal coordination which is the significant developmental phenomenon[14] regardless of the kind of phrase being coordinated, hence the need to have a separate

---

[14] Cf. Lust (1977) for an analysis of coordination in language acquisition using transformational theory. There are certain important differences, especially in the treatment of verb coordination.

label, with variables for the two phrases—X c X: all the following are marked as X c X, before doing any further analysis:

> boys and girls
> me and Pete
> the man and the woman
> all the fat men and three of the thin women ⎫ came
> it is old and dirty
> they went quietly and happily
> I washed and polished the car

And is the usual coordinating conjunction, though we may hear others, e.g.

> the man or the woman
> quietly but happily

and note the interesting Negative coordination

> (I saw) Billy, not Peter.

We do not distinguish *and* separately in transcription, for phrasal coordination; this is only done at clause level (under Conn at Stage V).

Above it was said that X c X makes *overt* coordination, i.e. an actual morpheme is present to express the link. This is usually opposed to *covert* coordination, where we know from the meaning or the intonation that coordination is present, e.g.

> I bought béer/crísps/and chèese/
> 'John the bùtcher arrived/

Here the nouns *beer/crisps* and *John/butcher* are being coordinated, without the use of a conjunction: these are not X c X, but are handled separately at Stage VI (NP Coord).

Once we have established an X c X, the methodological principle is to examine each X separately, to see whether there is any expansion at phrase or word level present. If there is not, there is no further analysis to do; if there is, the expansion is analysed in the usual way, e.g.

```
'cat and 'dog    rùn/
      S       15   V
 ─────────────
 X   c   X
X+S:NP
```

```
'boys and 'girls   rùn/
       S           V
 ─────────────
 X   c   X
 pl      pl
X+S:NP
```

[15] It would be possible to note these Xs as being two instances of 'N' at Stage I, but there are good arguments against this, e.g. these are plainly N, not 'N'; omitting the Determiner does not always produce a *less* complex NP (e.g. *the man and woman*) which a mark at Stage I would suggest; it goes against our general policy of marking expansions only.

the 'man and the wòman 'run/
```
                S
      _____
      X     c     X
      _____
      D   N       D   N
```
X+S:NP

the 'boy seemed 'very smáll/and ex'tremely dìrty/
```
      S     V                    C
   _____           _____
   D   N                 X      c         X
                       _____       _____
                       Int   X        Int     X
                  -ed                       -ly
```
XY+S:NP   XY+V:VP

Notes

(a) the analysis of mixed coordination, as in

I have béer/crísps/tomátoes/and chèese/
```
S  V                      O
         _____
         NP   NP     X    c    X
```
XY+O:NP

The analysis is not *beer-crisps-tomatoes and cheese*, with the first three items all being a single X, as is obvious when the NPs are expanded into *cold beer/salted crisps*, etc.   each NP is plainly a separate entity, and only the last is overtly coordinated to cheese.

(b) Note also the analysis of multiple coordination, as in

the 'lion and the 'tiger and the 'elephant looked wònderful/
```
                        S                        V        C
      _____
      X     c     X
      ____             _____
                       X     c        X
      _____       _____      _____
      D   N          D   N         D   N
                                          -ed
```
XY+S:NP

Each instance of a coordination is marked separately, from left to right, and *allowing for overlap*; then, the phrasal expansions are analysed in the usual way.

(c) Lastly, the special problems of the coordination of Verbs should be noted. As emphasized in *GALD* (44), verbs are the central, determining feature of clause structure. Apart from the immature clause patterns at Stage II (cf. p. 65), all clauses have verbs, either present or clearly elided. Indeed, a clause may consist only of a verb, and it is this which causes a point of possible confusion in relation to X c X. In the sentence *he is singing and dancing* we might argue for either of two analyses, as one clause (i) or as two (ii) (word-level analysis is ignored):

(i)   he   is   'singing and dàncing/   or
      S   V
      Pron Aux   X c X

(ii)   he   is   'singing and dàncing/
      S   V   and   V
      Pron Aux   v

(i.e. ellipsis of S+Aux in Clause 2)

Our view is that, unless there is a very clear prosodic break between the two Vs, the simpler analysis is (i). An example of such a break is:

    he is sìnging/——and dàncing/
    S   V   and   X

In cases where the break is minimal (he is sìnging/and dàncing/), the analyst has a problem, which he usually attempts to resolve on semantic grounds—is a single complex activity involved, or are there two separate activities. Sometimes one can find a neat contrast in the situation, as in *he washed and brushed his hair*: analysis (i) would be likely to mean his hair was being washed and brushed; (ii) would be more likely to mean he washed (himself), and then brushed his hair. If one cannot decide the issue on prosodic or semantic grounds, the sentence must be classed as Ambiguous.

The same arguments apply to the other inflected verb forms (e.g. *ran* and *jumped*), as they too operate as part of a larger clause structure. But what about the unmarked verb—*jump, go, walk*? Because these may occur in isolation, as single (imperative) clauses, usually with clearly different activities involved,[16] analysis (ii) would seem to be preferred, regardless of intonation, e.g.

    'look and (then) lìsten
    V_{imp} and V_{imp}

This would be analysed as clausal coordination at Stage V (see below). The alternative, to analyse this as X c X (i.e. a *phrase* structure and no more), would be very misleading.

(5) *c X*. Profiling here uses the same principle as above: marking first the coordination and then any other structural information, e.g.

    and John   and me   and the boy
    c   X   c   X   c   X
                      Pron   D N

---

[16] Not always. Note the contrast between *jump and shout* (at once), and *jump and* (then) *shout*. To avoid an ascent into epistemological problems, however, we analyse all of these in the same way, even where the two verbs are linked idiomatically, as in *go and see* (cf. *go to see*).

and jumping   and in there
  c   X $_{ing}$ c $\underline{X}$
                            Pr Adv

Notice that we cannot mark transitional information here, as there is only one element of clause structure involved.

(6) *Neg V and Neg X*. The scope of negation (i.e. which part of a sentence a negative word applies to) is a complex issue in linguistic analysis, nor are developmental norms well understood. What seems clear is that, after a period when the negative item stays outside clause structure, it then becomes integrated within the clause, generally being placed next to the item it negates. Because of the distinctive role of verbal negation in English (Neg V) we classify this separately from all other kinds of clausal negation (Neg X). In terms of profiling method, these categories are always marked in addition to whatever other information is present in the phrase, e.g. (clause/phrase levels only):

Neg V he isn't coming
        S   V   II C
          $\overline{\text{Aux Neg v}}$ III P (Aux)
                                  IV (Neg V)

        he can't be coming
        S   V   II C
          $\overline{\text{Aux Neg Aux v}}$ IV P (2 Aux)
                                  IV P (Neg V)

        he can't not come
        S   V   II C
          $\overline{\text{Aux Neg Neg v}}$ III P (Aux)
                                  IV PO

Neg X (I saw Smith) not hĭm/
                     Neg Pron   IV P (Neg X)
                                  III P (Pron)

        he saw mè/ not Jóhn/
        S V   O   III C
             $\overline{\text{X c X}}$ IV P
        Pron Pron Neg   III P (x 2)
                                  IV P (Neg X)

(7) *QVS and QXYZ*. As already mentioned, the use of inversion in *wh*-questions is later than in general questions, and does not take place all at once. At

one and the same time, therefore, a child might be experimenting with QVS and using his old strategy (QXY) with even longer utterances (QXYZ), as follows:

what is he doing   where your mummy is going now
 Q V S   Q   X   Y   Z
where is mummy   what books you did buy
 Q V   S   Q– –O S   V
                       =Q X   Y   Z   (cf. p. 76)

There is no separate label on the chart for the use of the QVX structure, once acquired, in more complex sentences, e.g.

what is mummy doing now
 Q V   S   A

If needed, further labels can be added, e.g. QVS (+X).

(8) +*S*. The important point to note is that for the S to be unambiguously analysable as a part of the imperative structure, it ought to be within the same prosodic contour, e.g.

'you 'sit 'down nòw/

The following would be analysed as two sentences:

yòu/—   'sit 'down nòw/
Social Minor   V   A   (=VX)
(Voc)

There will, of course, be unclear cases.

Word level

Several small but frequently occurring points of profiling method are needed here. There are also two orienting principles which need emphasizing:

(1) This column deals only with inflectional endings, not with lexical processes of word formation, i.e. the addition of prefixes, other suffixes, and the construction of compound lexical items (for this distinction, see e.g. Robins 1971).

(2) The order of acquisition given is not firmly established. The items towards the top of the list will emerge in advance of the items towards the bottom; but the appearance of any two adjacent items in a child may be the reverse of that shown.

-*ing*. This refers only to the -*ing* ending on verbs (what is often called the present participle ending). It does *not* apply to adjectives or nouns which also end in -*ing* (often historically deriving from verbs), such as *an amusing story, smoking is forbidden, my writing is awful*, and (to take a child example) *she's doing a chalking*. At Stage I in particular, it may sometimes be difficult to know whether a N or a V interpretation is required, e.g. P looks at picture of woman taking clothes out of a washing-machine, and says *washing* (=a Stage I Problem). The rarity of errors involving -*ing* in normal child language (cf. Kuczaj 1978) contrasts with the picture presented by most language disordered children. Note that so called 'stative' verbs in standard English (cf. *GCE*, 93 ff) are generally not used in an -*ing* form, e.g. *know* (*I am knowing), *see* (*I am seeing), *want* (*I am wanting).

pl. This refers to plurals of items used as *Nouns* only; other apparent plurals (e.g. *this/these, that/those, our* (= 'plural' of *my*), *are* (= 'plural' of *is*)) are not included. *One*, used as a headword, would be included because of the contrast between *a big one* and *big ones. All* nouns are included, whether regular or irregular. Cases such as *mices, mens*, are marked as plural, with the 'error' going under Stage VI (N irreg). In cases like *sheep, deer, postman* (which have phonologically identical singulars and plurals), context must be referred to to determine which number is involved.[17]

It was an ambiguous case of this last kind which led to a methodological suggestion that many Ts now adopt. In the sentence 'The post[mən] sorted the letters', it is unclear whether the noun is singular or plural; and if the accompanying context was inadequate, technically the whole sentence would have to be put in Section A, as Ambiguous. If P used many such sentences, this was felt to be unfortunate, as the whole of the Clause and Phrase structure is then lost, though this is quite unaffected by the decision concerning plurality. Under such circumstances, it is argued, one could profile the sentence, putting a questionmark (or some similar convention) under the plural box instead of the usual tick. Our feeling here is that it does not really matter which way one does it, as long as one realizes what one is doing, and works consistently. Ultimately, no information in the Ambiguous box is ever 'lost': it is always available for scrutiny sooner or later, after the clear sentences have been analysed; and if a lot of P's sentences are ambiguous in this way, then this scrutiny will not be long in forthcoming.

The same use of a questionmark could be introduced into any of the inflections below, e.g. is it -*ed* or -*en*, *gen* or *pl*?

-*ed.* One should remember here that -*ed* is solely a convenient abbreviation for 'past tense': it does *not* mean, 'only those past tenses which end in -*ed*'. All the following would be marked as -*ed*: *I walked/burnt/saw/went/took*; also *was/were/had/did*; also *I wanted, goed* etc. (though here an additional mark would have to be placed under V irreg at Stage VI 'Error').

-*en.* Likewise, one should remember that -*en* means solely 'past participle', and *not* 'only those past participles which end in -*en*'. It therefore includes: *I have seen/taken/walked/argued/gone/had/been/done/*; also *I have tooken* etc'. which are also V irreg 'Error' at Stage VI.

The distinction between -*ed* and -*en* is often unclear, especially with verbs which have identical forms for past tense and past participle (cf. *GCE*, 111 ff), e.g. *I got/ I have got, I looked/I have looked*. The analytic problem arises in cases such as

P   (*picks up a car*) I 'got a càr/
T   you've 'got a cår/

[17] In practice, this means (a) checking that more than one object is being referred to, and (b) checking that elsewhere in the child's language there is formal evidence of his controlling a singular/plural contrast, either in regular nouns, or by concord with Det, Pron, or V.

Should we attribute *-en* to P, or *-ed*? He is using a 'marked' verb form, so something must be noted. Context and T in this instance indicate that P is using the form *as if* it were *-en*, and we analyse it accordingly. Likewise, if it were:

P   I 'got a càr yésterday/
T   dîd you/

context and T would suggest the appropriate analyses to be *-ed*. But in cases such as

T   is the 'car in the bóx/
P   nò/
      I lòoked in thére/

it may not be clear from the context whether P has *just* looked, or whether he looked some time before; T has the option of saying *did you* or *have you*; the analysis is genuinely ambiguous, and should be marked as such (the questionmark device noted above is of no value here, as one would not know in which box to put it, in the Word column). In practice, additional clues occur, which would lead T to be able to make a decision, e.g. if in the above example P were then to say:

     I 'saw it 'under thère/

the use of *saw* would make us go for an *-ed* analysis for *looked*.

     3s. This is an obvious inflectional ending, but it must not be forgotten that there are irregular verbs which are also included under 3s, e.g. *does* ($=$/dʌz/ not /duːz/) *says* ($=$/sɛz/ not usually /seiz/), *has* (not *haves*), *was*. We also analyse *is* as 3s, and the reasons for this warrant discussion.

     The verb *be* in its present tense is the most irregular of all English verbs, and there is no obvious way of 'regularizing' it, to make it appear like other verbs (this is clear from the morphology literature of the 1940s, as several of the papers in Joos 1958 show). On the other hand, it holds a significant place in the acquisition of several clause structures (e.g. negative, interrogative, passive), and developmental errors in its use are worth noting. We therefore mark as much *be* information as we can, but only using categories *already needed* for other areas of our analysis, which means 3s for *is*, and Stage VI 'Error' (cf. p. 99) for any non-adult forms, e.g. *he be going, I are going*. Note that *he be's there* would be both 3s *and* Stage VI 'Error' (Tense).

     gen. As with *pl*, this category applies to nouns only, whether singular or plural ('s or s'). It does not apply to the possessive form of pronouns (*mine/yours/his/hers/its*).

     -est/-er. These refer to the expression of superlative and comparative within the word—usually with a clear inflectional ending. The periphrastic expression of comparison (viz. *as/more/most beautiful*, etc.) is handled in the NP (as Int X). Both adjectives and adverbs may be inflected in this way (cf. *GCE*, 286 ff for a discussion of the use of the inflection/periphrastic distinction). Irregular comparatives, where the inflection is not easily identified (e.g. *better, best, worse, least, more, most*) are also analysed as *-er* and *-est*.

-ly. This is the usual means of turning adjectives into adverbs (*quick→quickly*). The only problem arises with words like *hardly* and *really*: these look like Adj + *ly*, but they are not, as semantically there has been a change between adjective and adverb (*hardly* ≠ 'in a hard manner').

Stage V

There is little to be added to the theoretical discussion in *GALD*, 75–7, but a few detailed illustrations of profiling methodology may be helpful, and there is one obscurity in our original exposition which needs to be resolved. The most practicable procedure, we find, is to take care of the Sentence-Clause relationship first: once that is done, the structure of the individual clauses can be analysed in the usual way. For coordination, where the two clauses are 'equal' grammatically,[18] the procedure is as follows:

```
the 'boy sáng/ and the 'girl dànced/
  Clause      and     Clause              V C: Coord 1
──────────        ──────────              V Conn: and
  S  V                S  V
   etc.                etc.

òne 'boy will fáll/  or  twò boys 'will/
   Clause              c    Clause        V C: Coord 1
  ──────────            ──────────         V Conn: c
    S   V                  S   V
     etc.                   etc.
```

Go and look, etc., it should be recalled, are also handled here. For subordinate clauses, the easiest way of portraying the relationship is slightly different:

```
the 'boy sáng/    be'cause  he wànted to/
  S       V                      A               III C
                         ──────────────          V. Subord 1
                     s   Suþord Clause           V Conn: s
                           ──────────            II C
──────────                  S    V               phrase structure
  D   N                   Pron  V  Part             as above
      -ed                              -ed
XY + S:NP                XY + A:AP
```

```
'what   I   sáid/   was   the trùth/
        S           V        C               III C
      ──────────                              V S clause
    s   Subord Cl.                            V Conn: s
      ──────────                              II C
        S   V                 ──────          phrase structure
      Pron         Cop   D   N                  as above
            -ed 3s -ed
XY + S:NP         XY + C:NP
```

---

[18] Not always semantically: there can be a cause-and-effect relationship involved, as in *he died and he was buried*, where the reverse order is not acceptable. See further *GCE*, chapter 10, 661 ff on functions of *and*. With *but*, there is always a semantic dependency involved.

Note we may have a coordinating of subordinate clauses. With A clauses, each is counted as a separate main clause element, e.g.

he lèft be'cause he was tíred/ and be'cause it was làte/

| S V | A | | A | IV AAXY |

	Subord. Clause	and	Subord. Clause	V Subord 1+
				V Conn: *and*
	s S V C		s S V C	V Conn: s (×2)
	etc.		etc.	III C (×2)

With other clauses, the whole sequence is taken as a single element of clause structure—S, C, or O, e.g.

'what I sáid/ 'what I méant/ and 'what I'll ălways mean/ can...

	S			V	V S clause
	Subord. Cl.	Subord. Cl.	and	Subord. Cl.	V Conn.: s (×3)
					III C
	s S V	s S V	s	S A V	II C (×2)
	etc.	etc.		etc.	

the 'man 'said he would gò/

S	V	O		III C
		Subord. Cl.		V O Clause
				(N.B. no s)
		S V		II C
D N		Pron Aux v		phrase structure
		-ed		as above
XY+S:NP		XY+O:NP		N.B. the two
		X+V:VP		levels of element
				expansion

The four types of subordinate clause, S, C, O and A, are all placed in the Stage V Clause Column. The specific layout here is a matter of notational convenience only, and carries no theoretical implications. Because of the frequency of adverbial subordinate clauses, these are singled out for special attention, as Subord 1 ... 1+. This is the point which has caused confusion (cf. below, p. 248, fn. 31, and p. 199). It is by no means clear on the profile chart that the 1 ... 1+ line refers *only* to Adverbial subordinate clauses. It cannot refer to S/C/O clauses, as a sequence of such clauses is analysed as a *single* S, C or O. (This is because of their noun-phrase substitutability: a sequence of NPs constitute a *single* subject, not a series of subjects.) But we acknowledge that the term 'Subord', because of its general applicability to all types of dependent clause, is misleading as it stands: as a mnemonic, therefore, we recommend that 'A' be inserted after 'Subord' in that line. (This avoids the double-marking problem encountered by Bamford and Bench below, p. 249.)

C and O clauses are taken together, on grounds of frequency. Comparative clauses are quite unlike any other clausal pattern in the language, and need a separate classification. *Comp* stands for the 'compared element' (cf. *GCE*, 765 ff).

he is bìgger than the mán is/
S V   C   III C
          Comp s   S   V   V Comparative
                                                      V Conn: s
Pron Cop   D   N Cop   II C
  3s   -er   3s   phrase structure
     XY + C: NP   X + S: NP   as above

he is 'less hàppy than Jóhn/
S V   C   III C
          Comp   s   S   V Comparative
                                                      V Conn: s
Pron Cop Int   X   phrase structure
  3s   as above
          XY + C: NP

Conn. This refers to clausal connection only. Four types are distinguished. *And* is given separate mention on developmental and frequency grounds:[19] it is usually the first to appear and is then used everywhere! Other coordinating conjunctions (*but, or* and, formally, *for*) are placed under c. All subordinating conjunctions–adverbial (*because, when,* etc.), nominal (*who, what,* etc.), and relative (*who, that,* etc.)—are placed under s. Zero *that* (as in *he said he was*) is not given separate mention.

Other is a very broad category, in which we include any *overt* means of linking clauses *other than* that which is implicit in what has already been described further up the chart. If we take two clauses, and ask what is there in one which refers us forward or back to the other, there are several possibilities, some of which are illustrated here (see *GALD*, 50):

A man kicked a ball. *Then he* did *the same* with *another one*.

Pronouns and several determiners have this function, in addition to their roles in clause structure, as do ellipsis and comparative items. These have already been introduced onto the chart, so they are not marked again here. Under Other at Stage V are marked only those ways of showing clause connectivity *not* so far dealt with. Examples are (cf. *GALD*, chapter 10) those items which look like adverbials, but which have little specific meaning, and whose sole function is to relate clauses (they do not modify verbs in any way), e.g. well *I shall*; *what's that, then*; *so they did*. The majority of connectives (*conjuncts*), with specific meanings, are a later development (Stage VII under Sentence Connectivity), e.g. *first, later, also*.

[19] And on clinical grounds. See, for example, Naremore and Dever (1975) who, working with normal and ESN groups, show that *and* is a particularly important differential factor (92), along with the number of multi-clause constructions and hesitations.

It should be noted that the total under 'Conn' and under co-ordinate/subordinate clause structure may not tally. There are two structural possibilities which account for this:

(a) we may have a clause introduced by *and*, e.g.

T   so 'did you go to tówn/
P   yès/————and 'daddy 'saw 'Father Christmas/

Being linked to a clause, *and* is counted under Conn; but there is no corresponding mark under Coord, as two clauses are not being connected. This is in fact a very common occurrence, especially in Ps who have over-developed phrase structure, with no corresponding clause structure: having come to use *and* in phrases, they extend this into the beginning of whatever clauses they have acquired, producing an *and X——and Y——and Z* pattern.

(b) we may have an instance of clausal coordination with no overt connector, as in tags (e.g. *he'll miss it, won't he*) and comment clauses (*he came in, you see*). There are also P sentences, such as

he 'got his gún/'chased the màn/

This would be taken as Coord 1, and the 'Error' noted as Clause Coord in Stage VI (Other).

Tags. Both rhetorical and response-expecting tags are included here:

he's còming/isn't he/   (i.e. I'm telling you)
he's còming/isn't he/   (i.e. I'm asking you)

Negative and positive tags (e.g. *is he*, also with both intonations) are both included. On the other hand, tag statements, such as *he's a fòol/hé is/*, *'John should 'look where he's gòing/Jóhn 'should/*, are not counted as tags. All tags, whether question or statement, are analysed as Coordinated clauses as in the previous section (Coord 1, no overt connector); their clausal structural identity is then analysed further up the chart (viz. under VS), along with all relevant phrasal information, e.g.

          isn't   he
            V   S
Aux Neg V Pron
3s   n't
X + V: VP

(Note that the V is elliptical, therefore Aux not Cop.)

There is some recent developmental evidence that our putting tag questions into Stage V may be somewhat late, for many children: the Bristol Child Language Project has data which would place their main period of development much earlier, within the third year—perhaps as early as our Stage III (G. Wells, personal communication).

Exclamatory. This refers to specific clausal structures introduced by *how* and *what*, and should not be confused with the general notion of 'exclamations', which are analysed as Minor sentences. *How* and *what* are the only two question-words

which are used (in conversational English) with no VS inversion, and Q attached
to a NP (S, C, O or A) in initial position:

'what a 'nice dày it 'is/   'how wèll he 'talks/
    Q–C   S V   Q–A   S V

'what a 'lot of 'people càme/   'what a dày we've 'had/
    Q–S   Q–O   S V

Reduced exclamatory sentences (e.g. *how nice!*, *what a day!*, *what charm!*) are also
placed here, despite the fact that they display only a single element of clause
structure, as what we are noting is the development of any *how/what* structures
as such. We make no further clausal subclassification on the chart; but phrase/
word/transitional information is analysed in the usual way. *What* (*a*) NP and *how*
NP at phrase level are both Int X. Note the role of intonation in helping to distinguish an exclamatory sentence from a question:

T_1 'what chàrm/   (='isn't she wonderful!')
T_2 whàt 'charm/   (='I can't see any')

(There is, however, often ambiguity.)

    Postmodification. This is a notion which for us affects NPs only (though some
grammars do use a similar notion in the VP, with adverbials). Postmodification
may be phrasal or clausal.
    (i) *Phrasal.* The occurrence of a single Pr NP construction postmodifying the
Noun has already been introduced at Stage IV (NP Pr NP), e.g. *the man with a
hat, the funnel of the boat, the road to town, a present for John.* There is therefore
no need for us to have a slot for Postmod phrase 1 at Stage V, as this has already
been taken care of. We only need to mark constructions using *more than one* instance of Pr NP, e.g.

'Peter is a 'man in a 'hat in a hùrry/   (or ... *in a hurry in a hat*)

  S V   C
               Postmod phrase 1+

    Having marked this on the chart, the remaining constitutents of the Noun Phrase
are then marked in the usual way, viz.

a man   in a hat   in a hurry
 D N   Pr D N   Pr D N

Note that the possibility of confusion with adverbial phrases should not be overlooked (as with N Pr NP, p. 79).
    (ii) *Clausal.* Both finite and non-finite clauses (*GALD*, 48) may postmodify
the noun, singly or in combination. The procedure is to analyse all clause patterns

first, as in the following examples (the phrase structure of the earlier part of the NP is analysed separately):

```
the 'man who has fáinted/ is   in the gàrden/
     S                     V      A
        _____                              V Conn: s
           s        V                            V Postmod clause 1
___        _____   _____
D   N      Aux   v     Cop Pr D     N
                etc.
```

```
the 'man who(m) you sáw/ is ...
     S                    V                      V Conn: s
        _____                         V Postmod clause 1
           s      S   V
```

```
the 'bus which/that ar'rived lást/ is ...
     S                           V               V Conn: s
        _____                V Postmod clause 1
           s         V     A
```

The relative pronoun is usually omitted when it is the object of the subordinate verb, e.g.

```
the 'man you sáw/ is ...
     S         V
        _____                                  
        S   V                                    V Postmod clause 1
```

Here, no mark would be placed under Conn s.

A common pattern in learning to use relative clauses is to omit the pronoun in its subject role also, e.g.

```
'those are péople/'came to my pàrty/
    S    V            C
                _____
                   V      A
```

This would be analysed in the usual way at clause level, and the 'error' of not using the pronoun would be logged as a clause error at Stage VI.

Examples of non-finite postmodifying clauses are:

```
the 'man 'walking down the stréet/ is ...
     S                            V
        _____
           V            A                        V Postmod clause 1
```

```
the 'car 'parked in the stréet/ is ...
     S                          V
        _____
           V        A                            V Postmod clause 1
```

```
the 'way to dó it/ is ...
     S           V
        _____
           V   O                                 V Postmod clause 1
```

The same procedure applies if there is more than one clause, but note that, as above, the coordination, if used, must be counted as well:

the 'man who 'lost his càt/and (who) 'found an ówl/ is ...

S				V	V Coord 1; Conn:
Clause	and	Clause			*and*; Postmod
s V O		(s) V O			clause 1

Stage VI

Positive features (+)

GALD provides only a very brief outline of the data which would be analysed in their column, hence the following range of illustrations may be helpful. No new fundamental categories or structures will be found here: everything in the + column adds *extra* complexity to one of the categories or structures represented on the chart.

(1) *NP initiator*. Any part of the noun phrase preceding the Determiner— *all of the people, all the people, both my sisters, twice the amount, once a year, half a loaf.* These are all analysed as I D N, and logged on the chart as a 3-element Phrase (Stage III, Other) and under Initiator at Stage VI. Each item occurring before D is labelled as I, as follows:

almost all the people ...
  I   I D   N   (IV P O)

Several Determiners can also be found using an *of*-construction, e.g.

Some people saw me
Some of the people saw me
Enough bread was left....
Enough of the bread....

These are different from *all, both* etc., as the *of* is obligatory (contrast *all the people* with **some the people*). Such constructions can be analysed in several different ways. The analysis we follow is to take the semantic criterion to be the main one: both the sentences of a pair are saying the same thing—'someness' and 'enough-ness' respectively—hence we analyse them both as D N, and not as I D N:

some of the people
  D   N

(2) *NP Coord*. If coordination is overt, it will have been handled using the X c X convention. Stage VI is used when no morpheme of coordination is present, but the NPs are clearly related in this way, e.g. by intonational or semantic criteria. The clearest example is apposition (*GCE*, 620 ff), where (usually) two NPs have

the same syntactic functions, the same extralinguistic reference, and where one is omissible, e.g.

> John, the grocer, is coming
> The grocer, John, is coming
> John is coming
> The grocer is coming

Appositional structures are profiled in the following way:

$$\begin{array}{c} \text{Jóhn/the grócer/is còming/} \\ \underline{\hspace{2.5cm} \text{V}} \\ \underline{\text{NP} \quad \text{NP}} \\ \text{D} \quad \text{N} \end{array}$$

II C
NP Coord (VI)
DN at II

Another type of NP Coord is with lists of NPs, as with *the boy, the girl and the man went home*. X c X handles the NPs on either side of *and* (which is of course optional elsewhere, e.g. *the boy and the girl and the man went home*); each instance of a listing relationship between the other NPs is marked as NP Coord, as follows:

$$\begin{array}{c} \text{the bóy/ the gírl/ the 'man and the dóg/ 'went hòme/} \\ \underline{\hspace{5cm} \text{S} \hspace{2cm} \text{V} \quad \text{A}} \\ \text{NP}_1 \quad \text{NP}_2 \quad \text{NP}_3 \quad \text{NP}_4 \end{array}$$

III C
VI NP Coord (1 and 2)
VI NP Coord (2 and 3)
IV XcX (3 and 4)

The structure of each NP is then analysed in the usual way.

Note some of the less regular (but quite commonly used) types of NP coord:

cricket/my 'main 'weekend actìvity/is ...
my friend (,) Peter (,) is ...
we (,) all of us (,) wish ...
we both/each/all feel ...
I (,) myself (,) feel ...

(3) *Complex VP*. This category has already been introduced (p. 74) as the one used when more than one verb process is used in a single VP, e.g. Catenative + Aux, *he does want to go*. It is also used when still more complexity is introduced, as in

> I want him to go.
> I want the box working.
> He wanted (him) to help (the man) paint the house.

The NP between the Vs has a unique double-purpose role: it is simultaneously object of the first V and subject of the second. We do not, however, institute a separate category for this, but log the VP as a whole under Stage VI. The breakdown of the VP is then done in the usual way, e.g.

```
I  'wanted the old 'man to hèlp me/
S              V              O            III C
        V        NP        V              VI Complex VP
Pron          D Adj  N     Pron           IIP (VV)
        -ed                               phrase structure as above
        XY + V:VP
```

(4) *Passive*. Passive constructions are analysed in the usual way, with the 'overall' effect noted at Stage VI, e.g.

```
the 'cat     was 'bitten    by the dòg/
   S             V               A          III C
  D N          Aux v         Pr  D  N       VI Passive
             -ed 3s    -en                  phrase structure
                                            as above
XY + S:NP    XY + V:VP     XY + A:AP
```

Notes: (a) The agent is omissible in many passives, e.g. *the cat was bitten*, and some passives do not have obvious agents (e.g. *the house is sold*).

(b) Some constructions are midway between the passives and adjectives (e.g. *I was surprised by her attitude*; cf. *her attitude surprised me*, which suggests it is a verb, and *I was very surprised*, which suggests it is an adjective cf. *GCE*, 809).

(c) *get* can be used apparently as a passive auxiliary, e.g. *he got dressed, it's getting painted*; but there are several restrictions on its use and meaning (cf. *GCE*, 802–3) which suggests that it be taken as a full verb, hence the analysis:

```
he got dressed
 S     V
   V    V
```

(5) *Complementation*. In *GCE*, 'Complementation' is used in a broad sense, to refer to any elements of clause structure that are obligatory for the completion of verb meaning (thus including O_d O_i, V Part, etc. as well as Complements (C) in the narrow sense used so far). The basic complementation patterns have been handled at earlier stages, under SVO, SVC and SVA, and their associated phrasal expansions. There remain a few types of complementation pattern (abbreviated to Complement here) whose internal structure involves additional semantic or syntactic complexity than those already described, namely:

(i) More advanced copular constructions than *be* (Stage III), using such verbs as *appear (ready), feel (happy), look (sad), seem (right), sound (wrong), get (ready), go (wrong), fall (ill), run (mad)*. In addition to their 'linking' function, these verbs have a specific meaning, and they are thus rather different from *be*, hence it might be useful to add inverted commas to the label 'Cop', as a mnemonic, if a more detailed analysis of complementation were carried out, e.g.

```
he    fell   ill
 S     V      C
Pron 'Cop'
```

(ii) Constructions with Adjective and Prepositional phrase postmodification, e.g. *angry at* (*the man*), *happy for* (*her*), *bad at* (*swimming*), *pleased at* (*his answer*), *lucky in* (*love*), *aware of* (*the problem*), *busy with* (*revision*);

```
I    was  'bad at swimming/
S    V         C                         III C
PronCop  AdjPr    V                      III P ( × 2); VI Complement
              ing                        W
         XY + C:NP                       III T
```

(iii) Adjective + *that*-clause, e.g. *I'm sure* (*that*) *he'll come, it's obvious* (*that*) *he'll do it:*

```
I'm        'certain that he'll còme/
S V               C                       III C
        Adj.   Subord. Clause             VI Complement
                 s  S    V                V Postmod. clause 1
                                          V Conn: s
     Pron Cop          Aux v              II C
        'cop           'aux               phrase structure
             XY + C:NP                        as above
```

(iv) Adjective + infinitive, e.g. *He is slow to come, He is easy to see, I was cross to hear it:*

```
I    was  'happy to àsk/
S    V         C                          III C
           Adj   V                        VI Complement
Pron Cop                                  phrase structure
     -ed                                      as above
         XY + C:NP
```

(6) *Others.* This Stage has been studied very selectively, and the above categories are by no means a comprehensive account of the new areas of syntax being acquired. Patterns of clause sequence, complex prepositions (e.g. *in front of, on top of*—cf. *GCE*, 301–2), increased range of ellipses, and several other distinctive grammatical structures make their appearances, but none have been studied sufficiently for us to be sure of developmental norms. Placements at Stage VI or Stage VII Other must therefore be tentative.

Negative features (−).

The theoretical basis for the Stage VI 'Error' box is given in *GALD*, 78. Three aspects of the argument need re-emphasizing:

(1) Real or imaginary inverted commas should always be placed around the term 'error', in the context of child language development. We use this term (for want of a better) in an attempt to measure the distance still to be travelled by

P (once he has reached Stage V) to arrive at adult grammatical norms, and it there-fore means 'error from the viewpoint of the adult grammar'. 'Error' is not a pejorative term: on the contrary, the occurrence of errors, in this sense, is often the first sign that a child is making progress in the use of a grammatical system (as often pointed out in the case of irregular verbs, cf. Brown 1973). They are always child-initiated, i.e. are not part of adult input. *In all cases, errors are to be seen as a sign of development, not of failure.*

(2) There must be something physically present in the utterance on which to base the decision about error. If we did not have such a criterion, the notion of 'error' would go totally out of control, e.g. a Stage I child wants more milk and says *more*—this might then be analysed as a series of omission-errors for the sen-tence 'I want more milk' (Pron error, V error, N error etc.), which would plainly be absurd. On the other hand, in a child who says *me want milk* there is something *tangibly present* which can be marked as 'wrong', and this would legitimately be marked under Stage VI.

(3) The LARSP procedure analyses a construction as an error *only when there is independent evidence in P's usage that the grammatical system involved has begun to be acquired*. That is why the Stage is called 'Systems Completion'. To say that there has been an 'error' in Tense, for example, is to say (i) that P has begun to make Tense contrasts and (ii) that he is making errors in their use. It would not be enough to point to a verb being used inappropriately at Stage II (e.g. P says *daddy go* when daddy has already gone) and call this a Stage VI 'Error', if there were no evidence anywhere else that P had begun to develop tense forms (using Aux, *-ed*, *-en* etc.). As word order does not become well established until Stage III, and as grammatical systems such as Tense or Person do not begin to make their appearance until Stage III, the application of this principle thus means that few Stage I/II utterances would ever be analysed as containing 'errors'. For example, *daddy gone* would *not* be analysed as Tense error, nor *ball chair* as Prep error and Det error, nor *tickle dada* (meaning 'daddy tickle') as word-order error, nor *mummy daddy* as Coord error. On the other hand, once P has begun to develop his use of the various systems involved in these examples, then the analyst can detect a contrast (proportion correct v. incorrect), and any pattern of development here will have some clinical relevance.

How a child acquires a linguistic structure is unclear. What is known is that acquisition is not a single, sudden jump, but a gradual process, often taking several years. But the pattern of development involved is obscure. For instance, take the first occasion on which a child uses a feature, such as *-ed*. It is not known how far this feature is immediately available for other verbs, or whether there are restrictions involved. The work of Brown, Cazden and others shows that very quickly a new feature will be found over several lexical items, but how immediate this productivity is is not known. The process can only be plotted with ease in cases where a regular form is overgeneralized to irregular items, e.g. *goed, wented*— and these do not always occur (e.g. there is no irregular *-ing* form cf. Kuczaj 1978). Usually there will be more instances of a grammatical feature being used correctly than incorrectly in a sample–indeed, often there is no evidence of incorrect use at all, because only a limited and straightforward range of linguistic contexts are in use—*a box, a table, a chair* provide little scope for error; the problem arises over the uncountable nouns (*a wool, *a soap) which are less common, and which usually emerge later. Given the uncertainty of acquisitional norms in these matters, then, how are we to extract a workable procedure for handling the clear cases?

We use two criteria. To count as a Stage VI error, a feature must (a) contrast with a correctly-used feature from the same grammatical system at least once in the sample; e.g. *mummy daddy* (NN, but an attempt at XcX coordination) is an 'error' only if there is at least one instance of correct use of coordination—if there is not, we have no alternative but to take it as unproductive (classed under *stereotypes*); (b) contrast with a correct form from the same system which is the only possible or likely one in that context, e.g. *me like→I like; tickle dada→dada tickle, a wool→wool*. Note that *ball chair* would not be an error by this criterion, because the context is so unclear as to admit several competing possibilities for expansion— it is unclear what the error is (e.g. *ball is under the chair, is lying by the chair*). The longer and more complex the child's sentences get, of course, and the more determinate the context, the more a single error suggests itself, e.g. *the ball has rolled the chair*, where *under* is a clear Prep Error (cf. p. 216). For a child at Stage V, these conditions are usually such that the instances of error stand out clearly.

There is only one error type which is classified separately above Stage VI on the chart, and this is the lack of inversion with *wh*-questions (QXYZ) at a time when inversion (VS) has begun to appear elsewhere. We permit this exception in order to be able to show a clear developmental progression in the Question column, which otherwise would be broken.

Using these criteria, several grammatical systems emerge as being particularly prone to error, and a selection of these is given on the profile chart.

(1) **Pronouns**, e.g. *him got a ball, give it to she, I did see anyone*. The pronoun system is well established by Stage III, in its syntactic distribution and semantic function: the main problems lie in morphology, as the first two examples illustrate, and errors here may be heard from an early age. Each ungrammatical instance is counted once under Pron. For stages of Pronominal development, see Huxley 1970.

(2) **Determiners**, e.g. *a wool, building castle, I like cornet, boy is there, toys are in the garden*. All the common determiners are in regular use by Stage V, but at age 7 there are still problems in using the full set of contrasts (cf. Warden 1976, Maratsos 1976), and some take much longer (e.g. the *much/many* contrast).

(3) **Adjective sequence**, e.g. *an old big house, a wooden green brick, a big nice kiss*. Pairs of adjectives are in regular use from Stage III. Errors in the use of adjective sequences are uncommon in normal child development (cf. Richards 1979), and we have found fewer in clinical samples than our original sampling led us to expect.

(4) **Irregular nouns**, e.g. *mans, mices, mouses, sheeps, trouserses*. Plural nouns

are found from Stage III, and errors are accordingly quite common from a fairly early age.

(5) Tense. This is the label we use for *any* errors involving the basic Aux + V structure of the verb phrase (i.e. the auxiliaries *be*, *have* and *do*)—specifically, it includes both tense *and* aspect variation, e.g. *it be going, it was come, it did cut, it is go, I have went*. The basic patterns are established by Stage IV. *Notes:* (a) the *will/shall* forms are included under Modal, which is where the bulk of their function lies (cf. Palmer 1974); (b) *do* with contrastive stress is a normal adult possibility, e.g. it did 'cut/; (c) there are also *sequence* of tense rules, cf. **he saw me when I will come in*.

(6) Modal. Most modal auxiliaries are in use by Stage V (cf. 1.8 below), but it takes several years for their full syntactic and semantic restrictions to be learned. Most modal errors are semantic, e.g. (referring to past time event) *he may come here, please may you do this for me*, but some are clearly syntactic, e.g. *you bettern't do that, I used to couldn't do that*.

(7) Irregular verbs (other than *be*, *have* and *do* as auxiliaries) e.g. *goed, wented, tooken, seed*, copular *be* (e.g. *it be nice*). Past tense/participate verbs are found from around Stages II–III, and errors are quite common from after these Stages.

(8) Concord operates primarily between subject and verb, and possible errors are *the boy are, *the boys is, *we is going, **no one were coming*. Concord also operates between S and C (cf. **the boy was actors*), between S and reflexives (cf. *she hurt himself), between relative pronoun and antecedent (cf. *the man which came, *the box who was ...), and between quantifiers and nouns (cf. *two box, *many boy). *Note*: there is considerable variation in adult usage over some concord possibilities (e.g. *none was/were ..., everyone wants his/their. ...*): see *GCE*, 360ff.

(9) Adverbial position, e.g. *they inside are, **I lose always those*, **you go sometimes there*, **almost I've finished*, **we went then home*. Only a small range of adverbials have positional restrictions, and errors in their use tend to stand out. They could of course be subsumed under category (10).

(10) Word order, e.g. *neither I did, **the boy the man saw*, *the boy saw the man* (when context clearly warrants *the man saw the boy*), **he walked the hill up*.

(11) *Other*. A selection of errors which fall outside of the above categories, taken from the speech of several Ps is as follows: *the whole much (= 'the whole amount') (N type), **he tripped in the mat* (Prep.), *he fell off the ladder because he broke his arm* (clause sequence), **he kicked the car and broke* (subject deletion), **that is beautifuller* (comparison). Many Ps develop their 'favourite' types of error,

perhaps the result of a misdirected remedial strategy, in which case it may be useful to add the appropriate labels to this section of the chart. One (deaf) P's Error Box, after this treatment, looked as follows:

NP		VP		Clause	
Pron 4	Adj seq	Modal		Concord 11	
Det 16	N irreg 11	Tense	18	A position	
I 1		V irreg	9	W order 2	
		V part	4		
Other Prep 8		Cop 12			

Note that in all these cases, analysis of the sentence is first carried out in the usual way, e.g.

```
he walked  the hill  up
 S   V        O
   ‾‾‾‾          ‾‾‾‾
    V           Part
```

Once this is completed, the error is logged in the appropriate section of Stage VI.

Interpreting 'Errors'

The error box contains a great deal of potentially valuable information. It can indicate specific areas where P is currently attempting to make progress; it can give clear indication of the direction in which a particular period of structured remediation has been successful in promoting progress; abnormal patterns of Error can suggest weaknesses in the remedial method used; and so on. In interpreting Stage VI Errors, it is important to check totals in two dimensions: *outside* the Error box, to compare the total under VJ – with all other relevant totals further up the chart (e.g. – Pron cf. Pron; – Tense cf. Aux, 2 Aux, -ed, etc.); and *inside* the box, to check for any internal pattern, e.g. whether a problem is basically to do with VP, or NP, etc. Compare the following three cases:

(a)

NP			VP		Clause	
Pron	Adj seq	4	Modal		Concord 4	
Det	N irreg		Tense		A position 2	
			V irreg	3	W order 7	
Other						

(b)

NP			VP		Clause	
Pron	Adj seq		Modal	11	Concord	
Det	6 N irreg		Tense	1	A position	
			V irreg		W order	
Other Prep 14						

(c)

	NP		VP		Clause	
Pron	7	Adj seq	Modal	1	Concord	2
Det		N irreg 8	Tense	6	A position	
			V irreg	11	W order	
Other Adj Comp 4						

P in (a) had an underlying word order problem; in (b), P had particular problems with semantic categories within grammatical systems; in (c), P's difficulties were almost entirely in the area of morphology.

Given the criteria discussed above, we would not expect the error box to be much in evidence in normal children until Stages IV–V. This can therefore be an indication of the extent to which P's language is developing along normal lines. There are likely to be no marks in the error box while P is at Stage I or II; at Stage III a few may occur; and the figures should build up through Stages IV and V; Stage VI is the peak, and once reached, errors should begin to fall in range and frequency, until by Stage VII very few remain. Those which do remain are often surprisingly persistent: one normal 10-year-old was still saying *tooken* and *drawren*, but all other irregular verbs were correct.

It is also important not to confuse structural error with issues of sociolinguistic appropriateness or dialect variation. A Profile Chart is made for a single speaker, and therefore for a single social/regional dialect. This must be judged in its own terms, and P's language evaluated accordingly. Hence it would not be right to call *I ain't, he hurt me arm* errors: they may not be the standard language used for purposes of illustration in this book, and they may not be used by T, but this is a separate matter. Structurally, they may be the norm in P's linguistic background. And sometimes this norm diverges considerably from standard English, as with immigrant varieties.

Stage VII

It is unlikely that a P who has reached Stage VII would be systematically analysed using LARSP. We are unable at present to offer systematic guidelines for assessment or remediation here, in any case, as the acquisition research has not been done (for a review, see Karmiloff-Smith 1979). It is however useful to have the Stage represented on the chart, as often Ps at earlier stages do use sentences of the following kind, and they can thus indicate areas of particular strength or progress.

(1) Adverbial connectivity. Adverbials which are integrated into clause structure, modifying the verb (or some other elements) are called 'adjuncts' by *GCE* (chapter 8). The terms 'disjunct' and 'conjunct' are used for those adverbials which are not integrated into the structure of the clause: their primary role, in other words, is to interrelate clauses (or larger structures). The 'connecting' function of conjuncts is plainly seen in the following range of examples: *next, then,*

secondly, lastly, for a start, also, by the way, else, still, yet, anyway. Disjuncts often have an attitudinal emphasis, e.g. *probably, actually, surely, really, certainly, of course.* Use of the simpler lexical items may be heard from around Stage V, but the peak of development is much later—perhaps influenced by the extent to which such items are encountered in early reading and story-telling. These items are *not* analysed as part of clause structure, e.g.

    'I've 'got a 'new drèss/ànyway/
    S   V   O   I A conn

They are, in effect, the development of initiating *and*, c, s and Other at Stage V (cf. p. 89).

    (2) Comment clause. Sometimes whole clauses are inserted parenthetically into a sentence, without affecting the analysis of the surrounding structure, e.g. *you know, I mean, you see, I suppose, I'm afraid, as you say, do you think.* They usually have a separate tone unit, e.g.

    you knów/—I 'think it's rèady/
    'will he 'want a drìnk/do you thínk/

They have a limited potential for structural change (i.e. are idiomatic, or stereotyped), and are consequently not usually worth analysing further, e.g.

    it's grèen/ you sée/
    SV   C   Comm Cl

(The clausal coordination is however marked at Stage V, cf. p. 90.)

    (3) Emphatic order. Word-order variations for emphasis are very common in conversational English (see *GCE*, chapter 14), in addition to the use of intonation, common from a much earlier stage (e.g. *I want thàt dolly*), e.g.

Frèd his náme is/	
C S V	Stage III Clause Stage VII: EO
'that 'man I hàte/	
O S V	Stage III Clause Stage VII: EO
in the màrket I 'saw him/	
A S V O	Stage IV Clause Stage VII: EO
they are 'still thère/sóme of them/	
S V A A	

(In the latter example, the final phrase is of course part of the Subject, and is thus also NP Coord at Stage VI.)

Note also the common ASV/AVS patterns: *down we go, on they went, outside stood Jim, here are the boys, here I am, so did the other* etc. Some of these sentences may be heard in use very early, but usually as stereotypes.

(4) *It* clauses. The phenomenon of a *cleft* sentence (i.e. a clause divided into two parts, each with own verb) is a Stage VII development, e.g.

it was Mike who saw him,
it's thought he's coming,
it's next week's game he wants to see,
it was then I saw him.

These are analysed as SVO, etc. clauses in the usual way, with an additional mark against *it* in Stage VII. The final clause is analysed as a relative clause (Stage V), though there are important structural differences between these and relatives (cf. *GCE*, 953), e.g.

it was Mike who saw him
S V   C
    ‾‾‾‾‾‾‾‾‾‾‾‾‾‾‾‾‾
          s   V   O
it   etc.

Related sentences (e.g. the 'pseudo-cleft' sentence using a *wh*-clause, as in *what I want is a bath*) have already been classified under clause S in Stage V. Note that the *it* of simple sentences, e.g. *it's raining*, *it's a boy* is analysed solely as SV/SVC etc., and should not be classed as Stage VII *it*.

(5) *There*. Clauses beginning with 'empty', unstressed *there* are usually called 'existential' sentences, because of the meaning thus obtained (cf. *GCE*, 956 ff), e.g. *there are cows in the field*, *there's been a car stolen*, *is there any more bread?*, *there's a man I know who. . . .* Sometimes, other verbs than *be* may be used, e.g. *there came a time . . .*, *there stood a tree. . . .* All such sentences are analysed in terms of normal clause structure, with an additional mark under *there* at Stage VII, e.g.

there are cows in the field
S   V   C   A
there   etc.

(6) Other. The easiest way (sic) of assessing the extent of this category is to do a subtraction sum on the index to *GCE*: all the structures there, less those already described above, leaves the content of Stage VII Others! There are many common, but complex sentence types, e.g. extraposition sentences (moving a clause element from its normal position to the end of the sentence, and replacing it with *it*), e.g. *it's no use going home now* (cf. *going home now is no use*), *it doesn't matter what happens, you'll find it nice working here* (cf. *GCE*, 963 ff); verbless clauses (e.g. *when ready, it should be . . .*, *if ripe, you can . . .*); more complex indirect speech patterns (e.g. *he said he might*).

The remaining area of Stage VII, Syntactic Comprehension and Style are given only in outline, for reasons discussed in *GALD*, 82–3. Two points should be emphasized:

(1) Comprehension in the general sense is *not* referred to here, but only those cases where *syntactic production is clearly ahead of comprehension*, i.e. it is a

relatively late development. For example, in experiments of the kind referred to, children might *say* a doll was 'easy to see' (i.e. use the SVC/Stage VI Complementation construction), but fail nonetheless to comprehend it. The theoretical point is discussed by Clark *et al.* (1974), who give several illustrations. Common examples in P data are: the use of conjunctions such as *although, because, since* with the sense of little more than 'and'; the use of a passive construction without appreciating the 'reversed' agent/goal meaning; distinctions such as *buy/sell, teach/ learn, ask/tell*, which may 'sound' alright when P uses them, but where comprehension is lacking (e.g. *I want to tell you something*, where 'ask' is the meaning intended). All such sentences are analysed in the usual way, and the type of difficulty noted in some abbreviated form at Stage VII. In practice, there are few occasions in P samples where the need arises.

(2) Under 'Style' is placed any sign of a controlled use of the syntax of language varieties other than the 'mother-dialect' of the child. Evidence of such control is found as early as age 4 (cf. Sachs and Devin 1976), but most of the contrasts used then are based on grounds of frequency (e.g. using more questions in one social situation, less in another), and this is not what is included in the Stage VII category. This refers solely to the use of a new structure which falls outside of the normal conversational range of the child over the first 4 years or so. It thus includes: grammatical features of different dialects (e.g. *I ain't*, where previously *I'm not* was used), of different levels of formality (e.g. the learning of a more formal speaking style, e.g. *may I* for *can I*), of different subject areas (e.g. religious language, television advertising language) and of different media—in particular, the wide range of fresh constructions encountered in the written language. Such developments will particularly appear following the change from parent to peer-group orientation, and once the child begins school. As with (1), the sentences involved are analysed in the usual way, with a sociolinguistic note inserted at Stage VII.

The bottom line

(1) Total number of sentences. Add all clear sentences, i.e. *exclude* anything placed under Section A. Include sentences which are repetitions. Thirty-minute samples of the type described in *GALD*, chapter 5 produce between 100 and 200 sentences, for most normal children. In the context of language disorders, the figure can be either much lower than this *or* much higher (as with some linguistically hyperactive children—cf. Fig. 7, p. 107). Even a small sample of sentences (a dozen or so) can nonetheless be helpful, however, (cf. p. 22).

(2) Mean number of sentences per turn. T speaks to P, and P may or may not reply: this is a conversational *turn*. The three main types are: (i) P fails to reply; (ii) P replies with a single sentence; (iii) P replies with more than one sentence (i.e. there is spontaneous speech, in our sense). The figure in this box indicates the overall direction in which P is responding, and is arrived at by dividing the total number of sentences P uses (cf. above) by the total number of stimuli T

provides. If section B/C of the chart has been filled in, the information is automatically obtainable from the totals on the left of the page, viz.

			Totals
B	36	Questions	32
	21	Others	16
C			21
	57		69

69/57 = 1·2 sentences per turn

The smaller this figure, the more zero or Section A responses; 1·0 would mean no zeros, and no spontaneous sentences; the higher the figure, the more spontaneous sentences.

The only methodological point to note is that whenever P produces a turn consisting *wholly* of Section A utterance, the whole T–P interaction is disregarded. Any isolated Section A utterances within a turn are also ignored, the calculation being based on the residue.

(3) Mean sentence length. The total number of institutionalized words (items with a space on either side) in all clear sentences (i.e. excluding Section A and all self-corrections) is tallied, and divided by the total number of sentences. The minimum figure obtainable is therefore 1, for a 'pure' Stage I child. After this stage, however, there is no easy correlation between linguistic complexity and length.

(4) Other problems. Given the pressure under which most Ts have to work, it is inevitable that errors will be made in processing a sample of data—errors either of analysis or of profiling. It is hoped that the above pages will help to ensure a general consistency in the use of the procedure, but no-one can safeguard against performance errors, such as forgetting to analyse a structure as transitional information, or—having analysed it—forgetting to transfer it onto the chart. The workbook section of the present book is so designed as to focus attention systematically on each profiling operation in turn, in the hope that problems of this kind will be kept to a minimum. However, it may be reassuring to learn that a profile system tolerates a fair amount of error before it becomes misleading or unworkable. Given a chart on which, altogether, a hundred or more marks have been placed, the mistaken placement of a small number of these will be unlikely to affect our perception of the overall configuration, or our focus on the main gaps. We have found that a 10 per cent error is unremarkable, at the level of generality at which this profile is constructed; and it may be that sometimes the margin of error is greater. The important point is that 100 per cent proficiency is not a prerequisite of using this approach.

1.4

Interpretation and remediation

Interpretation

Once a profile has been constructed, it must be interpreted, and several comments about points of interpretation have already been made, in relation to individual Stages and Sections. Interpreting a complete Profile Chart involves the same 'differential' reasoning; but with more variables to take account of, a much larger range of possibilities emerges. It is also essential to use the profile in conjunction with the transcription, as decisions concerning the productivity of patterns (e.g. how much lexical variation there is in a structure) often need to be made. This is why so much space is given over to data, later in the book. In *GALD* (113–17), we outline some of the more frequently occurring profile patterns we have encountered, and several of these are illustrated in the case studies of later sections of the present book (see also Bax and Stevenson 1977).

The process of profile commentary may be seen from the following selection of four profiles, which illustrate patterns not so commonly encountered as those in *GALD*.

Sarah

Age 5;8; attending ESN(M) school, 15 minute sample of free conversation.

Assessment notes (Fig. 7)

(1) Very high number of sentences, produced at times with great speed; some conversational turns contained six sentences along with unintelligible utterances.

(2) Very short sentences; none more than 3 elements.

(3) One-third of P's utterances unintelligible or ambiguous.

(4) Predominantly spontaneous; also, response sentences tend to be shorter than spontaneous.

(5) Hardly ever fails to respond; no structurally abnormal responses; transcription shows a great deal of semantic randomness and irrelevance, in both response and spontaneous sequences.

(6) Stimuli bias to Others, as T tries to control P (*don't, no*, etc.), and glosses P's utterances; T has little chance, because of speed of P's responses, to redirect P using Questions.

(7) Half sentences are one element only (transcription shows that these often run together because of P's speed, and produce ambiguity).

SARAH   MAR '76   20 MIN.

A — Unanalysed

	Problematic
1 Unintelligible **88** 2 Symbolic Noise **/** 3 Deviant **/**	1 Incomplete **/** 2 Ambiguous **14**

B — Responses

Stimulus Type	Totals	Repet-itions	Normal Response								Abnormal		
			Elliptical Major				Full Major	Minor	Struc-tural	Ø	Prob-lems		
			1	2	3	4							
14 Questions	12		6	1	1			2		2	2		
64 Others	50	4	13	6	5			11			15		

C — Spontaneous 138   7   80   Others **58**

		Minor			Social **14** Stereotypes **/** Problems						

Stage I (0;9–1;6) Sentence Type

Major	Excl.	Comm.	Quest.	Statement			
		·V **5**	·Q· **/**	·V· **4** ·N· **58** Other **13** Problems **/**			

			Conn.	Clause		Phrase	Word

Stage II (1;6–2;0)

	VX	QX		SV **6**	VC/O **9**	DN **21**	VV	-ing **2**
				S C/O	AX **2**	Adj N **11**	V part **12** *	pl **20**
				Neg X **3**	Other	NN **14**	Int X **/**	-ed **/**
						PrN **4**	Other **2**	-en **/**

Stage III (2;0–2;6)

	VXY	QXY **/**	X + S:NP **2**	X + V:VP **2**	X + C/O:NP **4**	X + A:AP **/**	3s **/**
	let XY	VS **2**	SVC/O **15**	VC/OA **2**	D Adj N **/**	Cop **13**	gen **34**
	do XY		SVA **2**	VO_dO_i	Adj Adj N	Aux	n't **/**
			Neg XY	Other	Pr DN **2**	Pron **7**	'cop **/**
					N Adj N	Other **/**	'aux **11**

Stage IV (2;6–3;0)

	S	QVS	XY + S:NP	XY + V:VP **/**	XY + C/O:NP **2**	XY + A:AP **2**	-est **/**
		QXYZ	SVC/OA	AAXY	N Pr NP	Neg V **/**	-er **/**
			SVO_dO_i	Other	Pr D Adj N	Neg X	-ly **/**
					cX **2**	2 Aux	
					XcX **/**	Other	

Stage V (3;0–3;6)

	how	tag	and	Coord. **/** **/** ·	Postmod. **/** clause	**/** ·	
			c	Subord. **/** **/** ·			
	what		s	Clause: S	Postmod. **/** phrase		
			Other	Clause: C/O			
				Comparative			

(+)				(−)			
NP	VP	Clause		NP		VP	Clause

Stage VI (3;6–4;6)

Initiator **/**	Complex	Passive		Pron **4**	Adj seq	Modal	Concord **/**
Coord **/**		Complement		Det	N irreg **/**	Tense	A position
						V irreg **/**	W order **5**
Other				Other **Intonation 4**			

Discourse			Syntactic Comprehension	

Stage VII (4;6+)

A Connectivity	it			
Comment Clause	there **2**		Style * mainly sit down	
Emphatic Order	Other			

Total No. Sentences **200**	Mean No. Sentences Per Turn **2·5**	Mean Sentence Length **1·6**

Fig. 7   Sarah at 5;8—20-minute sample

(8) No Stage V structures, i.e. no complex sentence formation, either in clauses or phrases; developments at VI suggest P has a deviant order of development, having apparently 'jumped' a stage.

(9) No Stage IV clause structure.

(10) Very thin transitional structure; the only VP expansion is V Part (no VV or Aux used), and the V Parts are mainly one lexical collocation.

(11) Transcription shows the high phrase/word totals are boosted by a frequent use of a small range of lexical items—not technically repetitions or stereotypes, but the 'flavour' of the sample is that P is saying very little very often.

Remedial implications

(i) Check on extent of the attention/organizational problems other than with language. Is the language problem a reflex of this, or separate? How far is language being used in parallel with, e.g., motor activities?

(ii) Check on comprehension of Stage I/II structures especially.

(iii) Aim to develop a larger productive range of Stage I/II structures, avoiding stereotypes.

(iv) Need for fairly tight structuring of situations, to cut down on semantically irrelevant responses, and to promote more T control using Questions; aim initially to increase Response totals and cut down Spontaneous.

George

Age 5;1; attending ESN(M) school, 5-minute sample of free conversation.

Assessment notes (Fig. 8)

(1) Smooth-running dialogue, given the sample time; responds to all stimuli, but with few sentences per turn; long pauses, but T is ready to 'wait' for a response.

(2) High sentence length, which must be accounted for by Spontaneous Others; Spontaneous total quite high, compared with Responses.

(3) Question stimuli produce predominantly Minor responses; Other stimuli produce mainly 1-element elliptical.

(4) 'Reversed C' developmental pattern: clause structures at I and V, but continuous phrase structure down to Stage VI.

(5) Phrase structure almost entirely NP.

(6) Relatively high XcX; also NP coord at VI.

(7) Absence of verb development (at clause, phrase and transitional levels) means that Stage V strings will be of limited coherence; having begun to link clauses, this is likely to continue, with increasing fluency, but probable deterioration in intelligibility.

Remedial implications

(i) Work on VP, including X + V:VP.

(ii) NP responses to be structurally expanded by T; loose NP strings at V to be interrupted, with the aim of bringing the sequence under T control (esp. of Questions).

George 5;1   5 MIN.

A Unanalysed

		Problematic	
1 Unintelligible	2 Symbolic Noise	3 Deviant	1 Incomplete	2 Ambiguous

B Responses

				Normal Response						Abnormal		
				Elliptical Major				Full		Struc-		Prob-
Stimulus Type		Totals	Repet-itions	1	2	3	4	Major	Minor	tural	Ø	lems
12	Questions	12		3					9			
14	Others	14		12						2		

C Spontaneous | 14 | | 1 | Others | 13 |

Minor   Social 11   Stereotypes   Problems

Major   Sentence Structure

Excl.	Comm.	Quest.		Statement			
	·V· 1	·Q·	·V· 3 ·N· 7	Other 4	Problems 1		

Stage I (0;9–1;6)

	Conn.	Clause		Phrase		Word
VX	QX	SV 1	V C/O 4	DN 11	VV	
	2	S C/O 3	AX 7	Adj N 4	V part 1	-ing 2
		Neg X	Other	NN	Int X 3	pl 4
				PrN 7	Other	-ed 1

Stage II (1;6–2;0)

VXY	QXY	X + S:NP	X + V:VP	X + C/O:NP 1	X + A:AP 2	-en
let XY	VS	SVC/O	VC/OA	D Adj N 2	Cop	
do XY		SVA	VOdOi	Adj Adj N	Aux	3s
		Neg XY	Other	Pr DN 5	Pron 14	gen
				N Adj N	Other 3	

Stage III (2;0–2;6)

		XY + S:NP	XY + V:VP	XY + C/O:NP	XY + A:AP	n't
3	QVS	SVC/OA	AAXY	N Pr NP 2	Neg V	'cop
	QXYZ	SVOdOi	Other	Pr D Adj N 1	Neg X	'aux
				cX 1	2 Aux	
				XcX 5	Other	

Stage IV (2;6–3;0)

how		and 4 c	Coord. 1	1+ 1	Postmod. 1 clause	1+	-est
	tag	s 3	Subord. 1 3	1·			-er 1
what		Other	Clause: S		Postmod. 1 phrase		-ly 1
			Clause: C/O				
			Comparative				

Stage V (3;0–3;6)

	(+)			(−)			
NP	VP		Clause	NP		VP	Clause
Initiator 1	Complex		Passive	Pron 4	Adj seq	Modal	Concord
Coord 4			Complement	Det 3	N irreg 2	Tense	A position
						V irreg	W order 2

Stage VI (3;6–4;6)

Other | | | | Other Preposition 1 | | |

Discourse		Syntactic Comprehension
A Connectivity	it	
Comment Clause	there	Style
Emphatic Order 1	Other	

Stage VII (4;6+)

Total No. Sentences 40	Mean No. Sentences Per Turn 1·5	Mean Sentence Length 3·8

Fig. 8   George at 5;1—5-minute sample

Jeffrey

Age 7;11; attending ESN(S) school; 10-minute sample of free conversation.

Assessment notes (Fig. 9)

(1) Very little spontaneous use; responds to most Stimuli.

(2) Some repetition of Other stimuli (transcription shows that this was completely to intonational 'questions').

(3) Apparently developing clause structure, but transcription shows a fairly repetitive lexicon, with some probable stereotyping (e.g. *you know X* turns up 3 times, but with a different proper noun as *X*); also the SVOA total is entirely due to one verb.

(4) Very erratic phrase structure; DN and Pron are high, but transcription shows a limited use of lexical items.

(5) Balanced III/IV transitional line, suggesting a repeated sentence pattern (which transcription confirms).

(6) V Part is *put up* only; N in Pr N is proper noun only.

Remedial implications

The Stage III pattern looks false, considering the limited lexical range, and the gaps at I and II; therefore initial aim of I/II consolidation, by increasing lexicon and focusing on gaps.

Jannine

Age 8;6; normal school; left CVA 6 months prior to sample; 15-minute sample of free conversation.

Assessment notes (Fig. 10)

(1) Spread across Section A—one seventh of total utterances.

(2) Very high proportion of minor sentences as responses; suggests comprehension problems; otherwise a fairly good and normal pattern of development.

(3) High number of stereotypes.

(4) Use of initial conjunctions with no corresponding clausal coordination—pre-trauma carry-over?

(5) Low pronoun figure (cf. Subject omission, p. 29); also, low Aux and Cop.

(6) Apart from *-ing* (a puzzling omission), a well-developing word column.

(7) Isolated structural strength at Stage IV phrase level, with a wide range of lexical items.

(8) No Stage IV clause level.

(9) No initiating sentences (Questions, Commands, Exclamatory).

(10) See p. 28 for analysis of Section A.

Remedial implications

(1) Aim to eradicate phrase/word bias, and 'premature' coordination.

(ii) Focus on implications of Section A analysis (p. 29).

Jeffrey 7;11   5 MIN.

A	Unanalysed				Problematic		
	1 Unintelligible **2**	2 Symbolic Noise	3 Deviant		1 Incomplete	2 Ambiguous	**1**

B Responses

	Stimulus Type	Totals	Repet-itions	Normal Response							Abnormal			Prob-lems
				Elliptical Major					Full Major	Minor	Struc-tural	∅	
				1	2	3	4						
	26 Questions	**24**		**10**	**1**			**5**	**6**	**2**	**2**	
	21 Others	**21**	**4**	**9**	**3**			**4**	**6**			

C Spontaneous   **8**   **1**   **3**   Others   **5**

Stage I (C;9–1;6)	**Sentence Type**	**Minor**	Social **6**	Stereotypes	Problems

		Major		Sentence Structure				
	Excl.	Comm.	Quest.			Statement		
		·V· **1**	·Q·	·V·	·N· **6**	Other	Problems	

Stage			Conn.	Clause		Phrase		Word
Stage II (1;6–2;0)	VX	QX		SV **4**	V C/O **3**	DN **26**	VV **1**	-ing **6**
		1		S C/O **2**	A X **2**	Adj N	V part **3**	pl
				Neg X	Other	NN	Int X	-ed
						PrN **4**	Other	
Stage III (2;0–2;6)	VXY	QXY		X + S:NP **2**	X + V:VP **1**	X + C/O:NP **5**	X + A:AP **2**	-en
				SVC/O **7**	VC/OA	D Adj N	Cop **1**	
	let XY	VS		SVA **3**	VO$_d$O$_i$	Adj Adj N	Aux	3s
	do XY			Neg XY	Other	Pr DN **3**	Pron **17**	gen
						N Adj N	Other	
Stage IV (2;6–3;0)		, S	QVS	XY + S:NP	XY + V:VP **2**	XY + C/O:NP **2**	XY + A:AP **2**	n't
			QXYZ	SVC/OA **3** *	AAXY	N Pr NP	Neg V	·cop
				SVO$_d$O$_i$	Other	Pr D Adj N	Neg X	·aux
				only put up		cX	2 Aux	
						XcX	Other	
Stage V (3;0–3;6)		how	tag	and	Coord. 1	1	Postmod. 1 clause	1 ·	-est
				c	Subord. 1	1 ·			-er
		what		s	Clause: S		Postmod. 1 · phrase		-ly
				Other	Clause: C/O				
					Comparative				

		(+)			(−)			
	NP	VP	Clause	NP		VP	Clause	
Stage VI (3;6–4;6)	Initiator	Complex **1**	Passive	Pron	Adj seq	Modal	Concord	
	Coord **1**		Complement	Det	N irreg **1**	Tense	A position	
						V irreg	W order	
	Other			Other				

	Discourse		Syntactic Comprehension	
Stage VII (4;6+)	A Connectivity	it		
	Comment Clause	there	Style	
	Emphatic Order **2**	Other		

Total No. Sentences	**53**	Mean No. Sentences Per Turn	**1·07**	Mean Sentence Length	**2·6**

© D. Crystal, P. Fletcher, M. Garman, 1975 University of Reading

Fig. 9   Jeffrey at 7;11—5-minute sample

Jannine 8;6 — 15 MINS

A

Unanalysed			Problematic	
1 Unintelligible 4	2 Symbolic Noise	3 Deviant 5	1 Incomplete 4	2 Ambiguous 3

B Responses

Stimulus Type		Totals	Repetitions	Normal Response: Elliptical Major 1	2	3	4	Full Major	Minor	Abnormal: Structural	ø	Problems
46	Questions	40	1	10	2				25	3	2	
48	Others	46		8	1			7	30			

C Spontaneous

Spontaneous	Totals	Repetitions		
	21	1	7	Others 14

Sentence Type

Minor — *Social* 37 *Stereotypes* 18 *Problems*

Major — Sentence Structure

Stage	*Excl.*	*Comm.*	*Quest.*	*Statement*: Conn.	Clause		Phrase		Word
Stage I (0;9–1;6)		'V'	'Q'	'V' 2 'N' 8 Other 4 Problems					
Stage II (1;6–2;0)		VX	QX		SV 1	VC/O 4	DN 16	VV	-ing
					S C/O 4	AX 4	Adj N 3	V part 6	
					Neg X 1	Other	NN 4	Int X	pl 13
							PrN 3	Other	
Stage III (2;0–2;6)					X + S:NP 1	X + V:VP 1	X + C/O:NP 5	X + A:AP 3	-ed 6
		VXY	QXY		SVC/O 8	VC/OA 1	D Adj N 3	Cop 1	-en
		let XY	VS		SVA	VO_dO_i	Adj Adj N 2	Aux 1	3s 3
		do XY			Neg XY 1	Other 1	Pr DN 3	Pron 9	
							N Adj N	Other 5	
Stage IV (2;6–3;0)					XY + S:NP 3	XY + V:VP 4	XY + C/O:NP 3	XY + A:AP 2	gen 5
		+ S	QVS		SVC/OA	AAXY	N Pr NP 8	Neg V	n't
			QXYZ		SVO_dO_i	Other	Pr D Adj N	Neg X 1	'cop
							cX	2 Aux	'aux
							XcX 9	Other	
Stage V (3;0–3;6)	*how*		tag	*and* 6	Coord. 1	1 +	Postmod. clause 1 1	1 +	-est
	what			c	Subord. 1	1 +	Postmod. phrase 1 +		-er
				s 2	Clause: S				-ly
				Other 1	Clause: C/O				
					Comparative				

Stage VI (3;6–4;6)

(+) *NP*	(+) *VP*	(+) *Clause*	(−) *NP*		(−) *VP*	(−) *Clause*
Initiator 1	Complex	Passive	Pron	Adj seq	Modal	Concord
Coord 1		Complement	Det	N irreg	Tense	A position
					V irreg	W order
Other			Other			

Stage VII (4;6+)

Discourse		*Syntactic Comprehension*
A Connectivity	*it*	
Comment Clause	*there*	*Style*
Emphatic Order 1	Other	

Total No. Sentences	Mean No. Sentences Per Turn	Mean Sentence Length
107	1·2	1·9

© D. Crystal, P. Fletcher, M. Garman, 1975 University of Reading

Fig. 10 Jannine at 8;6—15-minute sample

Remediation

Descriptive and analytic skills of the kind involved in LARSP are a prerequisite for principled intervention, but they are not the same as intervention. One does not need to have a qualification in speech therapy or remedial teaching in order to understand, describe and analyse linguistic disorder: to be a language pathologist, in a strict sense, all one needs is clinical experience, plus training in the appropriate areas of linguistics and phonetics. But when it comes to *implementation* of one's analysis in clinical settings, then a great deal more is required—namely, the theory and practice of intervention and management—and it is this which constitutes the core of professional training. Language disorders are a linguistic problem; the language disordered patient is a therapeutic problem. There should therefore never be a conflict between the aims of linguist and remediator: the linguist's role stops short of implementing a remedial programme. Linguistic principles and findings must guide the planning of remedial work, but not its execution.

The factors which effect execution, and whose interaction needs to be understood in order to be assured of successful intervention, are well-known. They include the planning of the therapeutic environment, the structuring of situations, understanding the limitations of P in terms of attention, fatigue, behaviour, etc., the timing of intervention in P's day, the length and nature of sessions, and the frequency of intervention. All of this is in the nature of routine professional practice, though how much of this practice is based on solid theoretical foundations is difficult to assess. None of it, however, is the direct concern of the linguist or language pathologist (in the narrow sense).

These distinctions must be born in mind in any discussion of the remedial implications of LARSP, or similar procedures. At every LARSP course, we are asked such questions as: how long should T spend on a given structure? how long on one Stage before moving on to the next? how often should T profile P? Unlike the question 'What structure to teach next?' none of these questions has a linguistic answer. The answers depend on how things go in the clinical sessions, and ultimately it is T, and only T, who must decide when it is time to introduce a new structure, finish working on a structure, or Stage, or whatever. It is a decision that is partly intuitive, but it is also partly rational, and in this latter aspect linguistic factors will usually be taken into account. For example, presumably T would not move on from one Stage to the next unless there was a fairly consolidated look about the first Stage and signs of P attempting to use the structures spontaneously and/or to move on to more advanced structures. Another linguistic observation which may assist T in her decision to introduce a new structure is whether the new structure interferes with the patterns already in P's use, and which might even have seemed established. For instance, if T has been working with VO, expanding O into DN, she may be eliciting *kick the ball*, etc. with ease; attempting to expand O further, into D Adj N, say, may however have a harmful effect on the structure as a whole, with P perhaps failing to use D, or losing control of word order. The resulting deterioration in syntax would be a clear indication of the prematurity of T's decision. Other signs of prematurity may of course be nonlinguistic, e.g. increased distractibility, boredom, frustration.

What must not be forgotten is that there are no published norms for most areas of language acquisition. It is not possible, in the present state of knowledge, to say with precision what range and frequency of structures in a sample is normal in a statistical sense: this is the distance the subject has to move in order to be truly scientific. There are no theoretical difficulties in the way of developing these norms; the problem is solely an empirical one, with its associated methodological tasks (statistical, computational, etc.), and section 3.1 below indicates one direction in which research can proceed. In the meantime, T should keep in mind the importance of using *ratios* as indication of progress—such matters as the proportion of clause:phrase structures in use at a Stage, the proportion of adjacent Stage clause structures (e.g. Stage II:Stage III), the proportion of transitional features to clause structures, and so on. These are likely to be the true indices of development, rather than the totals for individual structures or categories. Strength of usage of a structure by itself is nothing: the strength may have come only at the expense of some other structure, which remains unused. Ultimately, all profile assessment, and all remedial strategies based on such assessment, are comparative exercises.

Similarly, there is unlikely to be a single 'best' method for eliciting a particular structure. There are certain general strategies, some of which are given in *GALD* (117 ff), but in the final analysis, everything depends on T's ingenuity in applying these principles to the materials available in a clinical setting, in interpreting P's behaviour so as to be able to select an efficacious stimulus, and in motivating P to work along the desired lines. Apart from these strategies, we have noted the importance of being aware of several more specific teaching principles, all of which have their origins in psychological, educational or linguistic theory. Some of these are:

(1) *Relating language to action.* Especially in the early stages of remediation, we note the greater success in working with language structures which have a clear and constant relationship to activities of P or activity roles between T and P (cf. Bruner 1975). For example, the use of dynamic verbs in forced alternative questions or commands, e.g. intransitive *walk, jump, dance, run, fall, clap* or transitive *kick, push/pull, wash, fight, kiss*: the use of the vocative + V structure as a precursor of SV, e.g. pìg/jùmp/ > 'pig jùmp/ > 'pig jùmping/. In these respects, using a new structure within a familiar action pattern (e.g. a parental game) seems more successful than trying to develop a new game to fit an individual structure. A particular strength of this principle is that it can be applied to pre-grammatical communication, as in the ritual games and noises illustrated by Bruner.

(2) *Making the problem real to P.* Particularly with Ps of good intelligence, we note a common reluctance to respond in artificial situations where the problem being posed may seem from P's viewpoint not really a problem at all. Questions which ask where an object is, or what colour, size, etc. it is may fall into this category; likewise, commands which make P act in apparently pointless ways. One

P informed us once that as T already knew where the duck was, he was not going to tell us! When this reluctance is noticed, we find it helpful to make the problem real, e.g. by 'blindfolding' T, or using a screen between T and P, or by using an 'intermediary' (e.g. a stupid puppet who gets things wrong, doesn't know where things are, etc. (cf. Lloyd and Donaldson 1976)). Apart from being an aid to decentration, the puppet technique also has the advantage of making P socially superior—a situation which can never be obtained in talking with an adult, no matter how pliable T allows herself to be.

(3) *Keeping P's language under T control*. In *GALD*'s discussion of remediation (124 ff, esp. points 1, 2 and 8), and also above (p. 4), we emphasize the need for P to be in control of T's grammar, and not vice versa. This means, in particular, selecting the right kind of structural reinforcement for P's utterances (cf. p. 57), and it is possible to become extremely skilful in building P's utterance into a sentence that relates to the teaching goals. With some types of child, however, the need for a more general strategy of control may make itself felt, e.g. with hyperactive or withdrawn children. In both cases, the treatment procedure may end up increasing P's anxiety, by attempting to make him do exactly what his condition does not permit him to do, viz. slowing the hyperactive child down (e.g. making him speak slowly, talk about one thing at a time) or making the withdrawn child open up (e.g. by plying him with forced alternative questions). We have found that by developing ideas we first met in the work of Marion Blank (cf. Blank 1973), T can often introduce an element of control with such children. In the case of Sarah, for example—a hyperactive child with acute attention difficulties and several behaviour problems (cf. p. 106)—attempts to elicit structured responses were regularly interrupted by irrelevant streams of speech. Sarah's attention would be caught by a picture of a banana on the wall, and she would be off (*me like them/want one of them/* etc.). Trying to bring her attention back to the task in hand rarely succeeded. Accordingly, T began to focus attention on the 'irrelevant' language: whenever P began to talk about bananas, T would stop the session and make P contrinue to talk about bananas for a fixed period, keeping her attention on the bananas until P was thoroughly fed up with them. At that point, it was noticeable how the prospect of an SVO drill along conventional lines began to appeal! This treatment approach resulted in due course in a much more controlled T-P interaction.

(4) *The importance of contrast*. The various grammatical features of English do not work in isolation, but always in contrast, e.g. singular v. plural, active v. passive, definite v. indefinite article, present v. non-present, one word-order v. another, etc. The famous principle of Saussure applies: 'in language, there are only oppositions.' What this means in practice is the need to devise contexts which will enable the contrast between the members of a grammatical system to be perceived directly and unambiguously. With some features, the contexts are easy, e.g. singular v. plural relates in most cases to the number of objects involved. With others, it is more difficult to show the contrast, e.g. past v. present tense, modal verbs, definite v. indefinite article. It is in devising ingenious contexts that most work needs to be done, and there are several suggestions on these lines in later sections.

But as a general rule, T should aim to avoid presenting single grammatical features, and should structure sessions so that contrasting features are juxtaposed. An example of this switch in emphasis would be moving from

  (a) Is that a cat > No/it's a dog/
to (b) Is that a cat > No/it's not a cat/it's a dog/

In (a) there is no clear point of structural contact between the negative and the question form; the parallelism is evident in (b). Another example would be the need to focus on the possessive system as a whole—*that's my car, that's your car, that's mine, that's yours*. Games can be devised in which T and P switch between all four forms. If only two are concentrated on (say, the first two), there is then the possibility that P will fail to see the contrast with the remainder of the system, and will treat the forms as in free variation, saying *that's mine car*, etc. Lastly, as P grows older, more structured substitution games can be devised, and in the visual mode, materials based on the lines of *Find a Story* or *Roll a Story* (Penguin Education) can be used.

The more a contrast can be made formally apparent, the easier it seems to be. This means avoiding homonyms (e.g. *swing on a swing, slide on a slide*), which can obscure a noun-verb contrast usually clearly marked in the language. Prosodic reinforcement (along with contrasts, gestures, facial expressions etc.) can be extremely helpful here, e.g. in the negation exercise above, using a fall-rise pattern (with its overtones of doubt) for the negative structure, viz.

  it's 'not a căt/it's a dòg/

or using the 'non-final' meaning of the rising tone to contrast with the 'final' meaning of the fall in a contrast involving the aspectual distinction, e.g.

  he's fálling/he's fálling/he's fàllen/ .

Likewise, if T can introduce lexical sets that are also plainly in contrast, such as antonyms, the point can be reinforced.

(5) *The role of definitions.* One of the most common strategies, used in both spontaneous conversation and standardized testing, is to ask P in effect to define a word. Not only 'What is (a) —?' and 'What does—mean?' are included: any question of the *What's it for?* type, or comments of the *Tell me some more about it* type are implicit requests for definition. It is therefore very important for T to be aware of developmental levels in children's defining ability. Litowitz (1977) describes five levels of definitional 'competence', in responding to sentences of the type 'What is X?'

Level 1: a non-verbal or semantically empty statement, e.g. pointing, *that, do like this* (plus gesture).

Level 2: word associations to the stimulus word, showing that a semantic field has been activated, but that no ordered form has been applied, e.g.

T	... shoe?	P	sock
T	... knife?	P	cutting

Level 3: concrete example of actual experience associated as a predicate to the stimulus word. This is a more complete semantic listing, but idiosyncratic to P, e.g.

T	... knife?	P	when you're cutting carrots
T	... bicycle?	P	you ride on and you fall off
T	... diamond?	P	people steal diamonds
T	... nail?	P	on your finger
T	... nail?	P	you could hammer in with wood for houses

Level 4: some awareness of a true definitional form, with P moving from individual experience towards general social information, especially using 'you could...' or 'when you...', e.g.

T	... knife?	P	a knife is when you cut with it
T	... apple?	P	you could eat an apple

Level 5: the true definition (in Aristotelian terms), specifying a class name plus defining attributes or properties (i.e. a Y is a kind of X). To begin with, these are lexically imprecise, e.g.

T	bicycle?	P	something you ride
T	... shoe?	P	a thing you put on your foot
T	... donkey?	P	an animal

But gradually P's taxonomies (that is, his awareness of the range of entities that belong in a class) improves, and we find

T	... knife?	P	a tool you can cut with

From a remedial point of view, it is important for T to assess the level at which P is operating before choosing her level of questioning and which mode of reaction to use. Making explicit the associative link between the items of level 2 (e.g. introducing the notion of 'wearing' between 'shoes' and 'socks' is a very different (and more difficult) task from generalizing P's experience at level 3 (e.g. 'do you only cut carrots with a knife?'). Semantic, syntactic and phonological (e.g. tonic placement) factors are involved. Conversely, a standard opening gambit, such as 'What's X for?', poses a much greater level of difficulty for P at the earlier levels than for P at levels 4 and 5.

(6) *Remediation and linguistic stages.* We are often asked whether remediation should always follow the chart's Stages. Might one not introduce the stages or features in a different order from the normal development? We do not do so ourselves, as we feel that the normal developmental path is at least a well-trodden path. We know something of the hazards that lie along it, and know something of norms of achievement if Ps are introduced to it. We have no objection to alternative routes being taken, as long as they are principled, e.g. related to some clear notion of cognitive complexity, auditory memory, motor skills, social function etc.

Above all, we recognize the central role of motivation in language learning, and have seen the ways in which individual development may be influenced by it. LARSP focuses on one aspect of language disability, but the best use of the procedure is made when it is interpreted and applied in the light of our knowledge of child development as a whole.

1.5

Micro-profile of Stage I

Michael Garman

General considerations

Given LARSP's morphosyntactic purpose, the 'thin' appearance of Stage I is understandable, but perhaps not as helpful as it might be, in relation to Ps who are at or approaching this stage of development. Two questions are frequently asked, which only a micro-profile can help answer: how can the LARSP approach be extended to Ps who are not yet at Stage I? are there guidelines for P's progression through Stage I into Stage II? Any answer to these questions will require, in the first instance, information about the normal patterns of linguistic development into and through Stage I, and it is on this point that the present section will concentrate. We shall be asking, in particular:

What are the stable patterns of vocabulary development just before syntax (i.e. at the one-word stage)?

Can any analysis be made of one-word utterances for a given child which will be relevant for (or foreshadow) the types of early constructions that the same child will use at Stage II?

As a great deal is known, in some detail, about the child's early vocalizations, can we use information from this area in furthering the child's grammatical development into Stage I?

Can we make use of relevant nonlinguistic information—level of cognitive development, gestures accompanying vocalizations, etc.?

During the formative years of LARSP, the bulk of language-acquisition research was directed at Stage II and onwards. Only a few researchers (e.g. Bloom 1973, Nelson 1973, Huttenlocher 1974) were beginning to carry out a micro-analysis of the earliest stages of vocabulary development and one-word utterances, and accordingly we had relatively little to say about Stage I in *GALD*. Now, as a result of several recent studies in this area, we can approach Stage I with increasing confidence regarding linguistic norms and patterns of development. This is, of course, not to anticipate the results of ongoing research; nor have we yet had much experience of applying a detailed Stage I analysis in assessment or remediation, either for the child who is not yet communicating at a Stage I level, or for the child who seems stuck at that Stage. But we do know more about what a Stage I micro-profile should look like, and this is what we are concerned with here.

The foreshadowing of Stage II constructions?

We look first at the P who is communicating at Stage I but seems reluctant to start combining elements. To what extent is it possible to analyse P's single-word utterances, classified as N, V, Adj etc., as attempts to foreshadow the SV, VC/O, AX etc. type utterances of Stage II? The commonsense view is to argue for continuity here. There seems little difference in principle or in method between the analysis of late Stage I and early Stage II utterances: the communicative functions of these utterances seem very similar, as do the kinds of contextual notes needed to elucidate them (cf. Bloom 1970). The question 'What syntactic construction does a given one-word utterance represent?' seems well-motivated, accordingly, and this has been the basis for viewing one-word utterances as *holophrases*, i.e. as single-word expressions of what are for the child whole sentences. There is a more cautious approach also, however, in terms of which we cannot talk of 'sentences' or 'syntax' until at least two elements are combined in construction.

What expectations of a Stage I child might we have if we adopted the holophrase approach and attempted to use contextual information to analyse his single-word utterances as foreshadowing the elements of Stage II constructions? We would expect, for example, that the child who seemed to rely a great deal on locative holophrases (i.e. a noun or an adverb in a locative sense, e.g. *garden* or *there*) would show a similar reliance on AX structures at Stage II (e.g. *Daddy garden, gone there*). We would also expect that holophrastic expressions of SVO constructions (i.e. a single-word utterance apparently representing S, V or O) would lead naturally to the use of SV and VO at Stage II. And further, we would expect that holophrastic negatives, possessives, questions etc. would progress naturally to their Stage II counterparts. Finally, a quantitative analysis should show, on the same expectations, micro-levels of development within Stage I, as certain 'sentence' types are acquired and stabilize in relation to others: and there should be a quantitative continuum across the boundary into Stage II. Rodgon 1976 is the main publication to address issues of this sort in recent years. Her analysis of the single-word speech of her subjects showed that 40 per cent of it or more could plausibly be analysed holophrastically (the rest falling under headings such as 'naming' and 'repetition') which were grouped together as non-holophrastic). Rodgon argued, accordingly, that 40 per cent of Stage I productions 'represents the first steps in the child's progress toward an understanding of linguistic relations, syntactic and semantic, in the adult sense' (94). And quantitatively she hypothesized that the proportion of holophrastic to non-holophrastic types would increase towards the end of Stage I, signalling the child's readiness to move into Stage II. This would follow from Bloom's (1970, 1973) assumption that at late Stage I there would be found *sequences of holophrases*, as an intermediate step between single-word utterances and Stage II constructions (cf. the examples cited in Clark *et al.* 1974).

But Rodgon's expectation was not borne out: no connection appeared between the proportion of holophrases to non-holophrases and developmental position within Stage I, or between the proportions of holophrases at Stage I and the proportions of holophrase sequences and true constructions of Stage II. Rodgon also hypothesized that 'it should be possible to train children to express in two words relations which they were already expressing holophrastically' (1976, 102). But training the SVO type did not have the expected effect (though this was the dominant type at the holophrase stage); and while the Locative and Possessive types *did* show a significant increase in combinatorial expression during the training period, this occurred independently of whether or not a child was expressing these relations holophrastically before training. These results have clear negative implications for any attempt to analyse Stage I utterances in terms of patterns of *syntactic* development. It seems difficult to draw reliable conclusions regarding the 'natural' (untrained) patterns of progression through Stage I; nor regarding how effective such training might be in facilitating the emergence of Stage II constructions. Hence it would seem wise to accept the view, expressed in Bloom 1973 for example, that there is no justification for treating single-word utterances as syntactic. But if this is correct, what other ways do we have of micro-analysing Stage I? Linguistically, there are two possibilities: (a) the nature of the vocabulary items used, in semantic terms (do they name objects, events, emotional states etc. ?); (b) the nature of the phonological system. We shall look briefly at both possibilities.

Vocabulary development

Two main approaches are evidenced in the literature. The first (e.g. Bloom 1973) tries to classify Stage I development in cognitive terms: what sort of concepts are expressed in early Stage I utterances, and how do they differ from those later on in Stage I? The second (e.g. Nelson 1973) tries an ethological approach: what sort of communication needs are served by Stage I utterances? One of the main conclusions of this work is that a child's word meanings may be just as immature as his word pronunciations, and that it is difficult to generalize from one child to the next. For instance, some early words may not be found in all children (as when items are used idiosyncratically by a family); they may have a larger scope (E. Clark 1973) or a narrower scope (Reich 1976) of meaning than the corresponding adult word; and antonyms may be synonymous for the child (e.g. preschool children have been reported as treating 'less' as meaning 'more', cf. Donaldson and Balfour 1968); and so on. Some idea of the plasticity of early vocabulary development may be gained by considering an example from Carter (1975): the child she studied had, at 1;0.22, a reaching-gesture accompanied by a freely-varying range of vocalizations of the [ma~me~mə~mai~moi] types. Gradually the gesture became less important, and the range of vocalizations split, around 1;4-1;5, into the [mou~mour] type and the [moi~mai] type. The first eventually narrowed into the adult word *more*, and the latter into *mine*, both around 2;0. This suggests that we shall have to make allowance for some fairly idiosyncratic strategies in normally-developing Stage I children.

Armed, but not alarmed, by such considerations, what sort of semantic classification might we make? A recent study by Benedict (1979) will help us both to review what has been researched in the last few years and to establish what current guidelines are available to us. Benedict looked at 8 subjects, aged 0;9 to 1;8, and tabulated their early vocabulary (the first 50 words) in comprehension (c) and production (p). To some extent her work builds on others' research, but it also extends and challenges some earlier views. Quantitatively, Goldin-Meadow *et al.* (1976) had argued that, in the course of vocabulary building around 2;0, (i) c precedes p, generally; (ii) the $c > p$ discrepancy is greater for verb-like elements than for noun-like; (iii) the discrepancy dwindles, as p increases, and disappears around 2;0. Benedict's findings basically extend those of Goldin-Meadow *et al.* to the earliest phase of vocabulary growth: she found the $c:p$ ratio to be around 5:1, with a 5-month gap between c and p at the 50-word level. Illustrating from just one child (Elizabeth) in the study, we have the following picture (Fig. 11). The mean interval for the group between 10–50 words in c was 2·69 months, a rate of 22·23 new words per month; in p the mean interval was 4·8 months, a rate of 9·09 new words per month.

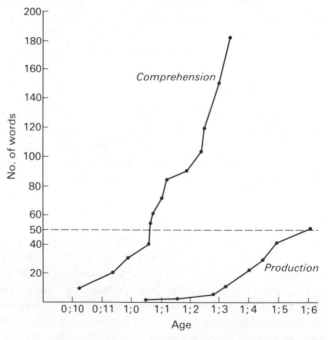

Fig. 11   Number of words, by age, for one child (after Benedict 1979)

Qualitatively, Benedict found that a system of semantic classification based on and rather similar to that used by Nelson (1973) was appropriate: the assignment of items to the following categories was based solely, of course, on the child's use of them (and not on their behaviour in adult speech):

A 1 Nominals (specific)
   2 Nominals (general)
B Action words: 1 Social-action games
              2 Events
              3 Locations
              4 General actions
              5 Inhibitors
C Modifiers: 1 Attributes
          2 States
          3 Locatives
          4 Possessives
D Personal-social: 1 Assertions
                 2 Social expressive

Benedict found (i) all the major word-types (A–D) were present from the start (as Nelson (1973) claimed); (ii) the largest classes were A2 and B1–5. Together, these accounted for 75 per cent of c and 69 per cent of p, at the 50-word level. This finding seems to neutralize the opposition between those researchers (McNeill 1970, Gleitman *et al.* 1972, Huttenlocher 1974) who claimed that 'object' words are dominant early items and those (Piaget 1962, Bloom 1974, Blank 1974) who stressed the role of early 'action' words. And, of course, Benedict suggests that the pattern for p (cf. Nelson 1973) is essentially that found also in c. There is, however, another important finding, which distinguishes c and p: (iii) in p there are about 3–4 general nominals to 2 action words at the 10-word level, and general nominals subsequently increase to become around 2·5 times as numerous as action words at the 50-word level (accounting for about 50 per cent of total vocabulary). On the other hand, in c the ratio is more like 5:1 in favour of action words over general nominals at the 10-word level, with each of these categories approaching the 35–40 per cent share of total vocabulary at the 50-word level. The general trend here, of course, is constant enough: that general nominals improve their share of both c and p vocabulary from the 10-word to the 50-word levels. This is the major developmental dimension, apparently, and it is a comparable upward movement in both c and p (Fig. 12). The pattern here seems to consist of a shift from

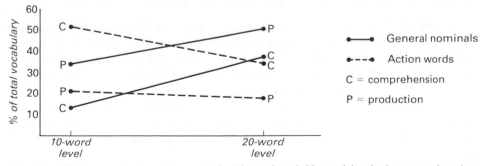

Fig. 12   The two major word types, at the 10-word and 50-word levels, in comprehension and production (after Benedict 1979)

action words to general nominals in *c*, and this then (cf. Fig. 11) can be seen as preparing the ground for the early and continued dominance of general nominals in *p* (around 5–6 months later).

The approach from the sound system

Just as we asked earlier, 'What syntactic construction does a given single-word utterance represent?' so we can now ask 'What early vocabulary development seems to be foreshadowed by particular patterns in sound production around the end of the first year?' And again we have to recognize that contextual notes will be crucial to our understanding of what is being built up: only in this way was Carter (1975), for example, able to document the unpredictable common derivation of *more/mine* in her child subject; and similarly Bruner (1974, 1975) has been able to demonstrate in what ways language can be argued to be an 'outgrowth of action' (see further on this below).

Turning, then, to the second of the two possibilities for a linguistic classification of Stage I, we may usefully take into account the work of Ferguson (1976), Crystal (1979) and Stark (1979). Ferguson recognizes 6 major steps towards the earliest linguistic sound system of the child:

(i) perception of speech v. non-speech (e.g. identification of tones of voice; differential response to parents' voices; and to voice noises v. handclaps etc.);

(ii) recognition of particular phonetic shapes/occasions of use (e.g. the child's eyes turn to clock in response to adult's *tick tock*, as early as 20th week);

(iii) cooing (experimentation with sounds, back consonants initially dominant);

(iv) babbling (cooing sounds diversify, leading to rich oral play: very different from adult sounds because of (a) vocal tract shape, (b) incomplete control of articulators, (c) independence of this type of vocalization from the phonological system of the adult language);

(v) pre-word (PW) (stable sound sequences, having child-specific form: meaning-relationship—i.e. there is no obvious adult model for PWs);

(vi) first words (FW) (stable sound sequences which are recognizably modelled on adult forms, with adult-based form:meaning relationship).

At the end of the first year of life a normally developing child will have perhaps a dozen or so PWs and one or two FWs. Babbling in a 'non-vocabulary' fashion will continue for up to another 6 months or so, alongside the strictly linguistic sound sequences of FWs. The coexistence of active PWs and FWs shows the child controlling two rather different sound-production systems: the babbling system (PWs) is unrelated to the phonology of the community language and relatively unconstrained, while the emergent phonological system of the community language is to be looked for in the small but increasingly dominant proportion of FWs.

It also seems likely that passive vocabulary is, from the start, in advance of the active: in terms of phonological representation, this will be expressed both in quantity and in quality. The child probably has a more advanced, phonological system in comprehension at the stage where, productively, he is relying on PWs (babbling) rather than FWs. These observations may be summarized as follows (Fig. 13):

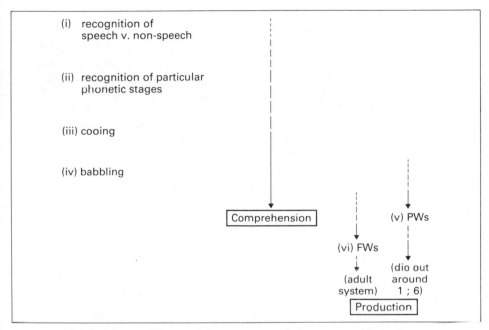

Fig. 13   Steps in sound perception and production prior to the start of a vocabulary growth (after Ferguson 1976)

Stark (1979) shows a largely similar pattern of development in terms of her own stages. The basic difference between her outline and that of Ferguson is that she has concentrated entirely on vocalizations, to the exclusion of considerations of perception. Thus she has nothing to say on Ferguson's point that the perceptual and vocalizing systems start off largely independently and gradually integrate. Stark, however, provides the stages and labels which we draw on most heavily for our characterization of vocalizations in the micro-profile; and it is worth point-ing out that she uses a more restricted sense of the term 'babbling' than does Fergu-son, as will be evident from the summary on p. 126. At Stark's stage 5, we make contact with Ferguson's (1976) PWs (alongside FWs).

But it is important to notice a further concept, identified by Dore *et al.* (1976—the 'phonetically consistent form' (PCF). Dore *et al.* point out that 'Investi-gators have employed one or both of two general criteria for identifying a child's initial word (Darley and Winitz 1961): (1) the approximation of phonetic form to forms of the adult language; and (2) consistencies of usage with regard to objects or situations' (18). PCFs do not meet either of these criteria, and yet are stable

Age	Stage	Vocalization types
to 8 weeks	1	Reflexive sounds—crying (has certain speech features) —fussing —vegetative sounds (has other speech features)
8–20 weeks	2	Cooing and laughter—combines the speech features of crying and vegative sounds. Back consonants dominant
16–30 weeks	3	Vocal play—longer series of comfort sounds disappear, replaced by single segments with steady C or V articulations, of considerable duration
25–50 weeks	4	Reduplicated babbling—series of CV syllables in which the C remains constant. Labial and alveolar stops/nasals, and /j/–glides frequent
0;9–1;6	5	Nonreduplicated babbling, and expressive jargon

in themselves and clearly potential precursors of vocabulary items in the full sense. The relationship between PCFs and the other categories recognized above is as follows:

PCFs—stable phonetic sequences, with little or no referential value, and no adult model;

PWs— stable phonetic sequences with consistent but idiosyncratic meaning;

FWs— adult-based forms, with adult-based meanings.

Finally, Crystal (1979) concentrates on the development of prosodic perception and production: most of the earlier stages in the development of prosodic control are incidentally handled by Stark (1979), while the post-0;6 development consists in the main of the consistent production of patterns which 'come to resemble pro- sodic patterns of the mother-tongue'. For Crystal, it is only at around 0;6 that we have the 'first sign of anything linguistic emerging' (though we ought to note that perception of adult prosodic contrasts seems to be established as early as 0;3– 0;4). Subsequent to the onset of LARSP's Stage I, the further development of pro- sodic factors (as set out in Crystal 1979) ceases to be of immediate relevance to us here (belonging more to a phonological than to a grammatical profile).

Cognitive development and other factors

Finally, we have to ask whether we can turn to stages in cognitive development, and/or in other relevant nonlinguistic behaviour patterns, for help in assessment and remediation. Corrigan (1978) has argued strongly for the view that, as far as cognitive development is concerned, we have to be precise as to what we are talking about when we investigate the degree to which cognitive stages of develop- ment tie in with linguistic ones. This is because a child may be simultaneously at one sensorimotor stage for one task and at others for other tasks. Corrigan took the Piagetian concept of Object Permanence and observed how it developed, in relation to linguistic development, in 3 children (aged 0;9, 0;10 and 0;11 at the start) as part of an 18-month longitudinal study. Her principal findings are:

(i) there is *no* general correlation between object-permanence ranks and length/complexity indices of language development;

(ii) there *is* a general correspondence between the onset of search for an invisibly displaced object (Object Permanence Rank 15) and the start of single-word utterances;

(iii) there *is* a general correspondence between the attainment of object permanence (Object Permanence Rank 21) and a spurt in the vocabulary growth of the children studied;

(iv) there is *no* distinction among vocabulary items along the line of the 'function' v. 'substantive' opposition as suggested by Bloom (1973), either in first appearance or in frequency (thus supporting Benedict 1979 on this issue).

The most important points for us are (ii) and (iii), since they seem to indicate areas where nonlinguistic assessment and remediation might be relevant to the nature of the linguistic system within Stage I. While it seems that language and cognitive development are not *directly* correlated, they are apparently each age-related, and hence in an indirect association: it seems likely that a developmental linguistic disorder may exist alongside an intact cognitive system, leaving the door open for cognitive training as a way into language.

Beyond this, however, it seems unwise to place too much faith in accounts of early cognitive development *in relation to language*, given the present state of research. But we surely ought to take account of the major early achievements that are reviewed in Bruner (1975): for example, the development of differential responding to people v. other entities; of the ability to maintain eye-to-eye contact; of responding with a smile or laugh to adult smiling or laughing; of the ability to imitate facial and manual gestures; and of the ability to follow an adult's line of regard. Bruner presents compelling evidence that much of what we think of as natural linguistic behaviour involves such actions and 'awarenesses' as these: joint attention, the ability to take turns in a joint enterprise, imitation etc. And Snow (1977), from a relatively independent field of research, reports that important developments take place before the end of the first year of life in the nature of the speech that adults (typically mothers) address to children. Clearly, eye-to-eye contact is a prerequisite for subsequent joint enterprises, whether imitative in structure or not, and whether linguistic or not.

Further, around the time reported for the ability to follow an adult's line of regard, Snow notes that mothers tend to respond to a variety of heterogeneous child vocalizations, including burps, as if they were contributions to a hypothetical discussion (e.g. 'Yes, what a nice little wind that was!', following a burp). This pattern continues, as a form of adult-dominated 'language' game, until the child is around 0;6: at this point, Snow reports a shift on the part of mothers to the sort of contribution that comments on objects and actions in the child's vicinity. It is as if mothers initially habituate their child to a to-and-fro 'language' situation (building in anything the child happens to emit), and then switch to a routine that will encourage the introduction of elements from the child's world into this conversational orbit. By this time, the child has started to enter into the turn-taking routine actively, and is becoming increasingly dominant in it. Further, Bruner reports that around this time a child will 'give' an object to an adult, but will apparently not see the adult as a potential partner (agent) in a to-and-fro 'object game'; that is, the child will not spontaneously release the object into the adult's hand. But the adult can initiate an object-interchange routine (paralleling the quasi-conversational routine reported by Snow) by removing the object from the child's grip and treating the child's subsequent reaching gesture as a response in a to-and-fro situation. The adult restores the object to the child, and an early 'joint action' turn is completed. (Carter reports that around this time the link between stable vocalizations and gestures is established, though in a preliminary way as yet.) A little later on, around the start of Stage I, the child may initiate a 'joint action' routine: and Bruner points out that this involves the child looking upon the adult as a potential agent. The child's responses subsequently grow more stable (Snow 1977) in relation to adult utterances, at around the time that Carter observes 'sensorimotor morphemes' (stable gesture-plus-vocalization complexes, with statable meaning). What follows from this stage is (i) an increase in the relative dominance of the vocalization component as opposed to the gesture in the child's overall communicative system, and (ii) an emergence of specifying objects by *name* as opposed to the gesture-plus-vocalization complex (on both of these points, cf. Carter 1975). And (i) and (ii) apparently take place alongside (iii), the attainment of the ability to search for invisibly displaced objects (Corrigan 1978). Finally, with Stage I nearly completed, and with the attainment of object permanence, Bruner (1975) reports that the child will frequently initiate an object-'joint action' game, by means of a word: the developing linguistic system, itself an outgrowth in part from early action routines, becomes integrated with such action routines.

This is, of course, a necessarily brief review of a large and complex research area, but it should serve its purpose of introducing the items we have recognized in our micro-profile of Stage I. On the profile chart, we have grouped together all these factors under the general heading of 'Behavioural Factors'; and those that relate to the child's contributions are set out down the left hand side, those relating to the adult's on the right.

The micro-profile chart

The bulk of the observations set out in this section have been incorporated, in summary form, in the micro-profile chart for Stage I which is set out here (Fig. 14): all that is required now is a brief description of its salient features, and some comments on the way that it may be used.

It will be seen that a pre-Stage I section is required, in addition to Stage I itself. The pre-Stage I section is concerned exclusively with developing patterns of vocalizations and perception of speech sounds: and these two systems gradually merge as the child develops structural constraints which process what it perceives and directly affect the nature of what it vocalizes. Even before this, however, the 'speech

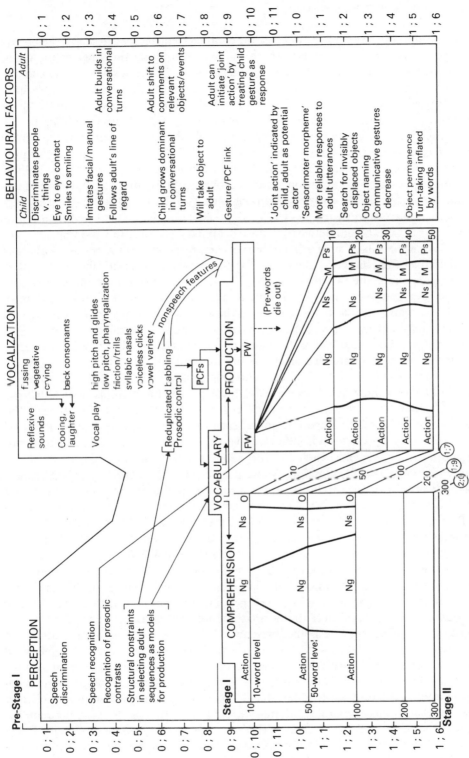

Fig. 14 Micro-profile chart of Stage I, with associated commentary

recognition' and 'recognition of prosodic contrasts' entries seem to mark the beginnings of a receptive vocabulary (note the line connecting this area of the chart with the FW line at Stage I). Under 'vocalization' we list the developmental characteristics that we look out for (though it should be noticed that the order of features recognized under the headings 'Reflexive sounds' and 'Vocal play' is not developmental). A number of features of vocal play and of reduplicated babbling fail to continue into speech and are not represented further in the chart (cf. the arrow labelled 'nonspeech features'). This leaves us with PCFs as the culmination of pre-Stage I perceptual-vocal ability on the production side (note the arrow linking the perception and vocalization systems around 0;5). In applying this part of the chart to pre-Stage I Ps who are vocalizing, one would attempt to 'place' their perceptual abilities and their vocalizations in relation to the items listed, and hence to arrive at suitable guidelines for pre-vocabulary vocalization training.

Turning to Stage I 'proper', the chart concentrates on the analysis of vocabulary rather than on syntactic categories, for the reasons discussed above; and it is organized under the two main headings of Comprehension (continuing the pre-Stage I perception column) and Production (continuing the vocalization column). PCFs continue into both PWs in the earliest vocabulary (which we consider as strictly outside the main vocabulary system that we wish to chart) and into FWs (which form the precursors of the main vocabulary system). The first level, quantitatively, on the Comprehension side is the 10-word line, at around 0;10: qualitatively, this is split up into Action, Ng (General nominal), Ns (Specific nominal) and Other (Modifier and Personal-social) categories (following Benedict 1979), a classification which may prove to convert straightforwardly into *GALD*'s 'V', 'N' and Other. The relative proportions of each of these categories within the total vocabulary at a given level is indicated in an obvious way by devoting corresponding amounts of space to each category along the relevant line. The 10-word line extends across into Production, where it is set at around the 1;1–1;2 age range, as indicated in the research literature: again the qualitative information is noted in terms of Action, Ng, Ns, and the remaining categories M (Modifier) and PS (Personal-social) are not conflated under Other here, since they are relatively more numerous than in Comprehension. Notice, though, that the 10-word line is not the first level recognized in Production: this is the FW/PW line (emerging from pre-Stage I speech recognition), following Ferguson's (1976) suggestion that early vocabulary is usually composed of a larger number of nonce-forms, which do not lead to the adult system, and just a few genuine first words. It is these latter which we assume to develop differentially into the word-classes recognized at the 10-word line; and we incorporate here Corrigan's (1978) observation that the ability to search for invisibly displaced objects is associated with the onset of single-word utterances. Benedict provides qualitative information on the production side for the 20-, 30- and 40-word levels also, and for the 50-word level on both Comprehension and Production. Notice that the 40- and 50-word lines are set close together on the chart, reflecting Corrigan's finding that the attainment of object permanence (at around this time) is associated with a spurt in vocabulary growth. Finally, Benedict's (1979) 100-word level information is included: and we have decided to indicate also the admittedly rather shaky evidence from Smith (1926) (cf. the discussion in McCarthy 1954) that the 100-word level in production is attained around 1;7. So also with the 200- and 300-word levels, which are (very tentatively) set at around 1;5 and 1;6 respectively in comprehension, and at around 1;9 and 2;0 in production.

The suggestion for assessment in this section of the chart is that where a P has some productive vocabulary its overall quantity should be assessed, and it should then be inspected for qualitative balance at whatever level is appropriate. Thus, if there are only 5 items in all, it will not be surprising to find that perhaps only one of these seems to represent an adult form; if there are 25 items, however, we should expect to find the sort of balance between different categories that is represented along the 20- and 30-word lines on the chart. In this way, a qualitative imbalance for a given quantitative level quickly becomes apparent, and the first step in remediation is to achieve a balance before proceeding. (It will, we hope, be clear that the practical use of micro-profiles such as this is in no way different from the more familiar profile used in *GALD*: the emphasis is on filling gaps, attaining quantitative norms where these can be recognized, and preserving balance in the system as it develops.) Our limited experience thus far suggests that appropriate training on the missing or 'thin' types of vocabulary items allows for subsequent quantitative increase of the *whole* system. This sort of procedure seems appropriate for carrying such Ps through Stage I once the initial development of word-classes is complete. In the cases where these classes have not yet been established (i.e. before the qualitative structure associated with the 10-word line of the chart), we distinguish two sorts of problem: (i) the number of items is fairly high (many more than 10), or (ii) the number is low. In the first type, we would first of all check for phonetic consistency of the forms (i.e., have PCFs actually been established at all?), and if all is well here, concentrate on differential-class training. In the second case, we are presumably more concerned with quantity: we check for PCFs, and then try to introduce just one or two FWs, while not wasting time in trying to eliminate PWs. Indeed, it might be a good strategy to encourage PWs by 'learning P's language' to begin with.

In conclusion, let us consider the type of P who still seems to stand outside 'the system'—the P who does not yet vocalize, or at least not consistently in any way that leads to placement on the chart. Where this sort of situation proceeds from largely nonlinguistic factors (as in elective mutism) we, as linguists, can of course recommend nothing. But it ought to be pointed out that the micro-profile can, like the larger profile, be used for comprehension work as well as for P's productions, and on written as well as on spoken language samples. The route into P's developing system has to be chosen by T. And, as with the larger profile, the further development of the chart described here will best follow from the ingenious use of it in a variety of situations by our good colleague, T.

1.6

Micro-profile of the Stage III Verb Phrase

Paul Fletcher

Widespread use of LARSP on children with language disability, over the last few years, has isolated the structure of the verb phrase (summarized in *GALD*, 54–5) as a specific area of difficulty (see Crystal and Fletcher 1979, and also Haber 1977), and has underlined the need for Ts to have a more detailed picture of normal development in this area, especially in the 'middle' stages, to augment the information already available from the Profile Chart. The present section will consider development in verb-phrase structure that can be linked to Stage III, in the main, although there will be some discussion of later developments.

The child's task: form and function

It might be useful at the outset to remind ourselves of the task facing the child in developing verb phrase (VP) systems (see further, Fletcher 1979). In the first place he has to learn the auxiliaries and inflections that make up the English verbal paradigm, the order in which they occur, and the cooccurrence restrictions that hold among them. The systems which make up the paradigm can be summarized as tense, progressive aspect, perfect aspect and mood.[20] Every verb form is marked for tense, either present or past, and in addition can be progressive, and/or perfect, and/or modal. The sentences on p. 133 illustrate the range of possibilities.

The child in learning the various verb forms has to appreciate that some forms have double marking (e.g. *be + ing*), others only single (e.g. past tense); that there is a fixed order of occurrence of items in the verb form. He also has to learn that some past tenses are irregular: that *am, is, 's*, are all forms of the verb *to be*; that the first auxiliary in the verb form is moved around the subject of the sentence to form questions (unless *who, what* etc. is the sentence subject); and that where there is no auxiliary, *do* is used instead, and tense marked appropriately; similarly, it is the first auxiliary of the VP to which the negative particle is attached. This is not an exhaustive catalogue of the syntactic and morphological facts he has to apprehend, but it will give some indication of the extent of the task, and would be one explanation for the long-drawn-out development of the VP in normal children.

[20] Voice is usually included as one of the systems relevant to VP structure (e.g. *GCE*, 73), but is omitted here as not relevant to Stage III syntactic developments.

tense only:	I fall	present
	I fell	past
tense and progressive:	he is falling	present
	he was falling	past, progressive
tense and perfect:	he has fallen	present, perfect
	he had fallen	past, perfect
tense, progressive and perfect:	he has been falling	present, perfect, progressive
	he had been falling	past, perfect, progressive
tense, modal:	he can dance	present, modal *can*
	he could dance[21]	past, modal *can*

There is another side to VP development, however, that has to be considered in accounting for the course of acquisition, or considering remediation for children with language disability, and that is the function(s) of formal markers. Not only formally, but also functionally, the complexities of the verb phrase are formidable. The first potential problem is the plurifunctionality of markers: for example, the *be + ing* form, usually described as the progressive, does indeed signal duration, or continuous action, as in *he's running*; but it can also be used to signal futurity, as in *John's coming* or *John's arriving tomorrow*. To take another instance, the past tense form primarily relates a previous event to the time of speaking, the time often being further specified by temporal adverbials, e.g. *I saw George yesterday, he left her last year*. But there is another important function of past tense which has nothing to do with previous time, and that is in sentences like *if George came, I'd leave*, where the past tense signals unreality. Examples of the multiple function of formal markers could be given for several other verb phrase forms. There is however another problem of functional analysis which needs mentioning: that for some of the semantic notions to which markers in the verb phrase refer, there are alternative means of coding. The modal notion of *possibility*, for example, often expressed in English by *might* (e.g. *John might be sleeping*), can also be expressed by adverbs without a modal (e.g. *maybe/possibly John's sleeping*), or by an alternative syntactic structure (e.g. *it's possible that John is sleeping*). Futurity can also be coded in a number of different ways (e.g. *John is coming (tomorrow), John will come (tomorrow), John is going to come (tomorrow), John comes tomorrow*).

What needs to be borne in mind, therefore, when we consider the development of the verb phrase in both normal and remedial contexts is that children are not necessarily going to use a particular verb phrase form with the same functions as adults. Indeed, as elsewhere in development, we might expect to find the form used with restricted function, or we might find it used in a wider range of situations than would be appropriate for an adult. To illustrate the two possibilities we can

---

[21] There are two interpretations for this sentence, of course. In one sense the past tense form of *can* refers to past time; in another sense the sentence refers to the *possibility* of the subject's dancing— he could dance if he tried, for example. The past tense forms of modals (like the past tense forms of main verbs—see p. 138) are not always used simply to refer to events previous to the time of speaking. In some cases (e.g. *shall—should*) the meaning of the 'past tense form' is quite different to that of its counterpart.

cite early past tense usage (at 2;2 or 2;3), where it has a restricted function, compared with adult usage, and its use about a year later, where it has an extended
usage. The first uses of past tense appear to be restricted to referring to a very
recent past event which has some concrete effect in present time, e.g. *spilt juice*,
broke cup, where the effect of the events in question is before the child's eyes (see
Antinucci and Miller 1976). About a year later, the child has extended the use
of past tense to refer to remote time, and is specifying the time at which the action
occurred, albeit vaguely, e.g. *I saw Granny last summer* (where *last summer* is known
to be inaccurate). In addition, he uses past tense in contexts which would normally
required the perfect—*I ate my dinner* instead of *I've eaten my dinner* at the moment
of completing the meal. Only later, as the perfect develops, does it take over this
over-extended function of the past tense form.

A further observation concerning the path of normal acquisition is that a child
will not necessarily stay within the confines of the syntactically defined verb phrase
when he wishes to modify the main verb in some way. It is at least as likely that
the child at early Stage III will say *maybe Granny come* as *Granny might come*;
the first is a SVA structure, the second SV with Aux marked at phrase structure.
Both however perform the same job for the child at this stage, stating his doubt
about Granny's coming. Though we can state in general terms what the syntactic
possibilities are for the child at any stage, we cannot predict which of the alternatives available to him he will take; and so we have to be aware that in certain
cases he will go outside the verb phrase as narrowly defined. While the number
of alternatives that lie outside the VP, or outside the set of auxiliary verbs, is not
extensive, nevertheless in any micro-analysis of the child's verb phrase development, they must be taken into account.

The micro-profile

One of the problems facing us in supplying more detail is the nature of the research
literature on verb-phrase acquisition, which is sporadic in its treatment. Nevertheless, enough can be gleaned from published and unpublished diary data and records
of spontaneous speech, and from accounts of specific VP areas (e.g. Bronckart
and Sinclair 1973, Harner 1976, Nussbaum and Naremore 1975) to make the exercise worth attempting. Table 1 illustrates such a micro-profile for the period
between 2;0 and 2;6, roughly the period covered by Stage III. It is in fact a synthesis
of the development of contrasts in the VP for some of the early diary literature
(especially of Hildegarde, a detailed account of whose language development
is given in Leopold 1949), several recent studies (see below), and my own diary
data.

Some of the features included in the micro-profile, particularly in the 'Other
Relevant Forms' column, have not been systematically studied, and their inclusion
is therefore tentative. The table is organized from left to right into columns labelled
according to the main verb-phrase systems: modals, the progressive, perfect,
present and past tenses, and the unmarked verb form (UVF), i.e. the lexical verb.
The righthand column is a miscellaneous listing of forms: marginal auxiliaries (e.g.

Table 1 The development of the VP at Stage III

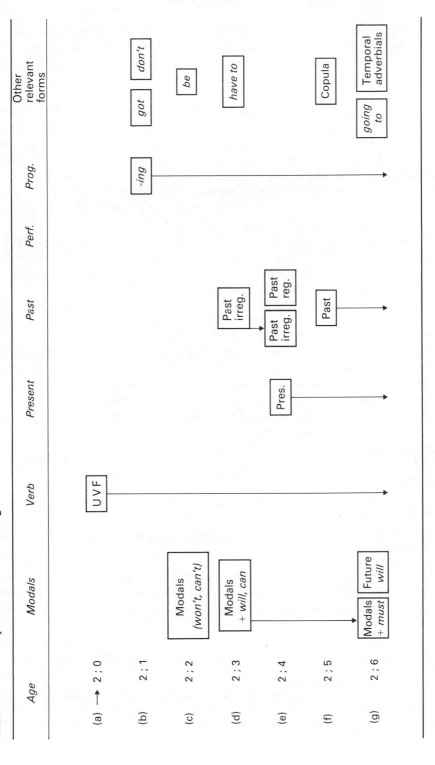

Age	Modals	Verb	Present	Past	Perf.	Prog.	Other relevant forms
(a) → 2 ; 0		U V F →					
(b) 2 ; 1						-ing →	*got* *don't*
(c) 2 ; 2	Modals (*won't, can't*)						*be*
(d) 2 ; 3	Modals + *will, can* →		Pres. →	Past irreg. → Past irreg. / Past reg.			*have to*
(e) 2 ; 4							
(f) 2 ; 5				Past →			Copula
(g) 2 ; 6	Modals + *must* / Future *will*						*going to* / Temporal adverbials

have to), particular analytic problems (e.g. *got*), copula and temporal adverbial. From top to bottom of the table, each line after the first, where the system includes simply the UVF, marks one or more additions to the set of V modifiers used by the child. These 'steps' in development are now dealt with individually.

(a) Leopold reports for H (aged 2;0) that on his return after a 6-week absence the most important change he noticed in her language was the increase in the number of verbs used—there had previously been very few. All are unmarked, and they are used not just as imperatives, but within sentences. Some examples of early sentences containing UVFs are: *my fix my dress, my get Papa's paper, Mama, scratch my back*. These examples include Stage III clause structures, but this step in development is first observed at the very beginning of Stage II, when SV or VO structures begin to appear (cf. Brown 1973, 317).

(b) The first verb modifier is generally agreed to be the *-ing* form, appearing without the Aux *be*.[22] There are some obvious reasons for this. (i) The *-ing* is phonologically salient—it is word-final, and consists of a VC syllable (unlike two of the past tense forms, /-t/ and /-d/, which are simply added to a syllable). (ii) The *-ing* morpheme, again unlike past tense, has only a single form in a dialect (interdialectal variation exists, of course, especially between /-ɪŋ/ and /-ɪn/). (iii) The *-ing* form can be suffixed to the majority of English verbs—only a small minority of stative verbs like *know, love, think, believe* tend not to occur with the progressive (and of these, many are unlikely to occur in the child's early vocabulary, which may be one of the reasons why overgeneralization of the *-ing* suffix does not occur— see Brown 1973, 303 and Kuczaj 1978 for discussion of this issue). (iv) The *-ing* form is relatively 'concrete' in meaning: input to the child will generally include *be + ing* forms as commentary on events going on in the child's immediate environment[23] *mummy's making a cake, daddy's painting the wall* etc.

The child's use of the minimal system he has at this point [UVF and *-ing*], can be illustrated by some of the data from Daniel at 2;0:

I watch you	(approaches observer, who is writing at a table)
I watching you	(as he is looking at what the observer is writing)
I watch you	(said over his shoulder as he moves away to do something else)

Here the *-ing* form is used, appropriately, to describe the (albeit brief) continuous action of watching; the UVF, the only other alternative he has in this rudimentary system, is used for anything other than continuous action, in this particular case

---

[22] It is necessary to point out that the use of many of these forms, including *-ing*, is variable at the outset and for a considerable period of time thereafter. That is, a form is sometimes omitted in an environment where its use in the adult language is obligatory. See Brown 1973, 255 ff, for a discussion of this aspect of language learning.

[23] Though there is at present no data available on this point, it would be useful to establish if mothers modified their input to children *functionally*, for instance by only using the progressive to refer to duration in the immediate context, and not to refer to the future. In this way input would directly influence the uses of formal markers by the child that we are able to observe.

both intention and completed action. The use of UVF for completed action can be seen again in this example from Daniel:

I doing poop   (when actually in the process)
I do poop   (said after he has finished, and stood up)

These functions (intention and completed action) are eventually to be taken over by *will* or *going to*, and past tense, respectively, but for the moment UVF has to serve.

The ORF column includes *got*, which turns up in examples like *my got my clothes* with, as Leopold points out, present meaning. No *get* form appears at this point, so it would not be appropriate to analyse this as a past form (cf. Brown 1973, 260). The other form included here, *don't*, has one example cited, *don't sleep*, and is also said to occur on its own.

(c) Like Daniel, and like the children from whom Brown derives his data, the first auxiliaries to appear are negative modals *won't* and *can't* at about 2;2 (cf. Klima and Bellugi 1966). Examples are given of *won't* on its own or with a verb, *I won't eat that*, and of *can't* on its own. Examples from Daniel at this point of development, however, show *can't* being used with verbs also, *can't do my zip up*. For Daniel, further, *willn't* was the negative form used in declarative sentences. These forms are, like -*ing*, perceptually salient (they are never reduced, as *can* and *will* are). They are useful for the child to express his unwillingness or his inability or difficulty in performing some action—often in a way in which an adult will not use a form. So Daniel uses *can't*, loudly and with feeling, when he is stuck in a large pot and unable to extricate himself. As we will see with their positive counterparts, which are the next development, it is perhaps the performative function of these forms for the child which is to be emphasized at this point. In the ORF column, the *be* form occurs in such examples by Hildegarde as *I be Nackedei*, presumably reduced from the parental *I'll be....*

(d) There are two developments at this point: the positive modals *will* and *can*, and some irregular past tenses. In addition *have to*, which though it is not syntactically defined as an auxiliary has a function similar to that of *must* in its 'obligation' sense, is cited for this stage also. The modal *will* has in the adult language a number of functions, of which volition and future reference are the most important. The function that *will* appears to have in early protocols is volition, but it is often closely tied to question-and-answer contexts, with the child replying *I will* to a question, or asking a question herself, *will you hold these*. These are the only inverted questions to appear at early Stage III, and these and declaratives with modals appear to be closely tied to action. The child may ask *can I blow candles out* when he wants to be lifted up to see a birthday cake, or may say *I can come in your bed* as he goes past his parents' room on his way to bed. In the first case the use of *can* results in him being lifted up; in the second case he suits action to the word by going into the room and clambering into the bed. There is obviously a complex of reasons for the appearance of some forms from a syntactically well-defined class before others. The modals which are closely tied to willingness, refusal and ability (in addition to the obligation of *have to*) to perform actions turn up early in the child's repertoire, and does not seem to be a coincidence.

Leopold's comment about the irregular pasts is that they 'begin to appear sporadically'. This is confirmed by Brown (1973), Ervin (1964) and others. As a good deal of section (f) below is devoted to past tense, I will not comment further on them here.

(e) Apart from the incorporation of some present tense forms, which for Hildegarde and Daniel begin to occur here, this step is included to underline the possibility that for some children the cooccurrence of irregular pasts with regular pasts, once these start to occur, may persist *without* the overgeneralization of the regular past tense ending to strong verbs. This latter pattern is certainly very common, possibly the most frequent strategy that English-speaking children follow. But there are children who for a short time have both irregular and regular pasts, and a recent analysis of the published Bristol project data indicates that some of these children maintain this distinction and do not go by the overgeneralization route. There is also evidence from other published studies (e.g. Kuczaj 1976, Fay 1978) that some children use yet another strategy for marking past tense on irregular (and sometimes regular) stems: they use *do*-support, with unstressed *do*, as in *he did 'come, he did 'show*.

(f) At this point there are several developments: the overgeneralization of past tense, already mentioned; the beginnings of the use of *be* with the progressive inflection; in addition the copula is now used more frequently. Some copula forms have been cited before, but the form was only used in isolated instances (e.g. at (e) a specific sentence *Mike was here*, used frequently, is cited). Past tense, in the examples given for Hildegarde and for others at this point in their development, is said to be used *aspectually*, that is to refer primarily to the nature of an action (its quality, duration, completion etc.) rather than to its place in time. Early past tenses appear to refer only to very recently past events which have an effect in the present: the child's still sketchy verb phrase maintains an aspectual distinction between complete and incomplete action via the past progressive contrast. The reason for the restriction on the use of past, it has been claimed (Antinucci and Miller 1976) is primarily a cognitive one: to be able to use past tense deictically, the child has to be able to build a *representation*, in the Piagetian sense, in memory, of the past events. To re-present past states of affairs will be easier for the child this young (or may only be possible for him) if the past event or process is limited to some present observable state. While this explanation is arguable, the data does seem to indicate that the child at Stage III does not extend past reference too far out of his current context, and it would seem sensible to take this into account when setting up a remediation programme. Contrasts of the *he's jumping/he fell* type, or *he's running up the hill/he ran down the hill*, if it is possible to supply appropriate accompanying pictures, would seem to be suitable to set before the child at the beginning.

(g) The next expansion of the system is intriguing with respect to tense. It is here that Leopold recognizes a use of *will* as a 'future tense', giving the example *don't hug baby Elinor, will cry*. This use of *will* is referred to as 'prediction' in *GCE*

(101), but whichever term is used, it is clearly a use of the modal distinct from its early performative function (see (c) above). Leopold notes that this use of *will* is becoming more frequent at this point, and that 'the support of an adverb of time seems to be felt as necessary' (31). Examples are *after a while, pretty soon, some day*. Correspondingly adverbs are used to support past tense, with *last summer* being used by Hildegarde for any past time reference. These adverbials continue to be few in number and relatively vague for some time, well into the child's fourth year. It is as if the child has realized that very often tenses in the adult language are supported by adverbials (Crystal 1966) and so includes an adverbial form, without having enough appreciation of time distinctions to make it semantically appropriate (for further discussion see Ames 1946, Weber and Weber 1976, Harner 1976).

What all this seems to suggest is that once the past/progressive contrast is established, work can proceed on a past/progressive/'future' *will* contrast,[24] possibly supported by simple adverbials like *yesterday, now, tomorrow*. The exact adverbials used will of course partly depend on the cognitive development of the child being taught: if it is felt that he understands more time distinctions than the average two-and-a-half-year-old, then of course more sophisticated temporal adverbials can be used.

At this point, in the middle of the third year, we have reached a point in VP development where some modal auxiliaries are used, and some contrasts established in the areas of tense and aspect. The development has been noticeably piecemeal, and some forms are used, and will continue to be used variably, particularly past tense. Several conditions affect this variability. The factors may be phonological—some verb stems plus past tense are apparently more difficult to pronounce than others (Derwing and Baker 1979). They may be syntactic factors—once the child begins to use complex sentences he may not at first follow sequence of tense constraints. There may also be semantic factors—past tense may initially only be marked on certain kinds of verbs (Antinucci and Miller 1976). The piecemeal development of past tense and other relevant forms will continue: modal auxiliaries will be learned one by one, and the perfect (*have* + past participle forms) will gradually emerge soon after the beginning of the third year, but will not be firmly established until around four.

The focus of this micro-profile, and the associated comments, has been Stage III. It will be apparent that much has been omitted that is relevant to the development of the verb phrase—the onset of double auxiliary marking, the problems of sequence of tenses, the passive voice, the syntactic problems of question formation, and so on. However, even from a brief account of the earliest steps in development, a great deal has been added to the initial specification of Verb Phrase on the Profile Chart, where Aux and Cop (along with the associated word endings) are the only items to appear. The micro-profile would seem to provide

[24] The *going to* form should not be forgotten. It is often more natural to use this to refer to the future *I'm going to Nana's tomorrow*, than to use *will*, particularly with the first person, as the latter is almost always then interpreted in its volitional sense.

considerable material for further remedial guidelines for the language disabled child, and at the very least a sense of expectation that remediation in this area is likely to be a slower and more complex process than in other areas of syntactic development.

Part 2

LARSP in clinical settings

2.1

Dawn House School

Corinne Haynes

Dawn House opened in October 1974 with eighteen children who were divided into three classes, mainly on the basis of educational and social compatibility. One period every day in each class was set aside for oral language work, but it was soon apparent that educational compatibility did not necessarily coincide with similarity in levels of spoken language, and that this discrepancy in expressive language ability made group teaching difficult for the tutor to organize, and an inefficient learning situation for the child.

As the school built up in numbers each term, this problem was exacerbated by new children entering with very undeveloped language and thus increasing the range of ability within the class. Experimentally we decided to establish small oral-language groups of three to five children, cutting across class boundaries and based only on oral language needs. These needs were determined by a battery of tests examining auditory skills of perception and discrimination; short-term auditory memory; comprehension (of vocabulary, content concepts and syntax); and expressive abilities in terms of vocabulary, content, syntax and phonological development. Assigning groups on this very wide scatter of abilities was not easy, and some arbitrary decisions were made; but after various trial and error procedures we established as the two most important determining factors:

(i) receptive v. expressive linguistic disability;
(ii) expressive linguistic level as measured by LARSP.

These categories produce reasonably linguistically homogeneous groups which work daily for a thirty to forty-minute session with a tutor who may be a teacher, speech therapist or aide. These groups work within the areas of listening and attention; comprehension; productive syntax; and uses of language. Phonological problems are normally dealt with separately. Each child has a language-group file with all possible areas of remediation listed including all the clause, phrase and morphological structures from the syntactic profile. This is used to keep a record of all the areas and structures worked on, with dates and comments. We have found this to be necessary, as the children progress at different rates and some adjustment of groups takes place every term. Detailed treatment notes remain in the language tutor's file, and tutors meet twice a term with each other to discuss problems and progress.

The most critical factor in determining the size of the group is distractibility, and any group containing a hyperactive child is not allowed to become larger than three children to one adult.

Remediation techniques for syntax are largely those outlined in *GALD*—modelling, drills and forced alternatives—but with the extra parameter of group interaction. In practice this means that modelling is increased as activities go round the group, with T stepping in to reinforce where necessary, and it becomes easier to exploit the game or drama situation. With some groups an element of competition can usefully be introduced, but on the whole we avoid this. We often also have speech therapy, teaching or social work students in school who can be added to the group in the role of 'stooge'—either getting things wrong, or failing to understand instructions until the correct structures are produced.

Daily language groups over a period of years create great demands for material and activities to ring the changes, particularly as our children all have learning disabilities. We are therefore building up a catalogue of ideas for remediation activities and games at all levels to which all the tutors contribute and on which they draw.

One further point concerns the way in which the profile is obtained. Most of the children who enter the school rapidly increase their communicability, even though linguistic skills are very poor. From these children we take a half-hour sample of data as described in *GALD* (but frequently having to reduce or abandon discussion of events outside the immediate experience). We then analyse and chart the data to the best of our ability. Some children, however, have persisting secondary emotional problems in speech situations for much longer, or are particularly verbally non-creative. We feel that the reduced utterances they produce, although typical of their performance in a one-to-one situation with adults, are well below their level of competence. For these children we have devised two alternative methods of drawing up the profile. The 'elicited LARSP' uses predetermined toys and pictures, and a question and answer format to elicit all the clause and phrase structures from Stage II to Stage IV of the chart. Beyond Stage IV elicitation is difficult, and for children beyond this stage we use an 'imitated LARSP' procedure, with structures from Stage II to Stage VI.

For purposes of comparison we have tried all three methods with some children. We find that both alternative methods, but particularly the elicited LARSP, correlate well with the spontaneously obtained data in indicating which stage has been reached, but provide incomplete information for planning a programme of remediation, giving no indication of pattern of balance of structures, or particular weaknesses.

According to the general level of structures, we assign children to groups and plan a programme of work designed to meet all the linguistic needs of all the children in that group. This may mean that some children will spend time working on structures that are already in their speech. Sometimes it is possible to stretch these children more, for example by including more phrase structures in their contribution, but generally we do not feel that any reinforcement is wasted. Also we do find some structures particularly difficult for all language disordered children—e.g. the development of the verb phrase, especially the use of tenses—and this increases group homogeneity.

Case study

Henry has a severe linguistic disability. Emotionally he is immature, fragile, and unable to accept failure. His learning disability is characterized by rigidity and inability to change his approach. Once embarked on a train of thought he finds it difficult to accept redirection, and this is apparent in the LARSP extracts.

He first came to DHS in October 1974 at the age of 8;5, with a history of failing to learn or to settle in the infant school, and having been rejected by another language school two years previously on the grounds of immature behaviour.

In outline, his developmental history shows: normal birth; one sister (two years older); slow development of normal feeding habits; delayed motor development (sitting at 0;10, walking at 1;6), but no clumsiness; no infant babbling; first vocalizations at 4; first words at 6. At one time he was thought deaf, and was seen by a teacher of the deaf between 2 and 3;6, when his hearing was found to be normal. Speech therapy (twice weekly) began at 5;6.

His first assessment on entry to Dawn House gave the following results:

Performance IQ (WISC)	—within average range
Hearing	—normal
Comprehension:	
EPVT	—SS = 88; percentile = 21; age equiv. = 7;5
RDLS	—over 6 yrs
Discrimination.	
Renfrew Picture Pointing	—within average range
Short-term auditory memory:	
ITPA Aud. seq. memory	—SS = 24; age = 3;10
Expression:	
Vocabulary (Renfrew Word Finding)	—correct 22; age = 6;8
RDLS	—age = 3;6
Renfrew Action Picture Test	—information $15\frac{1}{2}$ (= 3;6)
	—grammar 8 (below 3 yrs)
Edinburgh Articulation Test	—correct 38 (= 3;6)

By 1977 the picture of a child with severe expressive language disability was very clear. Test results during that year were as follows:

IQ (WISC)	—performance 93
	—verbal 62
Comprehension of syntax:	
Northwestern Syntax Screening	—30/40
Neale Reading Test	—rate 6;11; accuracy 7;3; comprehension 7;4

Discrimination:
  Wepman   —minus 2 (inadequate)
Auditory memory:
  ITPA (ASM)   —age = 4;0
Expression:
  Vocabulary (RWF)   —correct 47; age = 7;5/6
  Renfrew APT   —information 25 (= 5;6)
                    —grammar 23 (= 4+)
  Northwestern SS   —11/40
  ITPA Gram. closure   —19/33 (errors with pronouns, irregular
                    past tenses, irregular plurals,
                    comparatives and superlatives)
  EAT   —correct 50 (= 4;6)

Fig. 15 is an analysis of a 15-minute sample of speech taken in November 1974. It shows a clear phrase-level bias and verb weakness, but the picture is confused by the Stage VI Errors, which suggest uncertain productive control of some of the sentences used. At that time Sections A–C were not being routinely recorded, and are only partially calculated here. Extracts of the data on which these profiles are based are given as exercises 19 and 20 below (pp. 298, 300).

Henry's first full LARSP (Fig. 16) was in September 1975. At this time he joined a group of two girls, both less intellectually able and with severe phonological problems. The programme of work in the group was in all the general areas previously listed. The programme of syntactic remediation covered all the Stage III clause and phrase structures, with particular emphasis on the verb phrase *is + V + ing*. The copula was also selected for special attention, as the most frequently-occurring clause structure was the immature SC/O. Attempts were to be made to increase the range of phrase structures, thus giving more weight to utterances at the transitional level III to IV and so to Stage IV.

Henry's particular difficulties with the verb were soon apparent. He had abnormal, rather staccato intonation patterns and could not get into the swing of SVC or SVO by hearing and imitating the tune. We eventually found that by incorporating the Paget–Gorman signs (the system is generally used in the school) and limiting the choice of S to two or three, Henry was able to establish a motor pattern and begin to use SVC in the structured situation. Eventually he discarded the Paget signs, but this remains a vulnerable point, and the introduction of any new structures is likely to be met at first by deletion of Cop.

'Aux v' also proved problematic. Henry omitted Aux and used S + V + ing (*Daddy coming, me going*). It was found necessary for T to model each time immediately before Henry's turn. The most successful strategy was for T to make a semantically false description of an action, which Henry would then correct, e.g. T 'walks' a horse saying *the horse is sleeping*. Henry could correct this to *the horse is walking*.

Attempts were made to increase the importance of Aux by using strong modal forms *can* and *will*, and using toys and actions and question forms, e.g. *can the*

Henry 8;6 (Nov. '74)   A

A	Unanalysed						Problematic			
	1 Unintelligible **5**	2 Symbolic Noise		3 Deviant			1 Incomplete		2 Ambiguous **I**	

B Responses

					Normal Response							Abnormal		
			Repet-	Elliptical Major				Full		Struc-		Prob-		
Stimulus Type		Totals	itions	1	2	3	4	Major	Minor	tural	Ø	lems		
23	Questions	**16**		**4**	**2**			**I**	**5**	**3**	**7**	**I**		
10	Others	**7**							**6**	**I**				

C Spontaneous   **8**   **6**   Others **2**

	Minor			Social **10** Stereotypes **I** Problems				

Stage I (0;9–1;6) — Sentence Type

Major			Sentence Structure				
Excl.	Comm.	Quest.	Statement				
	·V·	·Q·	·V· **2** ·N· **8**	Other **(5)**	Problems		

Stage II (1;6–2;0)

		Conn.	Clause		Phrase		Word
	VX	QX	SV	VC/O **2 (+7)**	DN **3 (+2)**	VV **(3)**	-ing **I**
			S C/O **(3)**	AX **I (+4)**	Adj N **2 (+I)**	V part	pl **7**
			Neg X	Other	NN	Int X **(I)**	ed **3**
					PrN	Other	

Stage III (2;0–2;6)

	VXY		X · S:NP	X · V:VP	X · C/O:NP **I**	X + A:AP **(2)**	-en
		QXY	SVC/O **2**	VC/OA	D Adj N **(I)**	Cop	-en
	let XY	VS	SVA	VO₀O₁	Adj Adj N **(I)**	Aux	3s
	do XY		Neg XY	Other	Pr DN **I**	Pron **I (+3)**	gen
					N Adj N	Other **I**	

Stage IV (2;6–3;0)

	· S	QVS	XY · S:NP **2**	XY · V:VP	XY · C/O:NP	XY · A:AP	n't
		QXYZ	SVC/OA	AAXY	N Pr NP	Neg V	'cop
			SVO₀O₁	Other	Pr D Adj N	Neg X	'aux
					cX **I**	2 Aux	
					XcX	Other **I**	

Stage V (3;0–3;6)

		and	Coord. **I**	**I ·**	Postmod. **I** clause	**I +**	-est
	how	tag	Subord. **I**	**I ·**			-est
		c	Clause: S		Postmod **I ·** phrase		-er
	what	s	Clause: C/O				-ly
		Other	Comparative				

Stage VI (3;6–4;6)

(+)				(−)			
NP	VP	Clause	NP		VP		Clause
Initiator **I**	Complex	Passive	Pron **(I)**	Adj seq	Modal		Concord
Coord		Complement	Det	N irreg **I**	Tense **(I)**		A position
					V irreg		W order **(I)**
Other			Other				

Stage VII (4;6 +)

Discourse		Syntactic Comprehension	
A Connectivity	it		
Comment Clause	there	Style	
Emphatic Order	Other		

Total No. Sentences **31**	Mean No. Sentences Per Turn **0.9**	Mean Sentence Length

© D. Crystal, P. Fletcher, M. Garman, 1975 University of Reading

Fig. 15 Henry at 8;6 (Brackets refer to structures not found in the data extracts selected for illustration in this book (p. 298). Sections B and C figures are based on the extracts only.)

duck swim?, *will the boy fall?*, expecting the answers *yes he can* (*swim*), *no he won't* (*fall*) etc.

These were the problem areas. Work on sentence structures and other elements of phrase structure including pronouns proceeded slowly but smoothly. There were regular excursions outside the language group to try to increase carryover, e.g. going round school with a series of strange objects in a bag and the repetitive question *what is it?* Having so many Ts in one establishment means that there is always someone to practise on in return for similar services later!

By December 1976 there was evidence of slow movement down the Chart (see Profile C, Fig. 17). There was a definite increase in Stage III structures, a reduction of the immature SC pattern and some representation of Stage IV. But although the copula was beginning to be used, the only occurrences of Aux were in the *don't know* phrase, and it was felt wiser to log these as Stereotypes.

In January 1977 Henry joined a language group with one of the previous girls and two brighter, more responsive and creative boys, all at the same linguistic level of rather thin Stage III moving to Stage IV. Only one had normal sounding intonation, and he, like the others, had considerable problems with short-term auditory memory as well as a word-finding difficulty.

The plan for the syntactic part of their remediation was to work systematically through Stage IV clause and phrase structures, and for a many-pronged attack on the verb phrase to include verb–subject reversal in questions, simple past tense, and negative forms.

SVOO was the only sentence structure which gave Henry any problems. At first he could use only the direct object when describing an action which he had just seen take place, e.g. *you gave pencil*. It seemed possible that because all the group had witnessed the action there was no need to describe it fully. This was solved by introducing the 'birthday game'. Henry went outside the room and I would make a 'birthday present' of a small toy to one of the other group members, who would put it on his knee or under his chair, in sight but not too obviously. Henry coming back in would have two unknowns to discover and announce. e.g. *you give a ball to C*—and even eventually *you give S a book*.

In phrase-structure development, N prep NP proved to be a sticking point. A tinful of plastic animals was painted with different coloured stripes and spots, ties and bows. The game was to deduce by a process of elimination which one had been removed—the *cow with blue stripes* or *the sheep with a tie* etc. We found this needed constant reinforcement, or abnormal patterns were produced by Henry (and also by one other group member) (e.g. *the cow is blue stripes*). For this reason, it was decided to leave this structure for a while.

Because of the fluctuating presence of Aux in Henry's speech, Neg V was at first introduced using the visual reinforcement of word cards, colour-coded in the Lea (1970) colour pattern system, which is used for some written work at school. Thus a child might turn over cards from two face-down piles to ask 'Does X eat Y?'. The cards could be rearranged to produce the appropriate answer, and after a suitable amount of practice, the cards were discarded.

No attempt was made to introduce 2 Aux.

Henry 9;4 (Sept. '75)   B

<table>
<tr><td>A</td><td colspan="3">Unanalysed</td><td colspan="2">Problematic</td></tr>
<tr><td></td><td>1 Unintelligible 32</td><td>2 Symbolic Noise</td><td>3 Deviant</td><td>1 Incomplete</td><td>2 Ambiguous</td></tr>
</table>

<table>
<tr><td>B</td><td colspan="2">Responses</td><td></td><td colspan="6">Normal Response</td><td colspan="2">Abnormal</td><td></td></tr>
<tr><td></td><td colspan="2"></td><td></td><td colspan="4">Elliptical Major</td><td rowspan="2">Full Major</td><td rowspan="2">Minor</td><td rowspan="2">Struc-tural</td><td rowspan="2">∅</td><td rowspan="2">Prob-lems</td></tr>
<tr><td></td><td colspan="2">Stimulus Type</td><td>Totals</td><td>Repet-itions</td><td>1</td><td>2</td><td>3</td><td>4</td></tr>
<tr><td></td><td>160</td><td>Questions</td><td>143</td><td>6</td><td>52</td><td>5</td><td>1</td><td></td><td>1</td><td>72</td><td>11</td><td>16</td><td>1</td></tr>
<tr><td></td><td>15</td><td>Others</td><td>13</td><td>3</td><td>1</td><td></td><td>1</td><td></td><td></td><td>8</td><td>1</td><td>2</td><td>2</td></tr>
<tr><td>C</td><td colspan="2">Spontaneous</td><td>29</td><td>3</td><td>8</td><td colspan="2">Others 21</td><td></td><td></td><td></td><td></td><td></td><td></td></tr>
</table>

			Minor					Social 66	Stereotypes 5		Problems	

Stage I (0;9–1;6) — Sentence Type

Major — Sentence Structure

Excl.	Comm.	Quest.	Statement
	·V·	·Q·	·V· 7 ·N· 26 Other 19 Problems

			Conn.	Clause			Phrase		Word

Stage II (1;6–2;0)

	VX	QX		SV 4	VC/O 9	DN 8	VV	-ing 7
				S C/O 13	AX 10	Adj N 10	V part 7	pl 10
				Neg X 2	Other 1	NN 4	Int X 4	-ed 1
						PrN 12	Other	

Stage III (2;0–2;6)

	VXY	QXY	X + S:NP 1	X + V:VP 5	X + C/O:NP 7	X + A:AP 6	-en 1
	let XY	VS	SVC/O 4	VC/OA	D Adj N	Cop 1	3s 6
	do XY		SVA 3	VOdOi	Adj Adj N	Aux 5	gen
			Neg XY 2	Other	Pr DN 3	Pron 5	
					N Adj N	Other 1	

Stage IV (2;6–3;0)

	· S	QVS	XY + S:NP 3	XY + V:VP 4	XY + C/O:NP 2	XY + A:AP 4	n't
		QXYZ	SVC/OA 2	AAXY	N Pr NP	Neg V	·cop
			SVOdOi	Other	Pr D Adj N	Neg X	·aux
					cX 6	2 Aux	
					XcX 4	Other	

Stage V (3;0–3;6)

	how	tag	and 1	Coord. 1	1 ·	Postmod. 1 clause	1 +	-est
	what		c	Subord. 1	1 ·			-er 1
			s	Clause: S		Postmod. 1 · phrase		-ly 1
			Other	Clause: C/O				
				Comparative				

(+)				(−)			
NP	VP	Clause		NP		VP	Clause

Stage VI (3;6–4;6)

Initiator 1	Complex	Passive		Pron 1	Adj seq	Modal	Concord
Coord		Complement		Det	N irreg 1	Tense	A position
						V irreg	W order 1
Other				Other			

Discourse		Syntactic Comprehension	

Stage VII (4;6 +)

A Connectivity	it		
Comment Clause	there 1	Style	
Emphatic Order	Other		

Total No. Sentences 185	Mean No. Sentences Per Turn 1·06	Mean Sentence Length

© D. Crystal, P. Fletcher, M. Garman, 1975 University of Reading

Fig. 16   Henry at 9;4

Henry   10;7   (Dec. '76)   C

A	**Unanalysed**				**Problematic**	
1 Unintelligible **3**	2 Symbolic Noise	3 Deviant		1 Incomplete **4**	2 Ambiguous **2**

B Responses

			Repet-	Normal Response						Abnormal			
				Elliptical Major				Full		Struc-			Prob-
Stimulus Type		Totals	itions	1	2	3	4	Major	Minor	tural	Ø		lems
131	Questions	**127**		**39**	**14**	**5**		**10**	**57**	**2**	**4**		
37	Others	**36**		**1**	**1**	**1**		**4**	**26**	**1**	**1**		**2**

C | **Spontaneous** | **57** | **22** | Others **33** | | | | | | | | **2**

	Minor				Social **63**	Stereotypes **11**	Problems

Fig. 17   Henry at 10;7

© D. Crystal, P. Fletcher, M. Garman, 1975 University of Reading

Henry 11;1 (June '77)   D

<table>
<tr><td>A</td><td colspan="3">Unanalysed</td><td colspan="3">Problematic</td></tr>
<tr><td></td><td>1 Unintelligible 2</td><td>2 Symbolic Noise 6</td><td>3 Deviant 3</td><td>1 Incomplete 6</td><td>2 Ambiguous 4</td></tr>
</table>

B   Responses

Stimulus Type	Totals	Repet-itions	Elliptical Major 1	2	3	4	Full Major	Minor	Struc-tural	Ø	Prob-lems
			Normal Response						Abnormal		
119 Questions	114	3	23	7	4	2	5	68	2	2	1
28 Others	27	1	2	2			11	9	2		1

C   Spontaneous 44 | 1 | Others 43

		Minor			Social 76 Stereotypes 1 Problems				

Sentence Type

Stage I (0;9–1;6)

Major

Excl.	Comm.	Quest.	Statement (Sentence Structure)
·V·	·Q·	·V· 1 ·N· 9 Other 8 Problems	

Stage II (1;6–2;0)

			Conn.	Clause	Phrase	Word
	VX	QX		SV 6 VC/O 5	DN 30 VV 3	-ing 2
				SC/O 6 AX 7	Adj N 8 V part 9	pl 25
				Neg X 5 Other	NN Int X 4	-ed 12
					PrN 7 Other	

Stage III (2;0–2;6)

VXY	QXY	X + S:NP 5 X + V:VP 3 X + C/O:NP 6 X + A:AP 5		
let XY	VS	SVC/O 27 VC/OA 1 D Adj N 5 Cop 1
		SVA 12 VOdOi Adj Adj N 1 Aux 7
do XY		Neg XY Other 3 Pr DN 6 Pron 57
		N Adj N Other 1

Stage IV (2;6–3;0)

S	OVS 1	XY + S:NP 8 XY + V:VP 8 XY + C/O:NP 15 XY + A:AP 14
	QXYZ	SVC/OA 1 AAXY 2 N Pr NP 1 Neg V 3
		SVOdOi Other 1 Pr D Adj N 2 Neg X 3
		cX 5 2 Aux
		XcX 8 Other 1

n't 2
'cop 1
'aux

3s
gen
-en 1

Stage V (3;0–3;6)

how		tag	and 8 c	Coord 1 7 1·	Postmod 1 1·	-est
				Subord 1 1·	clause	
what			s 1	Clause: S 1·	Postmod 1·	-er
			Other	Clause: C/O	phrase	
				Comparative		-ly 1

(+)			(−)		
NP	VP	Clause	NP	VP	Clause

Stage VI (3;6–4;6)

Initiator 1	Complex	Passive	Pron 11	Adj seq	Modal	Concord 3
Coord 2		Complement	Det 4	N irreg	Tense 19	A position
					V irreg	W order
Other			Other			

Discourse	Syntactic Comprehension

Stage VII (4;6+)

A Connectivity	it	
Comment Clause	there	Style
Emphatic Order	Other	

| Total No. Sentences 185 | Mean No. Sentences Per Turn 1·3 | Mean Sentence Length |

Fig. 18   Henry at 11;1

In April, Henry's language group changed again, as the better members were making faster progress. In his new group, he was the more advanced member, a state which he prefers and in which he is more relaxed and productive. Work began on coordination and subordination of clauses using *and* and *but* as coordinators and, later, *because* as a subordinator. Henry made steady progress with coordination but had problems with *because* as a subordinator, needing a highly structured situation to produce his sentence and a great deal of reinforcement. After discussion with the authors of *GALD* in May, *because* as a subordinating device was discontinued and temporal adverbial clauses were introduced. However his cognitive difficulties with time have created problems here.

At the time of Henry's latest LARSP (June 1977, see Fig. 18), control of coordinating clauses is beginning to show, although he is still making more use of *and* and *and we* to hold the listener's attention than truly to coordinate clauses. The one subordinating device used is present in an incomplete utterance, *cos he might* — —.

Henry's progress has been as slow as his disability is severe. Using the LARSP method and profile has provided a systematic method of building up the whole range of his structures in a balanced way and establishing them meaningfully in his spontaneous language. It has also pinpointed some specific persisting problems which have received a considerable amount of attention with only limited success. We feel pleased with the hard-won progress he has made and feel that he has established a solid base upon which to build further.

2.2

John Horniman School

Ella Hutt

The children

The 24 children resident at the John Horniman School in Worthing have severe
language disorders of many kinds, but excluding those based primarily on hearing
loss, autism and low intelligence. They are admitted between the ages of 5 and
7, and most stay until they are 9. About three-quarters of them have expressive
disorders, and it is with these children that we have been experimenting with
LARSP for about two years. Their verbal comprehension on the Reynell scale,
and their attempts at spontaneous conversation, estimated subjectively, are on
average one year below that of their chronological age. But on the Reynell Expressive scale, including three aspects of expression (Language structure, vocabulary
and content), their scores range between 1;6 and 5. When only the grammatical
aspect is analysed, the average range is between LARSP Stages I and III, estimated
at 'grammatical ages' between 0;9 and 2;0.

The ways in which these children express themselves range from gross manual
gestures and/or grunts, to speech which—though its meaning can usually be understood—is inappropriate when compared to the children's intelligence and nonverbal competence. When it is encoded into a written form, it is even less acceptable. It is composed of strings of open-class words and a few prepositions and
possessives. They are usually in the right order, so the utterances are semantically
viable. But pronouns are substituted for each other, with object-pronouns pre-
dominating; there is no implicit tense distinction; most noun-determiners are
omitted, and so are all the parts of the verb *to be*. Negatives and conjunctions
are rare.

Possible reasons for these deviations are that the children are intelligent and
aware enough to want to express interesting information about people and things
around them, but have not yet been able to understand the relativity of 'I' and
'you'; they are uninterested in the differences between male and female, and are
unable to generalize the difference between the subject and the object of the verb:
there has been little need for them to distinguish the past or future from the present.
Because ownership is important, so are the words *mine/my*, and *yours/your*; but
the relative position of objects distinguished by *this* and *that* is not important, and
the subtle distinctions between demonstratives and articles, and between the

definite and indefinite articles even less so. The 'is-ness' of an object is so obvious that it is not worth remarking upon with the use of *is* or any of its counterparts. Because these children have a positive outlook on life, negatives are seldom necessary. Because the concepts of causality and purpose, conditionality etc. are not yet formed, conjunctions are not needed.

Sampling

As most of the children are not worried by a listener's inability to understand their speech, each one was seated at a desk with a cassette recorder in evidence, and invited to talk about a subject of his own choice. The adult asked questions only when the child's monologue was dying out, made a minimum number of comments, and made a written note of any ambiguous or unintelligible utterances. The session lasted for only 15 minutes, as this was considered long enough to obtain a viable grammatical sample. The children who found this approach difficult were given pictures to talk about, as were those already known to be virtually unintelligible. The sample was not taken until the child had been in the school for a few weeks. The sampler gradually learnt the wisdom of repeating any of the child's utterances which would not have been understood without the addition of visual clues such as pointing, gesture or signing.

When it was found that this type of sampling had to be followed by so many more hours' work to obtain each child's profile, a simple elicitation procedure was devised for use at six-monthly intervals, after the initial analysis on entry to the school. The sample still takes approximately 15 minutes to elicit, but to arrive at a usable profile takes only another 15, or, at the most, 30 minutes.

The elicitation procedure uses stimulus questions—mostly about pictures—and question-words, which the child uses as the first word of a longer utterance. These questions are designed to encourage speech and/or signing, and to discourage

Picture	Q Stimulus	Max. Reponse
Boy riding bike fast.	What's this boy doing?	SVOAA, e.g. The boy is riding the bike fast along the road.
Animals, of which at least 2, of different kinds, are standing, with the others in other positions.	Tell me which animals are standing.	NPcNP, e.g. The sheep and the pig.
At least 3 children in different positions, with the smallest in a describable position, e.g. under a table. (NB there must be another child of the same sex as the focused one.)	Tell me which child is the smallest.	NPPrNP, e.g. The girl under the table.

pointing. The aim is to elicit utterances up to Stage IV in complexity. Each stimulus is correlated with an expected 'maximum response', and a space is left for 'actual response', e.g. using a picture of a man giving an object to a girl, the expected response would be SVO$_d$O$_i$ (*the man is giving a present to the girl*, or the like); the actual response may be this, or some lower Stage structure, e.g. *man girl, giving to girl*, or part of a larger structure, e.g. *I see a man giving a present to the girl* (this last type being uncommon). Further examples of the stimuli used in the test are given on p. 154 (examples of actual responses are given on p. 158 below).

Transcription

The first set of samples were transcribed in full, that is, including both the child's and the adult's utterances. However, the latter we found to be an unwieldy addition to the amount of paper used, and when analysed in terms of Sections B and C, it was felt that they gave us in our situation no vital information which we did not already have after observing the child's verbal responses over a few weeks. We therefore did not use these sections in analysing samples. (In passing, it is noted that these 'rejected' sections *are* useful when analysing the minimal expression of the children with severe receptive disorders.)

Nor did we mark pauses, intonation and stress. No member of staff was proficient enough in transcribing intonation patterns. However, any immediately remarkable strangeness in intonation was noted, and questionmarks were written in appropriate places.

When most of the utterances are predictably short, they can be written in two columns, leaving four lines between each for the results of the four main analysis-scans. But when a transcriber expects more than a few longer utterances only two lines need be left, as the analyses themselves take no more space for long utterances than for short ones.

The transcription of utterances elicited in a test-format are written during the test, and only specific queries need be replayed later during the analysis process.

Grammatical analysis

The main emphasis during remediation is only as far as Stage V. Stage VI goals are relevant for only a few children, and if Stage VII were reached, we should suspect that the child should never have been placed at the school. So the analysis-form was redesigned: the top and bottom were omitted, and the space for recording Stages II to VI was expanded. No longer was it necessary to record in two or three subcolumns per section. Both clause and phrase elements were listed in one column each. It is now possible for those who can do small enough writing, and read it, to record specific examples of utterances. With this in mind we are planning to expand the space allowed in Stages II, III and IV, and/or to provide a supplementary sheet with detailed information recorded on a checklist about specific pronouns, copulas, auxiliaries (including modals), past tenses etc.

Although the actual number of most elements is recorded, it is considered that a subjective decision can be made on the necessity or otherwise of counting the number of DNs in Stage II when, say, there are examples of DAdjN and/or PrDN in Stage III. Information like this is redundant, and time need not be wasted in collecting it. Newcomers to the system, however, would be wise to count every item in the first few samples analysed, in order to rediscover the reason for this for themselves, and also to find what for them are easily-missed items. Among these are pronouns and parts of the verb *to be*; and the utterances which can be recorded in the very important transition stages between Stages I and II, and II and III. It is tempting to underestimate the importance of these utterances because they are amongst the most difficult to recognize.

Having tried several methods of recording the initial analysis of each utterance, the most economical is that of using pens of four different colours. With one the clause-elements are recorded (and sentence-connectivity, though this is rare), with another the phrase elements, with a third word-endings, and with a fourth the transition elements. They are written in the four (or two) spaces left for the purpose at the transcription stage, and the use of colour limits the number of possible items to be counted at the end of each scan, and thus speeds the process. The number of each type of element-group is recorded on the Profile Chart.

When the elicitation procedure is used, a tick shows the presence of an item, but even if a structure appears more than once, that is, both in the appropriate place and elsewhere, there is still only one tick. It merely shows availability, not frequency.

Profiling and interpretation

From an analysis of a spontaneous or elicited sample, one can judge whether a child has a consistent profile or not. While realizing that in any set of utterances there are generally more phrases than clauses, we have found that with these children phrase-structure is usually more advanced than clause-structure or the use of word-endings. (In passing, it is noted that children with receptive disorders who have received some grammatical instruction in the written medium (Remedial Syntax: see p. 165) have more stability in clause structure.)

It is important that an interpretation of a score-sheet is made only in close conjunction with the transcription of the sample or test.

Case study

In order to illustrate some of the above points, the following brief outline of one of the children may be helpful. Given the purpose of the present book, the profile data has been recast into conventional form.

Sam was admitted to the John Horniman School in August 1976 from an assessment unit. He was then shy, anxious and lacking in confidence. When he 'spoke' he opened his mouth but failed to use any voice. His communication system with his peers seemed to rely on punches and pinches. He was frequently observed holding his hand over his nose and mouth, especially when under pressure.

His postnatal history began with a period of six days in an incubator, and following this he spent the majority of the next three months in hospital due to failure to thrive. At the age of four he was admitted to hospital following a febrile 'blackout' and again later that year with pneumonia.

Both his first words and attempts at walking unaided appeared at the age of 1;6. His expressive language failed to develop at a normal rate despite therapy, so a recommendation was made for him to be admitted to this school at the age of 6;7. Assessments made in September 1976 showed: Merrill Palmer 6·5; Vineland Maturity Scale 4·4; RDLS VC 5·0–5·2, EL 1·7; WISC Full Scale 80; Peabody Vocab. MA 5·11. The (Bishop) Test for Reception of Grammar (May 1977) showed an uneven performance, with comprehension of word combinations being at the normal level, comprehension of reversible structures being at chance level (i.e. indicative of basic word-order difficulties), and comprehension of inflections and function words being somewhere between these extremes.

A 10-minute sample of Sam's spontaneous speech, made in November 1976, produced the following sentences:

house. yes. green. walking. (name of cat). running. horse.
?woman. pi (='water'). home. eat. drink. straw. yes. bird.
?cage. mum. (Unintell.) baby. fire. mummy. yes. bedroom. bed.
Guy (=name of child). Matthew. me. John.

Fig. 19 (Profile A) summarizes this data: see p. 295 for the data set out in problem form, and p. 318 for associated analysis and profiling information.

Fig. 20 (Profile B) summarizes a 15-minute spontaneous sample, made in May 1977. A selection of sentences is as follows:

house. red house. window. blue. tree sun in sun. tree. on the
grass. flower. red and blue. sun. stalk. blue one. yes. me.
digging. Mummy. in seed.

A complete list of the data is given on p. 296, and the associated analysis and profiling details are on p. 318.

Fig. 21 (Profile C) summarizes a further 15-minute spontaneous sample, made in September 1977. A selection of sentences is as follows:

playing. in the outside. Guy. making Guy bike. mend it. with hands.
yes. a letter. mummy. love from. Matthew. fly the aeroplane.
dentist. mummy tooth is broken.

A complete list of the data is given on p. 296, and the associated analysis and profiling details are on p. 320.

Fig. 22 (Profile D) gives in combined form the results of the structured language test, carried out in November 1976 and September 1977. The test responses are given on pp. 158–9 below.

Structured language test (preliminary version, Stages II–IV): Sam

	Maximum Response	Actual Response Nov. 1976	Sept. 1977
Clauses			
1 What's this boy doing? Tell me a long sentence about him.	SVOA	bike sit	the boy is on the bike
2 Tell me what this man is doing.	SVO_dO_i	(2 grunts)	the man is holding the cake
3 Tell me about this picture.	NegXY	sit—eat	the woman is looking at the dinner
Phrases			
4 Tell me which animals are standing.	NcN	baa—pig	sheep and pig
5 Where is the penny? (Tell me.)	PrDAdjN	in house	in the house
6 Tell me which child is the smallest.	NPrNP	baby	the girl is little
7 What would you have done if...	2 Aux	—	go to toilet
8 Tell me two things about this ball.	AdjcAdj	the ball is little	the ball is little the ball is big
9 Tell me which is the longest crayon. And whose is it?	NAdjN	me	blue one—John
10 Where are the matches? (Tell me.)	PrDN	in a box	on the box
11 Tell me which flowers you like the best.	AdjAdjN	red	I like the blue flower
12 (Pronoun, preferably third person.)	Pron		
13 What is he doing? (3 pictures: putting coat on, taking off, ringing up.)	V part	bed—walking (-*ing* signed)	dressing—taking off put on—telephone
14 How fast is he going?	IntAdv	walk (signed)	very fast
15 What is blue? (Tell me.)	DN	car	the car is blue
Word Endings			
16 What can you tell me about these two children?	-er	the boy walk	standing
17 What can you tell me about this boy?	-est	the boy a walk	the boy is standing
18 What does a bird (swimmer, postman, painter) do?	3s	[be—be—be]	fly—posting the letter—paint the house

	Maximum Response	Actual Response Nov. 1976	Sept. 1977
19 *a* This boy is eating an apple. He did the same yesterday. What did he do yesterday?	-ed	eat	yesterday he eat a apple
b They are looking at (or watching) the T.V. He did, etc.		—	yesterday look at the television
c She is opening a desk. He did, etc.		sitting (gesture)	yesterday open the desk
20 What has the boy just done?	-en	fall	fall
21 Whose (e.g.) shoe is this? (e.g. Guy's, David's, Matthew's, Louise's.)	gen	me	Max shoe—Guy boot
22 Tell me what are blue.	pl	car	the balls are blue
23 Tell me what he's doing.	-ing	—	(several examples)

Questions

I want you to pretend to ask some questions. I'll say the first word.
You say it again and then finish the question.

24 What		car (=QX)	the ball doing (=QXY)
25 Is		—	the ball in the car (=VS)
26 Where		—	is the pen (=QXY)
27 What kind		—	the pencil (=QX)
28 Who		—	is sitting on the chair? (=QXY) Mc.
29 How old		—	—
30 How		—	I sit on the chair (QXYZ)
31 Whose		—	is Miss Beaumont is sitting on the chair (QVS+)
32 Why		—	Miss Beaumont is sitting on the chair (QXYZ)
33 Which		—	Miss Beaumont chair (QXY)
34 How much		—	the chair (QX)
35 How many		—	chair (QX)
36 When		—	go to bed (QXY)

Comparing these profiles, three points stand out:

(i) The Stage I profile (A) develops down the Phrase column (B); this imbalance is beginning to be corrected in C, which shows a relatively more even distribution of structures across the chart.

(ii) There is a marked contrast between performance on the two tests, a Stage II–III pattern having become a III–IV pattern.

(iii) Comparing Test and Spontaneous results, the test results are predictably in advance of the spontaneous, but this contrast is more obvious for the November 1976 profiles than for those made a year later. The contrast between A and D (November) is striking, but because of its obviousness is perhaps not as interesting as the differential performance of C and D (September). C shows more Stage I and II (Clause) structure and a more well-developed Word column (i.e. the 'immature' clause patterns and the more 'tangible' morphological patterns, cf. *GALD*, 115). D (September) on the other hand shows a greater grasp of the more abstract structures at Clause level (Stage III, III transitional, IV) as well as a more balanced Stage II Phrase level. The Stage VI Errors, it should be noted, are almost all in relation to the Question task, and cannot readily be related to the task situation of Profiles A–C.

Remediation

In a school like this, remediation must be planned to achieve the greatest good for the greatest number of children possible. Time never allows for two adults to work with one child, and rarely for one adult with one child. Currently the most economical arrangement is to divide each class of nine children into three or four groups of two or three children, whose profiles match each other as nearly as possible. The adults leading the groups are the class teacher and the speech therapist, who in practice remediate the two most difficult groups; and one other teacher and the teachers' aide, whose two groups are the easiest. Each group meets for three twenty-minute sessions every week, and remediation is brisk and business-like.

The overall goal is to straighten each child's profile, before proceeding to further stages. Each remediator has a long-term plan, and the gaps in the profile provide a readymade list of goals for each child. They are ordered with the following criteria:

Clause structure should be at least as advanced as phrase structure and word-endings; phrase structure is next in importance, and word-endings the least.

Elicitation of statements should precede that of questions. (It must be borne in mind that the child who asks the initial questions of the teacher who models the replies is taking the part of the second adult in the ideal situation. The teacher's aim in asking him to do this is not to provide practice for him, but a stimulus for her own response.)

But is it absolutely necessary to make a profile at all? The first step is to teach a few intransitive verbs. A child to whom some are already available can be taught the words or signs for two or more people, and simple subject–verb sequences can be practised. A child who finds the next steps relatively easy is not wasting time.

Sam 6;10 (Nov. '76)   A (10 MIN)

A	**Unanalysed**						**Problematic**				
	1 Unintelligible /	2 Symbolic Noise		3 Deviant			1 Incomplete		2 Ambiguous		

| B | **Responses** | | | | | | Normal Response | | | | | Abnormal | | |

						Elliptical Major				Full		Struc-		Prob-
	Stimulus Type		Totals	Repet- itions	1	2	3	4	Major	Minor	tural	Ø	lems
		Questions											
		Others											

C	**Spontaneous**			Others	

		Minor			Social **3**	Stereotypes	Problems

Sentence Type

Stage I (0;9–1;6)	**Major**			**Sentence Structure**			
	Excl.	Comm.	Quest.	*Statement*			
		·V·	·Q·	·V· **4** ·N· **18**	Other **2**	Problems	

				Conn.	Clause		Phrase		Word
Stage II (1;6–2;0)		V X	Q X		SV	V C/O	DN	VV	-ing **2**
					S C/O	A X	Adj N	V part	pl
					Neg X	Other	NN	Int X	
							PrN	Other	-ed
Stage III (2;0–2;6)		V X Y		X + S:NP	X + V:VP	X + C/O:NP	X + A:AP	-en
			Q X Y	SVC/O	VC/OA	D Adj N	Cop	
		let X Y	VS	SVA	VO_dO_i	Adj Adj N	Aux	3s
				Neg X Y	Other	Pr DN	Pron **/**	gen
		do X Y				N Adj N	Other	
Stage IV (2;6–3;0)		· S	QVS	XY + S:NP	XY + V:VP	XY + C/O:NP	XY + A:AP	n't
			Q X Y Z	SVC/OA	AA X Y	N Pr NP	Neg V	'cop
				SVO_dO_i	Other	Pr D Adj N	Neg X	'aux
						c X	2 Aux	
						X c X	Other	
Stage V (3;0–3;6)	how	tag	and	Coord. **1**	1 ·	Postmod. **1** clause	1 +	-est
			c	Subord. **1**	1 ·			-er
	what	Other	s	Clause: S		Postmod. **1** · phrase		-ly
				Clause: C/O				
				Comparative				

	(+)				(−)			
	NP	VP	Clause	NP		VP	Clause	
Stage VI (3;6–4;6)	Initiator	Complex	Passive	Pron	Adj seq	Modal	Concord	
	Coord		Complement	Det	N irreg	Tense	A position	
						V irreg	W order	
	Other			Other				

	Discourse		Syntactic Comprehension	
Stage VII (4;6 +)	A Connectivity	it		
	Comment Clause	there	Style	
	Emphatic Order	Other		

Total No. Sentences **28**	Mean No. Sentences Per Turn /	Mean Sentence Length **1**

© D. Crystal, P. Fletcher, M. Garman, 1975 University of Reading

Fig. 19   Sam at 6;10

Sam 7;4 (May '77)   B (15 min.)

<table>
<tr><td>A</td><td colspan="4">Unanalysed</td><td colspan="2">Problematic</td></tr>
<tr><td></td><td colspan="2">1 Unintelligible 1</td><td>2 Symbolic Noise</td><td>3 Deviant</td><td>1 Incomplete</td><td>2 Ambiguous</td></tr>
</table>

<table>
<tr><td>B</td><td colspan="2">Responses</td><td></td><td></td><td colspan="6">Normal Response</td><td colspan="2">Abnormal</td><td></td></tr>
<tr><td></td><td colspan="2"></td><td></td><td rowspan="2">Repet-
itions</td><td colspan="4">Elliptical Major</td><td rowspan="2">Full
Major</td><td rowspan="2">Minor</td><td rowspan="2">Struc-
tural</td><td rowspan="2">∅</td><td rowspan="2">Prob-
lems</td></tr>
<tr><td></td><td colspan="2">Stimulus Type</td><td>Totals</td><td>1</td><td>2</td><td>3</td><td>4</td></tr>
<tr><td></td><td></td><td>Questions</td><td></td><td></td><td></td><td></td><td></td><td></td><td></td><td></td><td></td><td></td><td></td></tr>
<tr><td></td><td></td><td>Others</td><td></td><td></td><td></td><td></td><td></td><td></td><td></td><td></td><td></td><td></td><td></td></tr>
<tr><td>C</td><td colspan="2">Spontaneous</td><td></td><td></td><td colspan="2">Others</td><td></td><td></td><td></td><td></td><td></td><td></td><td></td></tr>
</table>

		Minor			Social **8**	Stereotypes	Problems

Stage I (0;9–1;6)	Sentence Type	**Major**				Sentence Structure		

| | | Excl. | Comm. | Quest. | | Statement | | |
| | | | ·V· | ·Q· | ·V· **7** ·N· **23** | Other **5** | Problems **1** | |

Stage II (1;6–2;0)

Conn.	Clause		Phrase		Word
V X / Q X	SV	V C/O **1**	DN **2**	VV	-ing **3**
	S C/O	A X	Adj N **2**	V part	pl **1**
	Neg X	Other	NN	Int X	-ed
			PrN **4**	Other **1**	

Stage III (2;0–2;6)

Conn.	Clause		Phrase		Word
V X Y	X + S:NP	X + V:VP	X + C/O:NP	X + A:AP	-en
Q X Y / VS	SVC/O	VC/OA	D Adj N	Cop	3s
let X Y	SVA	VO$_d$O$_i$	Adj Adj N	Aux	gen
do X Y	Neg X Y	Other	Pr DN **1**	Pron **1**	
			N Adj N	Other	

Stage IV (2;6–3;0)

Conn.	Clause		Phrase		Word
S	XY + S:NP	XY + V:VP	XY + C/O:NP	XY + A:AP	n't
QVS	SVC/OA	AAXY	N Pr NP	Neg V	·cop
Q X Y Z	SVO$_d$O$_i$	Other	Pr D Adj N	Neg X	·aux
			cX **1**	2 Aux	
			XcX **2**	Other	-est

Stage V (3;0–3;6)

	Conn.	Clause		Phrase		Word
how	and	Coord. 1	1 ·	Postmod. 1 clause	1 +	-er
	tag	Subord. 1	1 ·			
	c	Clause: S		Postmod. 1 · phrase		-ly
what	s	Clause: C/O				
	Other	Comparative				

	(+)			(−)			
	NP	VP	Clause	NP		VP	Clause
Stage VI (3;6–4;6)	Initiator	Complex	Passive	Pron	Adj seq	Modal	Concord
	Coord		Complement	Det	N irreg	Tense	A position
						V irreg	W order
	Other			Other			

	Discourse		Syntactic Comprehension	
Stage VII (4;6+)	A Connectivity	it		
	Comment Clause	there	Style	
	Emphatic Order	Other		

Total No. Sentences **58**	Mean No. Sentences Per Turn /	Mean Sentence Length **1·3**

© D. Crystal, P. Fletcher, M. Garman, 1975 University of Reading

Fig. 20   Sam at 7;4

Sam 7;8 (Sept. '77)   C (15 min.)

A	**Unanalysed**				**Problematic**		
	1 Unintelligible	2 Symbolic Noise		3 Deviant	1 Incomplete		2 Ambiguous

B   Responses

Stimulus Type		Totals	Repet-itions	Normal Response						Abnormal			Prob-lems
				Elliptical Major				Full Major	Minor	Struc-tural	Ø	
				1	2	3	4					
	Questions											
	Others											

C   Spontaneous | | | **Others**

Minor   Social *1*   Stereotypes **2**   Problems

Major   Sentence Structure

	Excl.	Comm.	Quest.	Statement				
Stage I (0;9–1;6)		·V·	·Q·	·V· **5** ·N· **12** Other **4** Problems				

Stage II (1;6–2;0)	Comm. VX	Quest. QX	Conn.	Clause		Phrase		Word
				SV **2**	V C/O **4**	DN **11**	VV	-ing **10**
				S C/O	AX **2**	Adj N	V part	pl **4**
				Neg X	Other	NN **3**	Int X	-ed **1**
						PrN **3**	Other	

Stage III (2;0–2;6)	VXY	QXY	let XY	X + S:NP	X + V:VP *1*	X + C/O:NP **2**	X + A:AP *1*	-en
	VXY	QXY VS		SVC/O **6**	VC/OA	D Adj N	Cop **3**	3s **y**
				SVA	VOdOi	Adj Adj N	Aux **5**	gen
	do XY			Neg XY	Other	Pr DN **9**	Pron **4**	
						N Adj N	Other	

Stage IV (2;6–3;0)	·S	QVS		XY + S:NP **5**	XY + V:VP **3**	XY + C/O:NP **3**	XY + A:AP	n't
		QXYZ		SVC/OA	AAXY	N Pr NP	Neg V	·cop
				SVO₁O₂	Other	Pr D Adj N	Neg X	·aux *1*
						cX	2 Aux	
						XcX	Other	-est

Stage V (3;0–3;6)	how	tag	and c s Other	Coord. 1 1		Postmod. 1 1 + clause		-er
				Subord. 1 1				
				Clause: S		Postmod. 1 phrase		-ly
	what			Clause: C/O				
				Comparative				

	(+)			(−)			
	NP	VP	Clause	NP		VP	Clause
Stage VI (3;6–4;6)	Initiator	Complex	Passive	Pron *1*	Adj seq	Modal	Concord
	Coord		Complement	Det	N irreg	Tense	A position
						V irreg	W order
	Other			Other			

	Discourse		Syntactic Comprehension	
Stage VII (4;6 +)	A Connectivity	it		
	Comment Clause	there	Style	
	Emphatic Order	Other		

Total No. Sentences	**53**	Mean No. Sentences Per Turn	/	Mean Sentence Length	**1·2**

Fig. 21   Sam at 7;8

Sam 6;10/7;8 (*Nov. '76 / Sept. '77*) D (*STRUCTURED TEST*)

A	Unanalysed							Problematic		
	1 Unintelligible 1/0	2 Symbolic Noise 1/0	3 Deviant I (□)/0					1 Incomplete	2 Ambiguous	

B Responses

				Normal Response							Abnormal		
					Elliptical Major				Full		Struc-		Prob-
Stimulus Type		Totals	Repet-itions	1	2	3	4	Major	Minor	tural	∅	lems
	Questions												
	Others												

C Spontaneous   Others

Sentence Type		Minor			Social	Stereotypes	Problems		

| | | Major | | | | Sentence Structure | | | |

Stage I (0;9–1;6)

	Excl.	Comm.	Quest.		*Statement*			
		·V·	·Q·	·V· 6/4 ·N· 7/3	Other 3/1	Problems		

			Conn.	Clause		Phrase		Word
Stage II (1;6–2;0)		VX	QX	SV 2/0	VC/O 0/2	DN 2/21	VV	-ing
			1/3	S C/O	AX 0/1	Adj N	V part 0/4	1/9 pl
				Neg X	Other	NN 0/3	Int X 0/1	
						PrN 1/2	Other 0/1	-ed
Stage III (2;0–2;6)		VXY	0/4 QXY	X + S:NP 1/1	X + V:VP 0/1	X + C/O:NP 0/2	X + A:AP 0/1	
		let XY	VS	SVC/O 1/1	VC/OA 0/2	D Adj N 0/1	Cop 1/1	-en
		do XY	0/1	SVA ˆ/1	VOdOi	Adj Adj N	Aux 0/4	3s
				Neg XY	Other	Pr DN 1/6	Pron 2/4	1/10 gen
						N Adj N	Other 0/5	
Stage IV (2;6–3;0)		· S	1/0 QVS·	XY + S:NP 1/1	XY + V:VP 0/3	XY + C/O:NP	XY + A:AP 0/1	n't
			QXYZ	SVC/OA 0/1	AAXY	N Pr NP	Neg V	·cop
			0/3	SVOᵢOᵢ	Other	Pr D Adj N	Neg X	·aux
						cX	2 Aux	
						XcX 0/1	Other	
Stage V (3;0–3;6)		how	and tag	Coord. 1	1 ·	Postmod. 1 clause	1 ·	-est
			c	Subord. 1	1 ·			-er
			s	Clause: S		Postmod. 1 · phrase		
		what	Other	Clause: C/O				-ly
				Comparative				

	(+)				(−)			
	NP	VP	Clause		NP		VP	Clause
Stage VI (3;6–4;6)	Initiator	Complex	Passive	Pron	Adj seq	Modal		Concord
	Coord		Complement	Det	N irreg	Tense 0/3 (19)		A position 0/2
						V irreg		W order (31,32)
	Other			Other ∅ Cop (21, 34).	2 Aux (31).			

∅ Subject (19₆, 36). ∅ Aux (14, 30, 36)

	Discourse			Syntactic Comprehension	
Stage VII (4;6+)	A Connectivity	it			
	Comment Clause	there		Style	
	Emphatic Order 0/3 (19) Other				

Total No. Sentences	/	Mean No. Sentences Per Turn	/	Mean Sentence Length	/

© D. Crystal, P. Fletcher, M. Garman, 1975 University of Reading

Fig. 22   Sam at 6;10 and 7;8—structured language test (Numbers in brackets refer to items of the test.)

He is gradually absorbing more about the concept of the method being used. The time will come when he finds a task difficult. This is when he begins to learn grammar systematically. He has to work harder. He enjoys the challenge. Further practice makes him more proficient. The reduction of clues makes the exercise more realistic. Before he incorporates the practised structure into his spontaneous production, he will have begun to practise another structure which had not previously been available. The process is like the waves rolling onto the sea shore. Each structure being used spontaneously is being closely followed by another which can be produced in a practice session when clues have been removed. In turn this is being followed by yet another which the child finds difficulty in producing, even when all the clues are present. This method can be used with or without a detailed profile for each child.

There are certain items on the LARSP chart which, although they add to a scorer's information, we have found to be of doubtful value to remediate. Some of these are: at clause level: SC/O; at phrase-level: AdjN (because, to be acceptable, the adjective would have to describe the plural form of a noun, and plurals need not be elicited till later in the scheme) and VV.

While it is understood that children with normally-developing language use pronouns, past tenses, past participles, noun plurals etc. incorrectly before generalizing the rules or their exceptions to correct them, we currently believe that children with expressive difficulties of any kind should be given correct models and taught to copy, practise and remember them at a comparatively much earlier stage. It has been found in grammatical and other areas that once an error has been established because it has been ignored or because no attempt has been made to correct it, it is extremely difficult to replace it with the acceptable version. This means that, particularly in the items mentioned, more practice than at first would seem necessary should be given to these children, in order that they overlearn each item rather than risk its being forgotten when new ones are introduced and supercede it.

Other methods to which spoken remediation is related

For a number of years two specific methods for language learning have been in use in the school, one written and one using grammatical manual signing. Both of these have facilitated the adoption of the spoken remediation procedure to be described.

Remedial Syntax is a method in which small slips of colour-coded card are used to make a sentence, which is then 'read', either by an attempt at speech, and/or by signing, and then recorded in a book and illustrated. Each colour is a code of a part of speech, e.g. nouns are orange, noun-determiners white, adjectives green, verbs yellow. The children learn the colour-patterns, e.g. 'white + orange + yellow + yellow', and 'white + orange + yellow + green'. They also learn to associate each written word with the object or action it represents, or with other colours, e.g. white always precedes orange, and never follows it. Pronouns and proper names are pink words, prepositions blue, adverbs and particles brown. The same colours are used for the cards involved in our current method for spoken remediation.

Although Remedial Syntax was designed for use primarily with the children with receptive disorders, it is also being used to a lesser degree with some of those with expressive disorders and, although they are never told the names of the parts of speech, all the children in the school are familiar with which type of word is written on which coloured card.

The *Paget–Gorman Sign System* can represent all common closed-class words and word-endings in addition to more than 3,000 content-words in English. It is used all the time with the children with receptive disorders; but most of the children in the school, by spontaneous imitation, learn how to sign, and they make as much use of the signs as individually necessary. Any spoken remediation method can capitalize on this bonus.

A remediation procedure based on LARSP

The grammar we teach must be semantically based. The meaningful elements in a simple sentence must permute in as many ways as possible, and their number increased; the quality of phrase structure must be improved; endings must be used to modify the meanings of open-class words; and the possibilities of ellipsis in speech must be introduced.

A verb is the kernel of an acceptable clause. So the children are taught to associate PGSS signs and written words with a few common intransitive actions which can be linked only with a subject until prepositions are used. They are permuted with all the available subjects, that is, all the children and adults within the classroom; and soon the actions of others in the building can be described. More concentrated practice in signing and/or saying the sentences can be given with two simple sets of cards.

The teaching-material is a big pack of cards which has evolved from very small beginnings. Each coloured card is 3″ square.

Verb cards and noun cards

On each yellow verb card is drawn a simple representation of the PGSS sign for a particular verb. A drawing of a sign is the only way in which a verb can be produced at random without a specific subject being present. The stem of the verb is written at the bottom of the card, so that the word finishes at the right hand edge of the card. The reason for this is that the card is placed on the left of a 3″ vertical × 6″ horizontal rectangle, on the right of which is written the verb-ending -*ing*. In order to allow for the changes in the written form of words with single consonant or -*e* endings, another faint consonant is added to the verb word, or the -*e* is crossed out faintly.

On each orange noun card is a simple drawing of the head of a person (man, woman, boy, girl) or animal (cat, dog, fish, bird). The drawings of the adult heads are at the top of their squares, and the children at the bottom of theirs; the females have hair, but the males have none. The children remember these conventions very quickly, but if they do not, it does not really matter, as syntactically the differences are unimportant. Cards representing other parts of speech will be described later.

The teaching technique described with reference to the first task, the elicitation of simple statements

The teacher-sequence which follows applies to all other examples of the production of statements or their parts, at all three levels, in clauses, phrases and words. The P in every case stands for the group of children. When P understands that people or animals can be permuted with actions, the cards are laid out on a desk in front of him. T sits opposite. Facing P is the array:

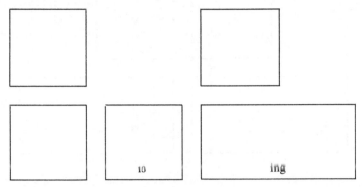

Above the two spaces are placed piles, one of 'actors', and one of intransitive verbs. One from each pile is turned over to fill the space, and a sentence appears. But as it is accompanied by a question, one card precedes the other. The verb card is turned over before the question, *Who is verb* (+)*ing?* Then the noun card is turned over so that the answer can be supplied. The method of elicitation is a modified form of modelled imitation. At first the most advanced P in the group is told to ask the question, e.g. *Who is coming?* (If necessary, T can help P with the question by signing it or writing it down.) T replies, *The man is coming*. P asks the same kind of question again, this time referring to another verb-card. T answers again. When Ps have listened to answers for long enough, the roles are reversed, and Ps in turn answer T's questions. If the question is to be *What is the* (noun) *doing?* the noun card is turned over before the question asked: then the verb card is turned over so that the question can be answered.

The questions can if necessary be simplified to *who?* or *what ... doing?* The answers can be simplified to a noun verb pattern with no *the*, no *is* and no-*ing*. With some Ps it is preferable that both question and answer utterances are complete, but the signing strings are reduced. Decisions about permutations like this can be made on the spot, according to the ability of P, and/or the expectation of T.

The first introduction of negativity should be in connection with present continuous verbs, though not necessarily as early as this. The type of questions changes from *who...?* or *... doing?* to a *yes/no* type, e.g. *Is the man running?* A pile of *yes* and *no* cards provides the cue to the answer. If *yes* is turned up, an extended answer is *Yes, the man is running*, or *Yes he is*, with an emphatic *is*. It should be made clear here that the subject and auxiliary are reversed in order to produce a question. At first they can be changed over but this is too cumbersome a process to do quickly. Once the principle is grasped, the word *is* can be written twice on a horizontally rectangular card. When the question is asked, the one on the right of P is covered by the subject-card. Before the spoken answer is given, the subject-card is slid over to cover the *is* on the left. The *is* card itself does not slide about if fixed to the desk with plastitak.

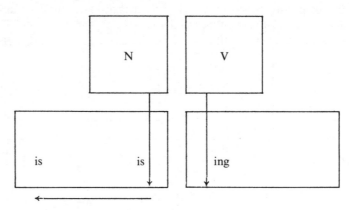

Progressions—(1) sequence of difficulty

It would be impossible to make the same definite sequence of practice designed to be suitable for every P. It is only possible to indicate progressions in each aspect. These can be dovetailed for each group of children who unknowingly dictate the next step. For instance, given a set of pseudo-transitive verbs, they can make acceptable sentences with no object. But eventually one of them completes the sentence in a different way, that is, not only with a verb but also an object, thus setting an example to the other children who usually need no encouragement to follow it. The way is then open for the progression from *What is the man doing?* to *What is the man eating?* and thence to transitive verbs, when the first question can be *What is the man making?* with the answer, ... *a plate*. The second can be *What is the man doing?* with the answer, ... *making a plate*. The last question *What is happening?* is answered by the complete statement *The man is making a plate*.

(*a*) *Verbs.*   The use of a main verb is vital to a clause; auxiliaries are considered at phrase level; and verb-ending modifications are among the earliest to appear in normal development. They are relevant to all three sections, and of paramount importance. Once the use of *is* (phrase level) is firmly established, *are* is taught. At first, the indeterminate *they* may be used to describe any pairs or larger groups of people or animals. Then the plural pack is shuffled with the singular pack, and the alternatives *is* and *are* are shown. When names of people in the environment are used as alternatives to *the boy* etc., a child sometimes turns up his own name. He is taught to use *am* in this context. If a child is too confused by this demand, all names of children in the group are removed before the next session, and not replaced until this extra item can be tolerated, and easily incorporated.

Some children may need extraneous clues for a full understanding of the need for the past tense (word level). So an introductory item, e.g. *last Thursday*, precedes the subject when *was* and *were* are first introduced. They can usually be taught together. The concepts of singularity and plurality have been established from *is* and *are*, and this concept of tense difference is a different aspect, which still includes singularity and plurality.

Later the time clue may be removed from the beginning of the sentence and replaced at the end. But by this time each child can choose his own time-element. This is an effective test of whether he understands the difference between past and present. Past historic forms should be introduced soon after this. As the most common verbs have irregular forms, there is no extra card with the regular *-ed* ending. Instead, another yellow card is fixed behind each verb card by a staple at the top. At the bottom of the back card is the past tense word. The first time it is introduced, the new past-tense forms should be included in the question, e.g. starting with *Who ran?* rather than *What did John do?* Most children do not need to look at the past tense word in response to the first question. But when it is necessary, for example, after the second type of question, the child lifts the top card and 'reads' what is underneath. It has been noticed that several children who do not know the past tense of a verb, and who cannot decode it from its written or printed form in other contexts, can remember the word when they see it on the back card. Gradually each child remembers it without looking.

The future tense can be approached by the colloquial *going to*. An appropriate time phrase can be placed at the beginning of the sentence in early practice, e.g. *next week*, but later can be removed, and a self-chosen item can be added to the verb by the child. The variation *I* (or *we* or *they*) *want to* can be introduced here. Until the third person singular form of the verb is taught, no people or third person singular pronouns can be used.

Lee's (1966) sequence in her plan for *Developmental Sentence Scoring* has been used as a basis for the progression in auxiliary verbs. The next subsidiary verbs to appear are *can*, *will* and *may*. It is more appropriate to use these with transitive verbs, as the doubt implied when these words are used as questions is more often related to the object than the verb itself, e.g. *Can/will/may she (get the dinner)?* When the negative aspect is introduced with these verbs, the step from *can* and *not*, and *will* and *not* to *can't* and *won't* follows fairly soon, at approximately the same time as the positives *could*, *would*, *should* and *might*. Later, *couldn't* and *wouldn't* are joined by *must*, *shall*, *ought to*, and *have/had/has to*. At approximately the same time comes the need for the use of *don't*, *didn't* and *doesn't* in negative statements. It is however important that practice in past tense forms should precede practice in *did*, *do* and *does* questions, which in their turn should be fully established before *didn't*, *don't* and *doesn't* questions are introduced.

Next comes the past participle (word level) which, in normal development, is used at roughly the same time in the present and past perfect (e.g. *I have eaten, I had eaten*) and the passive (e.g. *it is/was eaten*). It is questionable whether the *-en* forms should be introduced before or after the forms which match the ordinary past tense. It is probably better to practise the new construction with known forms of the verb, e.g. *washed* and *painted*, then proceed to a selected group of *en* verbs, e.g. *grown, done, given*; and finally to mix the two types.

The third person singular of the present simple tense (word level) is not in common use. It should be practised with the verbs on which it is most often used, and which are followed by fairly simple direct objects, e.g. *likes, loves, wants, uses*. The inclusion of *says, thinks, hopes* etc. presupposes an ability to form noun-clause objects. This may be possible, especially if the introduction of the *-s* form has been delayed. When the *-s* is used easily by a group of children, its use can be generalized by occasional practices with the other verbs, but with the addition of a choice of the three adverbs *always, sometimes* and *never* in an initial or medial position, e.g. *everybody always sits; sometimes he eats (bananas); she never makes dresses*.

The use of two auxiliaries together (phrase-level), *would be -ing, must have -en* etc., are useful semantic starters. They almost always invite a subordinate clause. The adult can judge whether a child has internalized the meaning of a modal verb by the way in which he follows it by another phrase or clause. It is at this stage that subordinating conjunctions can be permuted along with the rest of the parts of speech. But this must be done carefully. It is usually wiser to provide a choice of conjunctions rather than a random selection. Some of the verbs can be eliminated from the packs to reduce the number of nonsense sentences. Or an unsuitable conjunction picked at random from the top of a pile can be rejected to the bottom of the pile. In the latter case, there should be several copies of each conjunction in the pile, to avoid frustration.

(b) Nouns and pronouns.   These are the subjects and objects of simple sentences, at clause level; they are preceded by determiners and/or possessing nouns, and/or adjectives, and/or prepositions to form noun phrases. A suggested logical progression, partly based on Lee, is given in the diagram on p. 171. In general the object pronouns are introduced before their corresponding subject pronouns; and the second person precedes the (first and) third. Possessives must not follow too closely on plurals, to avoid confusion between them.

(c) Noun determiners.   It seems in practice that *the* is the most useful determiner to introduce first, as it can be used for both singulars and plurals. For the same reason *my* and *your* can be introduced soon, probably first in the object position or before animate subjects. When all the subjects are singular, *this* and *that* provide interesting alternatives, and most children learn quickly to understand their relative meanings. *A* can substitute for a singular *the*, leaving *an* till later; and *some* for a plural *the*. *His* and possessive *her* need a judicious introduction, usually in the object position, but preferably several weeks before or after the object pronouns *him* and *her* are first used, or even the subject pronouns *he* and *she*. Children find difficulty enough in remembering to use *she* instead of *her* in the subject position,

| Subjects | | possessives | Objects | |
nouns	pronouns		nouns	pronouns
name singular person or animal			name singular thing	
	it this you that			it you
				me her him
men women children boys girls cats, etc.			plural things (regular)	
	he she it	singular e.g. Mary's— the boy's—	plural things (irregular)	us them
	we these they those			somebody everybody
the man and the boy	somebody everybody	somebody's everybody's		mine his hers theirs ours }also used in subjects
		plurals e.g. the boys' the men's		

without our adding to it and eliciting, for example, the error *she dog* in place of *her dog*.

Lee groups together the other less frequent determiners, *our*, *their*, *these* and *those* with the initiators *some (of the)*, *all (of the)*, *a lot of (the)*, *the other*, *another*, followed by *both* and *every*. These appear in LARSP Stage VI, which is beyond the immediate goal of the work described in this Chapter.

(*d*) *Adjectives.* Those which appear the highest in frequency lists are those which can apply to both people and things, or those which describe gross differences, e.g. *big* and *little*. It is useful to be able to use the same selection of adjectives as complements to names, people and things, before using the groups which are applicable mostly to people or mostly to things. Care should be taken to extract uncomplimentary adjectives, e.g. *silly*, *noisy*, before using the complimentary ones to describe people with specific names.

Progressions—(2) gradual removal of clues

Assuming that P has been given and has used all possible clues, and achieves near 100 per cent success, the task is then made more difficult by the gradual elimination of the clues, that is, of noun determiners, parts of the verb *to be* etc., and the word endings; and all signing, which has been used both by the teacher as a second visual aid to P's memory, and by P as a kinesthetic aid. Some Ps can remember visual images of words which have been removed, and they nod in the direction of each written word and each space as they say each word. The surest way to remove this clue is to ask P to turn his chair round, with his back to the desk. If necessary T can move to face him. This means that no cards at all are visible, and the way is open for T to ask P similarly structured questions about people in pictures, and about people he knows. The memory of the structure of the expected answer is still fresh enough in his mind, so he usually succeeds. Of course the real test of his acquisition of a new structure is whether he uses it in another context, and later with another person, either in answer to a question, or as a spontaneous statement.

A structured walk implies the necessity for application of what has been learnt in the classroom. It may be round the school building, or slightly further afield, the only requirement being that people can be seen doing a variety of actions. Most structures can be practised, and Ps soon seem to grasp the notion that this is no ordinary walk. Once each structure can be produced easily in a mobile situation, they can base their remarks on a grammatical structure just as easily as on spontaneous interest. As the response structure has been well practised, it is T who starts asking the stimulus questions. Later in the walk Ps are encouraged to do more questioning. And having talked about happenings in the present continuous tense, the meaning and function of the past continuous can be emphasized by sitting down at the end of the session to remind each other of what was happening, e.g. *What was the man holding?*, *What were the birds eating?* It can be pointed out to any child who argues that the man is probably still holding the bag, or the birds are still eating the bread, that this is an uncertain fact now, but was certain when it was happening, hence the need for the past tense here. It is probable that children whose language therapy is given in a school clinic would not need to be taken on such walks, as they would have more frequent opportunities for spontaneous practice when mixing with children with normally-developing language.

Progressions—(3) the elicitation of questions

When P is familiar with any specific statement structure, he can be encouraged to ask the corresponding question. He has been listening to its model throughout the time he has been answering it. It is wise when changing roles to change chairs too, so that the questioner is in the position of T, and addresses the questions to the other children and the teacher who has changed places with him. At first P finds questioning much more difficult than he thinks it will be, so T can help him by signing the words for as long as necessary. Not all the Ps in a group are ready for this progression at the same time, which allows the less advanced ones to gain more practice in making statements before it is their turn to become questioners.

Other formats

It is important that no child sees the practice-sessions as ends in themselves. In the same way the use of the cards must be flexible. The pile-format is only one method of random selection of cards. Others are those of pelmanism, rows of cards, and specially drawn pictures, e.g. to elicit the preposition *in*.

Pelmanism—some examples of the use of pairs of cards. Each child picks up two cards in turn. The first one picked up should be the first word which is said. In the first three examples, each child who picks up a 'positive' pair keeps it.

(i) Aim at the use of *is* and/or *not*. Use any pack of coloured pictures of objects (i.e. not the line drawings of objects on orange cards) and the adjective pack (having removed any which would always be inappropriate), e.g.
Stimulus: *Is the ball red?*
Response: Either, *Yes, it is (red).*
Or, *No, it'(i)s not (red) (It'(i)s blue).*

(ii) Aim at verb and particle, and/or *can* and *can'(no)t:*
S   *Can you get up?*
R   *Yes, you can (get up) (off the chair).*
or
S   *Can you ring down?*
R   *No, can'(no)t (ring down).*

(iii) Aim at verb and object, and/or *can* and *can'(no)t:*
S   *Can you post a letter?*
R   *Yes, you can (post a letter).*
or
S   *Can you write a picture?*
R   *No, you can'(no)t (write a picture).*

(iv) Aim at the use of the possessive. In this example, every child who remembers to say or sign the possessive, may keep the pair:
S   *Whose cake (is it)?*
R   *Mary's (cake).*

Rows. This is essential for some items, e.g. *-est* and *-er*.

adj	
adj	er
adj	est

The pile is upside down, and the top one is turned over. It is moved down the column twice, leaving a space for the next one:

S   *What is big?*
R   *A car is big.*

S   (While the adjective is moved down to the next row)
    What is bigger?
R   *A bus is bigger (than a car).*
S   (While the adjective is moved down to the last row)
    What is biggest?
R   *A ship is (the) biggest.*

The concepts of comparatives and superlatives are first taught with the same adjective used three times, e.g. *cold, colder, coldest;* other common adjectives which can be treated in this way are *hot, dirty, fat, loud, sweet, pretty.* But semantically it is important to use some adjectives in pairs of opposites, e.g. *short* and *long*, producing the sequence *short, longer, longest;* or *long, shorter, shortest.*

'In'.   Two sets of cards are used. Those in the bigger set are the same size as the main pack. Drawn on each of these is an object which can contain other objects or people, e.g. a bag, a house, the sea. A horizontal slit is made in each card. The smaller set of cards are half the width of the others, and slightly shorter. Drawn on each of these is a person or object which can be contained. Each one can be pushed into the slit of the bigger cards. The following sequences can take place (the piles are separate):

S   (After the bigger card is turned over) *What's in the...?*
R   (After the smaller card is slotted into the bigger card) *The....*
or
S   (After the smaller card is turned over) *Where is the ...?*
R   (After the bigger card is turned over) *In the....*

In another exercise, each of the smaller cards is already slotted into one of the bigger cards. The same sequence as above can be reversed, but the past tense used, e.g. *What was in the...?* etc.

Planning a session

It is important to have one aim only per exercise. In each 20-minute session there are a number of ways of ringing the changes, in order to retain the maximum attention. The same goal can be pursued through the whole session, but via different formats. When further practice is needed in a specific item, and yet the children may have become bored with it, the pressure can be removed from it by changing another element in the sequence, e.g. if T's aim is to improve the use of the past tense, she asks P to use a pronoun in the reply, e.g.

S   *Did the woman run?*
R   *(Yes). She ran.*

When concentration is required for another element, the original goal is more easily reached. Or, the same grammatical goal can be pursued, and the levels of difficulty, and therefore the amount of challenge increased, by the removal of clues. Two or three different items may be practised. Then they should come from different columns in the analysis, i.e. clause-level, clause and phrase-level combined; and word-endings.

Because visual clues are present, there should be the minimum of errors in the item being practised. If errors are made in another aspect, they can usually be overlooked. If not, the correct version can be spoken casually by the teacher. But if one of the children remarks upon the error, it should be acknowledged but dismissed. There are rare occasions when it should be followed up, especially if it worries the child who made the error. The children's attitude in the session is based on the idea that it is a game which is enjoyable, but which helps to improve their ways of talking. They are usually prepared to change later in the session to an exercise which practises another type of element which they find difficult.

The complete pack of cards

The main pack consists of three to four hundred cards, representing most of the words on the John Horniman School first-level vocabulary. As there are so many nouns, some have been omitted. Those retained are those which can be possessed. The reason for this choice is that all 'possessible' nouns can be used in other syntactic contexts, but the opposite is not true. 'People' nouns are on cards of a slightly different orange colour from that of 'object' nouns. The three types of personal pronouns (e.g. *I, me, mine*) are on pink cards of three slightly different tones. On the cards are:

simple drawings of people, animals or objects;
simple drawings of PGSS signs of verbs, prepositions and adjectives: each word is also written small at the bottom of the card;
large words are written on the cards which represent all the other closed-class concepts, i.e. noun determiners, pronouns, modals and (other) auxiliaries (including the negative elliptical forms of the most common, e.g. *can't, didn't*), *not, yes* and *no* (several of each).

The reasons for not drawing the PGSS signs for these words is that they are very common, and their written form must be learnt as soon as possible for reading purposes. *Small words* are written at the bottom of the cards representing conjunctions. The reasons for a reduced size of word are that they are introduced much later in the scheme when reading ability probably includes them; and sometimes it is essential that they are chosen and not produced at random. They take up less room when they overlap each other vertically.

The complementary pack consists of all the endings for open-class words, i.e. for verbs (*-ing, -en, -s, -'s, n't*), for nouns (*-s, 's, s'*) and for adjectives (*-est, -er, -ly*). The colour of each word-ending card corresponds to that of the open-class word it follows. Each card is twice the length of the square which is laid on top. This ensures that the child sees the two morphemes as one word. Both verbs and adjectives whose final letter is a single consonant or an *-e*, have the second consonant added faintly, or the final *-e* crossed out faintly. There is no need to point out the reason, but children who ask can be given the explanation, and some of them apply it to their written work in the classroom.

The backs of the cards

It is sometimes necessary for T to know something about the word on the card before it is turned over, e.g. when singular and plural subjects are mixed, the question must vary between *Who is . . . ing?* and *Who are . . . ing?* Various hieroglyphics on the back of the cards give this kind of information. A thick dot indicates a singular, and a thick line a plural. If these are put on the same place on each card, e.g. the top left-hand corner, the pack can be re-sorted more quickly, both so that all the cards are facing the same way, and so that they return to their original piles. Noun determiners and pronouns are marked in the same way as nouns. Other information given on the backs of the cards is:

for verbs:	intransitive, pseudo-transitive, transitive
	irregular past, or ending in sound *-t, -d, -id*
	(*e*)*n* past participle or not
	whether the questions *where?*, *when?*, or *why?* can be asked
for adjectives:	applicable to people and things, e.g. *big*
	not applicable to people, e.g. *long*
	not wise to apply to names, e.g. *silly*
	colour
for prepositions:	whether they can answer the questions *where?* or *when?* or both.

Storage

Only one person can satisfactorily use each complete set of cards. Specific subsets are combined for a specific group of children, and it is a waste of time to refile all the cards after each session, as the same set is often used for several consecutive sessions. They can conveniently be stored upright in small boxes, the sets being kept together with rubber-bands. The following sections have been found to be practicable:

people and animals:	singulars
	easy plurals and hard plurals, e.g. *men, women, a boy and a man* etc.
pronouns:	proper names
	subject
	object
	possessive, e.g. *mine*
auxiliary verbs:	*is, am, are, was, were*
	want to, going to
	will; positive modals; *has to* etc.
	do, does, did; *don't, doesn't, didn't*
	some negative modals
	have, has, had; *been*
main verbs:	intransitive
	pseudo-transitive
	transitive

adjectives:	for things *and* people
	for things alone
	for people alone
	numbers
non-human nouns:	singular
	plural
prepositions	
adverbs	
not and *n't*	
conjunctions:	coordinating
	subordinating
noun determiners	

A final section in a box can contain all combinations of sets in current use.

Use of the cards with other types of children

So far, descriptions of the card method have referred to children with expressive language disorders. It is hoped that they will also be used with the smaller number of children with primarily receptive disorders. They are accustomed to 'reading' the written sentences they compose with either signing and/or spoken words. In the LARSP method they are presented with readymade sentences, and it should help them to absorb the colour patterns more effectively if they see each one repeatedly in a quick unhindered sequence. When they are working primarily with their own written words, other kinds of activities are interposed, i.e. matching each concept with a written word, remembering the colour pattern, and copying the result.

There is no theoretical reason why a modified form of the card method should not be used with children with other handicaps, e.g. low intelligence, provided that a simple enough type of symbol can be drawn and understood. Bliss symbols are a possible example. Bigger, but fewer cards could be used according to the potential ability of the group.

Effectiveness of this type of remediation

So far it has not been possible to provide any objective validation. But subjectively it is considered that this method of remediation is more effective than those already used in John Horniman School. Previously we have relied on specific individual and/or group practice given by the speech therapist in her sessions; on different kinds of practice, with an emphasis on written grammar, in the classroom; and on various kinds of corrections given by other adults in the children's environment. These approaches are still used, but probably more as supplements to the spoken, systematically structured one described here. All remediators are working with the same kind of basic information, and in the same broad progression.

During the parts of the programme in which the children are encouraged to complete sentences in their own way, many different grammatical forms are generated. The starter is the sequence of two or three cards in which the same number of concepts are thrown together. This triggers the children's imaginations, and often they produce more than one sentence, or even a complete short story, including rationalizations of any group of concepts which they consider to be inappropriately clustered.

In addition to the improvement in the children's grammar, this method carries with it a number of bonus effects. The ability to read closed-class vocabulary is increased. So is the vocabulary itself. One group, although using the possessives *his* and *her* appropriately, was totally unaware of the existence of the word *their*. They had never 'heard' the word before, but were able to use it correctly after very few examples.

The children gain incidental practice in the use of the Paget-Gorman Sign System. It is reasonable to suppose that 'kinesthetic feedback' is at work. The more signing they do, the more the children are able to remember the feel of a grammatical structure in addition to the visual pattern.

Reading is another skill which is practised incidentally. The words describing all concepts except the nouns are written on the cards, either alone or in association with the drawing of the sign. This ensures that the spellings of most of the common morphemes, i.e. all the closed-class words and all the word endings, are read frequently and should become more readily recognizable in other contexts.

The spontaneous writing of some children has become freer and greater in quantity. Written ellipses are more often used correctly, as in *He's telling you that the dog's box isn't here.*

2.3

The Nuffield Hearing and Speech Centre

Elspeth Paul

The Nuffield Hearing and Speech Centre is the Department, within the Royal National Throat Nose and Ear Hospital, concerned with the diagnosis and care of children who have some form of language disorder.[25] The range of disorders is extremely wide and includes hearing loss, mental retardation and many more subtle but linguistically crippling conditions. The speech therapists and doctors work in close cooperation, and for many years it has been policy for a speech therapist to do a joint clinic with the Centre's Medical Director. The speech therapist assesses the child's comprehension, expressive language, articulation and prosodic features, with the doctor taking a detailed case history. Medical staff, speech therapists and parents discuss the findings, and future management is arranged. Children from all over the country attend for assessment but some are unable to have speech therapy at the Centre as they live too far away. There is a small residential unit for children with particularly severe forms of disability. They attend as weekly boarders and receive intensive help from teachers, speech therapists and nursery staff.

LARSP was first introduced at the Centre in 1975, after a series of visits by the authors to discuss analytic techniques and case studies. In July 1976 the Department of Post-Diploma Studies in The National Hospitals College of Speech Sciences ran a course on the Routine Use of LARSP, and this proved most helpful as it consolidated the use of the technique. We feel it was beneficial to be able to discuss details of the procedure directly with the authors over several visits rather than to learn the use of LARSP solely from the book.

The first analysis attempted was of a three-year-old with normal language. In many ways this proved to be the most difficult analysis, as the amount of language was so much greater when compared to the children attending for speech therapy. But apart from the necessary practice, an additional benefit of encountering analytic complexity in the normal child is the way in which knowledge of the developmental stages is reinforced.

Members of staff who were taught traditional grammar at school found LARSP

[25] I am most grateful to Mr Martin, Medical Director of the Nuffield Hearing and Speech Centre, for reading this manuscript.

easier than younger members who had little or no grammar in English language teaching. Quirk and Greenbaum (1973) was found useful in explaining grammatical structures and this was used as a reference book when difficulties in analysis were encountered.

For several weeks the speech therapists worked together at staff meetings analysing a child's language. After three or four analyses had been completed it was felt better for each person to analyse a sample of language individually, and then to compare results.

At first the main problems were to do with spending too long on the transcription of the taperecordings; overcoming disagreements and reaching a consensus on the actual analysis of a grammatical structure; and becoming familiar with the terminology and abbreviations used on the chart. It took some time for therapists to appreciate the need for transcription discipline: initially, when transcribing a recording, they would puzzle for too long over an utterance which was difficult to understand, only eventually coming to realize that it should be entered in the unintelligible section and only reconsidered if felt to be an important part of the recording.

Use of LARSP at the Nuffield Centre (1976–7)

The practice has been to use LARSP routinely with certain well-defined categories of children, the majority of whom have delay in their use of expressive language. It is usually a morning's work to transcribe and analyse a half-hour's recording. We have found it better to transcribe the tape as soon as possible after the recording, but it is usually more convenient to leave analysis to be completed at a later stage.

The staff of the Nuffield Centre have been asked by speech therapists working in other clinics to analyse their samples of children's language for them. This is not feasible in a busy department, and it is in any case of more value for each speech therapist to carry out her own analysis and plan of remediation.

It has been felt for some time that the existing techniques of assessment of expressive language disorder and its remediation need to be expanded, and we are of the opinion that LARSP has helped to give a clearer picture of specific difficulties in syntax. In terms of implementation, we do sometimes use the procedure when a child is referred to us for full assessment. It has been used, for example, with deaf teenagers and it is found that their spoken language is often limited to Stage III (cf. chapter 2.5 below). However, because of the time involved, it is not found to be practical to carry out many analyses for assessment only, and we feel accordingly that the main value of the procedure is as a basis for remediation.

Several ways of implementing the use of LARSP in the weekly or monthly speech therapy sessions in the residential unit and in the assessment clinic have been discussed. In the clinic, as one might expect, the use of pictures for SV, VO, SVO etc. produces very stilted language, especially with the deaf children. They so often need such structured teaching of language that very stereotyped sentences were evoked. Although this is useful, in order to evaluate what structures have been learnt formally, it is not a good guide to their spontaneous use of language. We have found that the most natural language is elicited from a play situation, using carefully graded and selected test material of common objects and miniature toys, a longstanding feature of the assessment procedure at the Centre and one which could readily be adapted to the requirements of LARSP, as outlined in *GALD*, chapter 6. In the screening of expressive language in the clinic, the speech therapist notes down examples of speech heard and this is checked against as detailed a description as possible obtained from the parents. We have found that the two usually correspond quite well and there is a reasonably good correlation with the results of more detailed analysis for the range of children whom we usually see. The therapist becomes accustomed to this form of observation and finds, for example, an SVO- or a QXY-type sentence as easy to identify as a phonetic contrast such as [ʃʌn] for [sʌn]. On the clinical assessment form there is now a chart for the therapist to fill in structures heard in clinic. The therapist notes down structures heard at each stage rather than having most of the structures listed.

The main pitfall that has been found is in mentioning age levels as if they were absolute entities. For example, a 13-year-old with a profound hearing loss might be at Stage IV coming on to Stage V and therefore at the approximate age level of 2;6–3;6 years. If this is quoted out of the LARSP context, however, it is easy to forget how relatively advanced this is: if one fails to realize that the main syntactic development is complete by 4;6–5 years, one might well conclude that the child is at least ten years behind—and we have often encountered this reaction. It is however more accurate to say that the child in this example is two stages below completion of syntactic development, in the process quoting examples of his actual language and itemizing missing or abnormal patterns.

The participation of parents in language remediation

As most children seen are of pre-school age, often 2–3 years old, it is the policy of the department to involve the parents in therapy. Because many travel from considerable distances, children are usually seen once a month for an hour. Following this, parents are expected to follow a programme of therapy at home so that in effect treatment is daily. A particular methodological problem therefore is how to implement the use of LARSP by working through the parents.

With children having virtually no verbal expression, the outline of therapy is governed by the profile chart: at Stage I, nouns are followed by verbs, and then adjectives and adverbs are introduced. At this stage parents usually work easily with their child and readily accept the need for 'action' words and 'describing' words, if the build-up of sentences is explained.

Once children reach Stage II, the degree of explanation required varies according to the educational background of the parent. There have been parents with a good understanding of traditional grammar who welcome a more 'scientific' approach. However, some of the parents, although understanding the theory, cannot easily implement the techniques of eliciting different structures. They need many examples of games, and the speech therapist has to ensure that there is not too much pressure put on the child. Parents without any knowledge of grammar usually realize that there is something wrong with the way words are put together and accept help with eliciting two- or three-word utterances. However, it is only in the very first stages that monthly therapy is found to be acceptable, and we have found that once Stage II is started more regular weekly help is essential.

Whether the child is attending weekly or monthly, the parents have to be present throughout the therapy session so that they can understand the techniques being used and see when an utterance is accepted. One important and perhaps surprising difficulty is to demonstrate that a less than 'perfect' form is permissible at times. The therapist should observe the parents working with the child and then correct any mistakes in management. It has been found that some parents managed better without a detailed explanation, which only served to confuse them. For example, it might be sufficient to mention only that the child needs help with words like *in* and *on*, if working on Pr Adj N, without going into details of developmental strategy, or how this structure relates to others. The parents can then more readily grasp the purpose of the games. We have noted that the earlier structures are easier for parents to grasp than later stages. In our case, this causes no problem as most of the children attending are at Stages I, II or III. A notebook explaining the specific games, and a handout giving very general remarks on the structures being worked on, are given to the parents. Copies of pictures used in the clinic session are given when appropriate; or, if the child is better with common household objects or toys, this is demonstrated to the parents.

A basic outline of material needed for LARSP has been drawn together in a file giving ideas for eliciting different structures. Relevant pictures, e.g. the outline drawings from ICAA, are filed under appropriate headings. In this way the therapists pool their ideas, and difficult structures like QXY are discussed so that a series of games can be given to parents. The work on this continues, fresh difficulties are encountered and new ideas evolve.

The use of LARSP at the residential unit

The residential unit is for around 12 children, aged about 4–6 years, who have severe speech and language difficulties—often with additional problems of mental and social handicap, motor coordination or deafness. They attend as weekly boarders; the year is divided into four terms. Staff include three teachers, a speech therapist and several nursery nurses. At the unit every effort is made to ensure that the parents are aware of their child's range of abilities and difficulties and to involve them in the remediation programme. They meet the staff each Friday to learn the Paget–Gorman Sign System and discuss the therapy. No home practice is expected other than suitable modification of the patterns of communication to help their child. Most of the children are at Stage I or II on admission, and few develop sufficient language to be beyond Stage IV when they are transferred to other schools. The work in the classroom and in speech therapy is closely linked, so that the staff are working on the same structures. The Colour Pattern Scheme is used to help reading and writing, and this can reinforce the speech.

If it is decided to carry out a linguistic analysis on one of the children, certain difficulties become apparent. During the recording of data the child signs as well as speaks. Copious notes are sometimes needed to aid the transcription of the tape e.g. if a child says [sɪʔɪ] for *sleeping* but signs |sleeping|, remembering the *-ing* ending, this is scored appropriately on the profile chart. Spoken words are always insisted upon as well as signing. All the staff, teachers, speech therapists and home care staff use PGSS, and at times a recording has been made by the nursery nurse primarily responsible on the home side to ensure a more relaxed response from the child. Frequency of recordings for analysis varies from child to child. Sometimes one recording at the start of the term can provide work for the whole term.

When reassessing (depending on the child) the therapist sometimes concentrates on clause, phrase, word and connectivity scans only, and does not complete the upper part of the chart. With some children, whether attending the Nuffield Centre for weekly therapy or in the residential unit, the degree of spontaneity and type of response is not a problem. The therapist has a good knowledge of the child's ability in this area and no formal assessment of it need be carried out. Similarly, during the course of reassessment, this section is not completed each time, but only for every second or third assessment.

Even in the absence of recognizable spoken language, we have found that therapy is best planned on the basis of LARSP. Nouns, then verbs, are introduced using PGSS, and a basic vocabulary has been compiled for this. At this stage PGSS is a most useful therapeutic tool, and the teachers and therapists work on the same vocabulary list, in the classroom, in the speech therapy sessions and in the more formal Paget sessions. Similarly for later stages, the appropriate linguistic structures are taught throughout the school day, the home care staff continuing to apply them unobtrusively during the child's play times, at meals and whilst getting ready for bed.

A case study

This case history is of a child who is at the residential unit. William was referred to the Nuffield Hearing and Speech Centre in November 1974 at the age of 3;1. At this time, he had few words and a very limited amount of vocalization. Birth was normal and there were no postnatal problems. All milestones were achieved normally except for speech. He was the younger of two children. There was no family history of speech disorder. Hearing was within normal limits. When assessed by the clinical psychologist in the department, his IQ was in the 80s. He had specific motor coordination problems in the speech apparatus. On assessing his language using the Reynell Developmental Language Scales, his comprehension was found to be within normal limits.

Monthly therapy was arranged. Initially therapy was aimed at increasing the range and amount of vocalization. Tongue and lip movements were extremely limited, and he dribbled frequently; therefore therapy also necessitated motor work.

No recordings were made initially, as the words he did use were poorly articulated. Therapy was planned to elicit structures at Stage I, so nouns were first

William 5;0   A

A	Unanalysed				Problematic		
	1 Unintelligible **15**	2 Symbolic Noise		3 Deviant **I**	1 Incomplete		2 Ambiguous

B Responses

				Normal Response							Abnormal		
			Repet-	Elliptical Major				Full		Struc-		Prob-
Stimulus Type		Totals	itions	1	2	3	4	Major	Minor	tural	Ø	lems
27	Questions	**26**		**20**	**I**			**2**	**2**	**4**	**2**	
17	Others	**16**		**10**				**3**	**3**		**I**	

C Spontaneous   **15**   **5**   **12**   Others **3**

		Minor		Social **5**	Stereotypes		Problems

| Stage | Sentence Type | Major | | Sentence Structure | | | |

Stage I (0;9–1;6)

	Excl.	Comm.	Quest.	Statement			
		·V·	·Q·	·V· **15** ·N· **35**	Other **I**	Problems	

			Conn.	Clause		Phrase	Word

Stage II (1;6–2;0)

Comm.	Quest.	Conn.	Clause		Phrase		Word
V X	Q X		SV **2**	V C/O	DN	VV	-ing **9**
			S C/O **2**	A X	Adj N **I**	V part	pl
			Neg X	Other	NN	Int X	
					PrN **I**	Other	-ed

Stage III (2;0–2;6)

Comm.	Quest.		Clause		Phrase		Word
V X Y			X + S:NP	X + V:VP	X + C/O:NP	X + A:AP	-en
	Q X Y		SVC/O	VC/OA	D Adj N	Cop	
let X Y	VS		SVA	VOdOi	Adj Adj N	Aux	3s
			Neg X Y	Other	Pr DN	Pron	
do X Y					N Adj N	Other	gen

Stage IV (2;6–3;0)

Comm.	Quest.		Clause		Phrase		Word
			X Y + S:NP	X Y + V:VP	X Y + C/O:NP	X Y + A:AP	n't
· S	QVS		SVC/OA	AAX Y	N Pr NP	Neg V	'cop
	Q X YZ		SVOdOi	Other	Pr D Adj N	Neg X	'aux
					cX	2 Aux	
					XcX	Other	

Stage V (3;0–3;6)

Comm.	Quest.	Conn.	Clause		Phrase		Word
how		and	Coord. **I**	I ·	Postmod. **I** clause	I +	-est
	tag	c	Subord. **I**	I ·			-er
		s	Clause: S		Postmod. **I** · phrase		
what		Other	Clause: C/O				-ly
			Comparative				

(+)			(−)		
NP	VP	Clause	NP	VP	Clause

Stage VI (3;6–4;6)

NP	VP	Clause	NP		VP	Clause
Initiator	Complex	Passive	Pron	Adj seq	Modal	Concord
Coord		Complement	Det	N irreg	Tense	A position
					V irreg	W order
Other			Other			

Stage VII (4;6+)

Discourse		Syntactic Comprehension	
A Connectivity	it		
Comment Clause	there	Style	
Emphatic Order	Other		

Total No. Sentences **57**	Mean No. Sentences Per Turn **1·3**	Mean Sentence Length **1·1**

© D. Crystal, P. Fletcher, M. Garman, 1975 University of Reading

Fig. 23   William at 5;0

introduced. As he built up a vocabulary, verbs were attempted by using forced alternatives. The method proved not to be helpful initially, as the length of utterance confused him. It could however sometimes be used in shorter form to elicit nouns (e.g. *Is it a book or a ball?*), without repeating the full sentence.

Despite the limited vocabulary, work was undertaken on joining two elements—*no*+Noun and *more*+Noun, as he had begun to use both these words. He started conjoining spontaneously, rather than in a structured situation only, in August 1976. Progress was so slow, however, that admission to the unit was discussed then arranged for September 1976.

Initially he made slow progress with PGSS, as his motor coordination made signing difficult. But once he had settled into the unit and began to realize that his attempts at communication were of some avail, he became less aggressive. He started using PGSS purposefully and this greatly aided his vocal communicative efforts.

The basic vocabulary was introduced in the classroom and in his speech therapy sessions. Although he had started conjoining some items, his grasp of structures at Stage I was not felt to be secure enough to continue with Stage II immediately. Only later were two-element structures introduced in a systematic way.

In October 1976, the first recording was made for analysis. He signed at the same time as speaking, and in this way the therapist could more easily understand his speech. Without this, many of the words in the transcripts below would otherwise have been unintelligible. The session was on a reasonably formal basis as this was the only way to elicit language. An extract from this session follows, with the profile (Fig. 23, Profile A) based on the session as a whole.

T	'who is this/	*looking at pictures*
P	gìrl/	
T	gírl	
P	sîtting/	
T	'sitting on a cháir/ —	
	'what's the 'girl sìtting ón/ —	*P signs*
	'that's rìght/	
	whát is she 'sitting on/	
P	gìrl/chàir/ — —	
	bòx/	
T	bòx/	
	'good bòy/	
	whò is it/	
P	wàsh/	
T	nò/	
	whò is it/	
P	gìrl/	
T	a gìrl/	
P	àrm/	
T	gírl/	
P	àrm/	

T	'what is she dôing/
P	wàsh/
T	'washing hér/
P	àrm/
T	gòod/——
	who is it/
P	bàby/
T	yès/
P	(1 syll.)
T	báby/
P	bòy/
T	'what is the 'baby dòing/——
	thât's 'right/
P	sìt/
	sìtting/
	sìt/
T	on thé/
P	flòor/
T	flòor/
P	er
T	gòod/
	'who is thìs/
P	màn/slêeping/
T	gòod/
	a 'man 'sleeping ín/
P	bèd/
T	m̀/
	'who is thìs/
P	'mummy sìtting/
T	gôod/
	'clever bòy/——
	'what ìs it/
P	dìrt/
T	it's dìrty/
P	m̂/
	wàsh/
T	we'll 'have to wàsh it/ . or rùb it/
P	yēah/
T	'what are you going to dò this 'afternoon/
P	oùt/
T	you're 'going tó/
P	wàlk/
T	wàlk/
	m̀/
	'what èlse are you 'going to 'do/
P	er
T	m̀/
P	bòok/

P signs

T	a bôok/
	ôh/
	'read a bòok/
P	yèah/
T	and 'are you 'going to màke 'anything/
	'what will you màke/ - - — —
	'what will you màke/
P	bòat/
T	you're 'going to 'make a bòat/
	'very gòod/

From this data, it can be observed that many Questions and Prompts were essential in order to elicit language. A significant portion of the data is Unintelligible, and one-third of the spontaneous utterances are self-repetitions. At Stage I William was far better at nouns than verbs, and SV had been introduced before VO. There seemed to be a developing Stage II pattern, with both clause and phrase structure represented, but he used no questions, not even by intonation. On four occasions in the extract he gave a structurally abnormal answer, and he often confused *wh*-question forms.

The plan of therapy was accordingly to work on both questions and statements. Under the first heading, work was planned for Q, leading to QX. Under the latter heading, therapy would focus first on the use of verbs, then introducing VO, while consolidating SV. At phrase level, DN was to be introduced and further work given on Adj N and Pr N. Finally, there was to be work on V Part and Int X. No work was planned for VV and NN. This plan of therapy provided work for eight months. (Therapy was also directed throughout this time at increasing the number of sounds of articulation.)

Present state of linguistic development

The following extract is from a recording of William at 5;9.

T	what is it/	*looking at shopping*
P	to'mato grôw/	
T	tomâto/	
	it's gròwn/	
	yès/	
P	mum — 'mummy bùy/	
T	'mummy 'buys whàt/	
P	chôcolate/	
T	dóes she/	
P	for mê/	
T	'what are thòse/	
P	'strawberries mê/	
T	stràwberries/	
	who èlse 'has 'strawberries/	

```
P    mê
T    who èlse/
P    Jànet/
T    yès/
P    (1 syll.)
T    'that's a lèmon/
P    lèmon/
     (sucking noise)
T·   yès/
     it's sòur/
P    banàna/
T    banàna/
     'what's thìs one/
P    juìce/
T    'fizzy juìce/
     yès/
     it's lemonàde/
P    mê/
T    do you lìke lemonáde/
P    yès/
T    do you 'have it at hǒme/
P    yès/
```

Looking at this transcript and the associated chart (Fig. 24, Profile B), it can be seen that William is now clearly at Stage II; there has been a considerable increase in the range of structures used. The recording for the second profile was made nine months after the first by one of the nursery nurses. The time between analyses had been unusually long, but as the child had very severe difficulties progress had been slow, and there had been no need of a further profile at an earlier point. There are still a number of unintelligible utterances. However there are some spontaneous sentences and he is responding more readily to Other stimuli as well as direct Questions.

No question-words appear in the recording sample, but there are questions by intonation. When questions were checked later it was plain he could use *what* and *who*. He is now using SV and VO more, and at phrase level there are a wider range of structures. He is beginning to manage three words together, as is shown at the transitional stage between Stages II and III, the object being expanded (e.g. *wet his face*). One example of D Adj N was heard.

The current plan of therapy is to concentrate on question-forms, as they still cause difficulty. He also needs help to build up the word level structures: he can manage -*ing* and plural *s*, but their use is variable. Now he has more structures at Stage II, work is to be given on expanding S and O, and the plan is to proceed to SVO at Stage III as soon as possible.

The teachers and speech therapist will continue to work together using PGSS. As far as elicitation is concerned, it is now possible to use forced alternatives to supplement the use of modelling, expansion, and cueing.

William 5;9   B

A **Unanalysed**   **Problematic**

1 Unintelligible 13 2 Symbolic Noise 1 3 Deviant   1 Incomplete   2 Ambiguous

B **Responses**

				Normal Response							Abnormal		
				Elliptical Major				Full		Struc-			Prob-
Stimulus Type		Totals	Repet-itions	1	2	3	4	Major	Minor	tural	Ø		lems
57	Questions	45	2	29				4	11	1	5		
36	Others	36	10	24				2	10				

C **Spontaneous**   25   4   21   Others 4

	Minor				Social 21		Stereotypes		Problems	

Sentence Type

Stage I (0;9–1;6)

	Major				Sentence Structure					
	Excl.	Comm.	Quest.		Statement					
		·V·	·Q·	·V· 10 ·N· 38		Other 10	Problems			

Stage II (1;6–2;0)

				Conn.	Clause		Phrase			Word
		V X	Q X		SV 5	V C/O 3	DN 4	VV		-ing
					S C/O 1	A X	Adj N 3	V part 1		2
					Neg X 1	Other	NN	Int X		pl
							PrN 9	Other		-ed

Stage III (2;0–2;6)

		V X Y	Q X Y	X + S:NP	X + V:VP	X + C/O:NP	X + A:AP			-en
			Q X Y	SVC/O	VC/OA	D Adj N 1	Cop		-en
		let X Y	VS	SVA	VO_dO_i	Adj Adj N	Aux		3s
				Neg X Y	Other	Pr DN	Pron 5		gen
		do X Y				N Adj N	Other		

Stage IV (2;6–3;0)

				X Y + S:NP	X Y + V:VP	X Y + C/O:NP	X Y + A:AP		n't
		· S	Q V S	SVC/OA	A A X Y	N Pr NP	Neg V		·cop
			Q X Y Z	SVO_dO_i	Other	Pr D Adj N	Neg X		·aux
						c X	2 Aux	
						Xc X	Other	

Stage V (3;0–3;6)

			and	Coord. 1	1 ·	Postmod. 1 clause	1 ·	-est
	how	tag	c	Subord. 1	1 ·			-er
			s	Clause: S		Postmod. 1 · phrase		-ly
	what		Other	Clause: C/O				
				Comparative				

(+)				(−)			
NP	VP	Clause		NP		VP	Clause
Initiator	Complex	Passive		Pron	Adj seq	Modal	Concord
Coord		Complement		Det	N irreg	Tense	A position
						V irreg	W order

Stage VI (3;6–4;6)

Other   Other

Discourse   Syntactic Comprehension

Stage VII (4;6+)

A Connectivity	it	
Comment Clause	there	Style
Emphatic Order	Other	

Total No. Sentences	106	Mean No. Sentences Per Turn	1·2	Mean Sentence Length	1·1

© D. Crystal, P. Fletcher, M. Garman, 1975 University of Reading

Fig. 24   William at 5;9

Second case study

This case study is of a boy, Nick, who attends the Nuffield Hearing and Speech Centre. He was referred in November 1975 at the age of 7;1. He had had speech therapy for six months prior to the referral.

The birth and postnatal period were normal. There was no family history of speech and language difficulties. Milestones were achieved normally; he started babbling at the usual age and his first words were at 1;4. His speech was always difficult to understand and he became very frustrated. By 4;6 he was joining two to three words together but according to his mother there were no 'proper' sentences.

He was assessed by the clinical psychologist at the Nuffield Centre and he came in the dull-normal range on the intelligence scale. Hearing was within normal limits, but he had a very poor auditory memory. Verbal comprehension was found to be within normal limits except for a difficulty in retaining longer instructions.

Expressive language was at Stage III. Articulation was assessed using the Edinburgh Articulation Test and he scored 25. The errors were mainly omissions of final consonants and simplification of consonant clusters. Vowels and most initial consonants were accurate. Rhythm was jerky and intonation patterns limited.

Speech therapy was arranged on a weekly basis. Initially, this was directed at work on his phonemic system, as until his speech became more intelligible, transcription of the recording would have proved almost impossible.

In April 1976 a recording was made for analysis. As is seen from the chart (Fig. 25, Profile C) he was at Stage IV, with three coordinate clauses at Stage V. Typical sentences at this point were:

'I got 'three sister/
'fish and dòg/
'that dùck pond/
I 'take her oùt sómetimes/and 'dog 'nearly bèat her/
I 'got 'one of them cár/
'what thàt/

He was quite spontaneous in conversation and he responded well to both Questions and Others in Section B. Several of his repetitions were of Stage IV structures. By this time only nine utterances were unintelligible. The low occurrence of word-endings was accounted for by the fact he still omitted final consonants on many occasions. Question-forms were poorer than clause- and phrase-level structures.

Initially structures not heard on the tape were checked and it was confirmed that $VO_d O_i$, the copula and VS questions caused great difficulty. Therapy was started on the use of the copula by using forced alternatives: *is* and *is not* were contrasted, e.g. *Is the cup green or is the cup not green?* The full form was used as he could not easily manage the abbreviated *'s*. (This form was introduced separately once his articulation had improved.)

Work on $VO_d O_i$ was given. Selections of pictures were used for O_d and O_i and he had to select items for each part of clause structure, e.g. *Give the book to the boy*.

Nick 7;6

<table>
<tr><td>A</td><td colspan="4">Unanalysed</td><td colspan="3">Problematic</td></tr>
<tr><td></td><td>1 Unintelligible 9</td><td>2 Symbolic Noise 1</td><td>3 Deviant</td><td></td><td>1 Incomplete 3</td><td>2 Ambiguous</td></tr>
</table>

<table>
<tr><td>B</td><td colspan="2">Responses</td><td></td><td></td><td colspan="4">Normal Response</td><td colspan="2">Abnormal</td><td></td></tr>
<tr><td></td><td colspan="2"></td><td></td><td></td><td colspan="4">Elliptical Major</td><td colspan="2"></td><td></td></tr>
<tr><td></td><td colspan="2">Stimulus Type</td><td>Totals</td><td>Repet-
itions</td><td>1</td><td>2</td><td>3</td><td>4</td><td>Full
Major</td><td>Minor</td><td>Struc-
tural</td><td>Ø</td><td>Prob-
lems</td></tr>
<tr><td></td><td>67</td><td>Questions</td><td>58</td><td>1</td><td>34</td><td>4</td><td></td><td></td><td>2</td><td>13</td><td>5</td><td>4</td><td></td></tr>
<tr><td></td><td>23</td><td>Others</td><td>19</td><td>5</td><td>10</td><td>3</td><td></td><td></td><td>1</td><td>5</td><td></td><td></td><td></td></tr>
<tr><td>C</td><td colspan="2">Spontaneous</td><td>39</td><td>3</td><td>2</td><td colspan="2">Others 37</td><td></td><td></td><td></td><td></td><td></td><td></td></tr>
</table>

		Minor			Social 18	Stereotypes		Problems	

Stage I (0;9–1;6) — Sentence Type

Major

Excl.	Comm.	Quest.	Statement			
	·V· 2	·Q· 1	·V·	·N· 6	Other 5	Problems

		Conn.	Clause		Phrase		Word

Stage II (1;6–2;0)

			VX	QX 6		SV 10	VC/O 16	DN 38	VV	-ing 4
		1			S C/O 5	AX	Adj N 8	V part 10	pl
					Neg X 3	Other 6	NN	Int X 9	
							PrN 1	Other 1	

Stage III (2;0–2;6)

VXY	QXY 4	X + S:NP 8	X + V:VP 15	X + C/O:NP 11	X + A:AP 5	-ed 5*
let XY	VS	SVC/O 17	VC/OA 8	D Adj N 1	Cop 1	-en
do XY		SVA 7	VOdOi	Adj Adj N 2	Aux 22	3s
		Neg XY	Other	Pr DN 7	Pron 32	gen
				N Adj N	Other 1	

Stage IV (2;6–3;0)

· S	OVS	XY + S:NP 3	XY + V:VP 2	XY + C/O:NP 3	XY + A:AP 2	n't
	QXYZ	SVC/OA 5	AAXY	N Pr NP	Neg V 9	'cop
		SVOdOi	Other	Pr D Adj N	Neg X	'aux
				cX 7	2 Aux	
				XcX 5	Other 1	

Stage V (3;0–3;6)

how	tag	and 3	Coord. 1 3	1 ·	Postmod. 1 clause	1 +	'st
		c	Subord. 1	1 ·			-er
		s	Clause: S		Postmod. 1 · phrase		
what		Other	Clause: C/O				-ly 2
			Comparative				

Stage VI (3;6–4;6)

(+)				(−)			
NP	VP		Clause	NP		VP	Clause
Initiator	Complex		Passive	Pron 4	Adj seq	Modal	Concord
Coord			Complement	Det	N irreg	Tense	A position
						V irreg 1	W order 2
Other				Other Aux 7		Cop 14	

Stage VII (4;6+)

Discourse		Syntactic Comprehension
A Connectivity	it	
Comment Clause	there	Style * all got
Emphatic Order	Other	

Total No. Sentences 125	Mean No. Sentences Per Turn 1·4	Mean Sentence Length 2·8

© D. Crystal, P. Fletcher, M. Garman, 1975 University of Reading

Fig. 25   Nick at 7;6

Nick 8;6

A	**Unanalysed**				**Problematic**		
	1 Unintelligible /	2 Symbolic Noise 3	3 Deviant		1 Incomplete /	2 Ambiguous	

B **Responses**

				Normal Response						Abnormal		
				Elliptical Major				Full		Struc-		Prob-
	Stimulus Type	Totals	Repet-itions	1	2	3	4	Major	Minor	tural	Ø	lems
	32 Questions	32		8	2			12	10			
	15 Others	14		1	1			10	2			

C **Spontaneous** 49 | 2 | Others 49

		Minor			Social 12	*Stereotypes*	*Problems*	

Sentence Type

Stage I (0;9–1;6)

Major				Sentence Structure			
Excl.	Comm.	Quest.		*Statement*			
	·V· 1	·Q·	·V·	·N· 2	Other	Problems	

				Conn.	Clause		Phrase		Word

Stage II (1;6–2;0)

VX	QX 5		SV 12	VC/O 9	DN 14	VV	-ing 8
		S C/O 6	AX	Adj N 3	V part	
		Neg X	Other 1	NN	Int X	pl 2
				PrN 7	Other	-ed 11

Stage III (2;0–2;6)

VXY 5	QXY 1	X + S:NP 5	X + V:VP 6	X + C/O:NP 17	X + A:AP 3	-en 1
let XY	VS 1	SVC/O 22	VC/OA 2	D Adj N 2	Cop 2	
		SVA 1	VO_dO_i	Adj Adj N	Aux 15	3s 1
do XY		Neg XY	Other	Pr DN 1	Pron 54	gen
				N Adj N	Other	

Stage IV (2;6–3;0)

· S	QVS	XY + S:NP	XY + V:VP	XY + C/O:NP	XY + A:AP	n't 5
	QXYZ 2	SVC/OA 8	AAXY	N Pr NP	Neg V 4	
		SVO_dO_i	Other	Pr D Adj N 2	Neg X 4	'cop
				cX 2	2 Aux	'aux 1
				XcX 2	Other	

Stage V (3;0–3;6)

how	tag	and 1	Coord. 1	1 · 1	Postmod. 1 clause	1 ·	-est
		c	Subord. 1	1 ·			-er
		s	Clause: S		Postmod. 1 · phrase		
what	Other		Clause: C/O 1				-ly
			Comparative				

	(+)				(−)		
NP	VP		Clause	NP		VP	Clause

Stage VI (3;6–4;6)

Initiator	Complex		Passive	Pron	Adj seq	Modal	Concord
Coord			Complement	Det	N irreg	Tense 2	A position
						V irreg	W order 2
Other				Other Aux 8			

Stage VII (4;6+)

Discourse		Syntactic Comprehension	
A Connectivity	it		
Comment Clause	there	Style	
Emphatic Order	Other		

Total No. Sentences 95	Mean No. Sentences Per Turn 2·0	Mean Sentence Length 2·5

© D. Crystal, P. Fletcher, M. Garman, 1975 University of Reading

Fig. 26 Nick at 8;6

Question forms were weak so work was started on QXY, which he was using but with unstable word order.

His parents had virtually no knowledge of grammar, but they were aware of their son's difficulty in putting words into sentences. His mother was present at most of the treatment sessions to ensure that she understood exactly what was being taught. Games were written out so that practice could be given at home. Several examples were required for each structure to keep his interest. The correct syntax was also written down so that his mother knew exactly what to expect from him.

Several other recordings were made for analysis, but the upper part of the form was not completed, as it was felt that it did not provide further information. The clause, phrase, word and connectivity scans only were completed. For some of the recordings no transcriptions were made, but the tape was listened to for the structures that had been receiving attention. Test situations were also recorded when forced alternatives were given to evaluate how easily he managed the different structures.

After one year's therapy for syntax and articulation a smaller sample (95 sentences) produced a chart as in Profile D (Fig. 26). The main progress was in the use of questions, although he still made errors (e.g. *where it go*). Word endings were used more frequently and fewer errors were made. There were fewer 'immature' structures at Stage II, and a wider range of structures at Stage IV (this time, with no repetitions to 'inflate' the figures). Predictably, because of his continuing difficulty with the auxiliary verb, no 2 Aux structures were used. There were eight omissions of the auxiliary verb in contexts were it would normally be expected. The main omission on the chart was subordinate clauses, but when tested later it was established that he could use one subordinate clause in a sentence. There had been considerable work given on subordinate clauses prior to the analysis and he could use them easily within a structured situation.

The fluency of his speech had greatly improved and it was felt that once the use of subordinate clauses, questions and the auxiliary verb were consolidated, further therapy for syntax would not be immediately necessary.

2.4

The Audiology Unit, Reading: a preschool group

Mary J. L. Auckland

This chapter deals with the use of LARSP in the Audiology Unit of the Royal Berkshire Hospital, where a number of disciplines involved in the speech and hearing field work together.[26] The work falls into three main areas at the preschool level of communication: assessment, research and remediation. Bamford and Bench show in their section (3.1) how LARSP has been used as a research tool. It is proposed to concentrate here on the use of LARSP as a clinical tool for assessment and remediation of a group of children.

The Unit provides intensive speech therapy individually and in groups. Children eligible for intensive therapy at the Unit are preschoolers who cannot benefit from once-weekly therapy. In the past, the feeling has been that such young children with severe language-learning problems could only benefit from individual therapy, but judging by the lack of literature, group therapy has not been thoroughly considered.

Group therapy is obviously attractive to an understaffed profession in terms of time-saving. It allows more children to be seen on a more intensive basis. But there is far more to the consideration of group therapy than these practical points. What is it, then, that group therapy can offer? To generalize our experience: individual therapy can promote steady progress in selective linguistic skills, whereas group therapy often produces more dramatic changes affecting a wider range of communication skills. An interpretation of the selective improvements gained by individual therapy may be that the child is being taught very specific language skills in relation to one person, the therapist. It is a controlled, ungeneralized, formal approach to language learning; it must be so for the child who cannot gain from the apparently haphazard linguistic environment utilized by his eloquent peers. The group situation is not so sensitively monitored, particularly in relation to the degree of control over the actions, interactions and utterances of other members of the group. In this sense the child experiences a greater variety of communication in action, but still more organized than his previous experience of language. For example, a child who uses few commands towards his therapist, when

[26] Grateful thanks go to Marielle Coghlan, Christine Scott and Jane Sparke for their backing and very hard work throughout; not forgetting the patience and valuable support of SC.

guided, seems to have few scruples in 'bossing' his peers (see also the comments in *GALD* (155) on questions towards therapists).

Our experience then, has led us to expect different results from individual and group therapy. Results are more definable from individual therapy, or (perhaps it should be said) more testable because of recent developments in assessment materials. Progress in a group is often of a different nature and this makes it more difficult to assess. There are vague subjective impressions from therapist, mother and nursery teacher, 'it seems as though he knows what he wants to say more', 'he mixes so much better with the other children', etc. There are few tests developed in relation to these areas of social and linguistic competence, so progress is not accurately identified and may remain unacknowledged. Thus any debate regarding the merits of individual versus group therapy has measurable evidence on one side only.

If we accept that both forms of therapy have something to offer, and what they offer is different, it may be that they are complementary and not in competition. Practically, it would be very time-consuming to offer two forms of therapy where one may suffice. The earlier question 'what is it that group therapy offers?' may become modified to 'can the benefits of group and individual therapy be combined?' That is, can the measurable aspects and remedial decisions of individual therapy be used within group therapy? To carry this through, one would attempt to take a group of children, combine their assessed abilities, and make remedial decisions as for an individual. We would not necessarily have any better measure of the less definable benefits of group therapy, but we would see whether we could produce results we had thought could only be brought about by individual therapy. We decided to attempt to evaluate therapy for a group of children in this way.

The children

The children were selected for the group in the normal way; that is, therapists within the Health Area put forward children they felt would gain from group therapy. The suitability of children was discussed by the Unit therapists who were going to run the group. The majority of the children were patients of the Unit therapists, but there was still a considerable variety of reasons for putting children forward (e.g. because the child had reached a plateau in individual therapy and needed a 'boost', or because a child appeared to be acquiring language but not its social uses). Criteria as to suitability were very loose at this stage, as children could still after assessment be eliminated from consideration for group therapy. Comprehension of over a three-year level and an ability to produce three-word utterances were base-line requirements. Children who had any behavioural problems or separation problems (mothers were not present during the group) were considered, as long as their numbers remained in the minority. In fact none of the children put forward were rejected after assessment. We took the first 14 children, and as none were rejected on assessment, we were left with this rather large group.

The children consisted of 2 girls and 12 boys between the chronological ages of 3;2 and 5;1. Verbal comprehension age range 2;10 to 5;5. There were practical problems in completing the post-therapy assessments for 3 of the children—consequently the data of only 11 children is presented here: 9 boys and 2 girls.

The assessments

We identified eight areas in which we wanted information

1 attention
2 symbolic processes
3 auditory skills (hearing, discrimination, recognition)
4 comprehension (verbal and visual)
5 speech functions and social behaviour
6 expression (syntax and manual expression)
7 vocabulary (receptive and expressive)
8 phonological systems

Each child was assessed a fortnight before the group commenced. The areas were assessed separately, although there is considerable overlap between some, e.g. (1) and (3), (2) and manual expression, (4) and (7). Where possible, the assessments were made by the child's own therapist. This was more important for the shy and/or unintelligible. The assessments had three purposes: to ensure the range of ability was not too great; to show us which areas required remediation; and to act as a 'before' test in a before-and-after test comparison.

We had difficulty in finding assessments that would not only give us levels for comparison, but would also give clear remedial directives. This, and our previous success with LARSP for individuals, influenced our choice in its use, against briefer syntax screening tests. It is not proposed to go into the assessments used for other areas, and they are only mentioned here to show how syntactic skills compared with other areas and also to stress that not all the group's time was spent on syntax.

Once the assessments had been completed, an average was calculated for each area to give a group profile. Using a group profile is probably the biggest single factor influencing remedial decisions which differentiates group therapy from individual therapy. No remedial decisions were based on the assessments of individuals. It is tempting to do so because averages hide individual problems; but had we not used group profiles we would have been administering individual therapy en masse rather than real group therapy.

Not all the assessments used give results directly comparable between areas. We were able to compare assessments that gave age scores to give us some idea of priorities of remediation. These assessments are compared in Fig. 27.

LARSP is not an assessment that gives a standardized age score, so it must be stressed that the syntactic level is only an average of roughly-estimated age levels. Whilst stressing its indeterminacy, it must be said that we feel it does give a true picture of the group's syntactic level in relation to other areas.

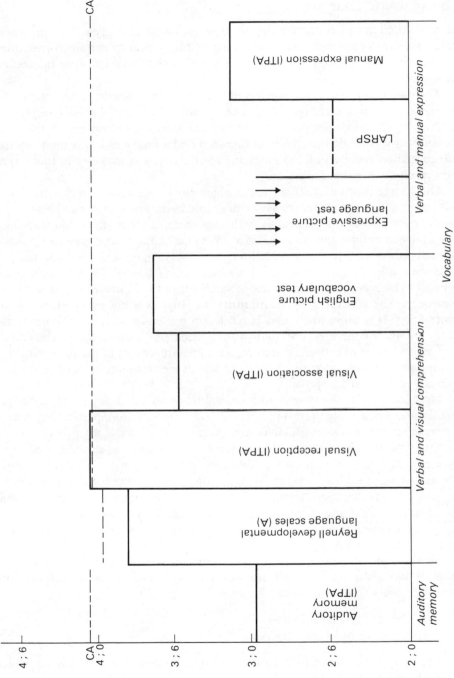

Fig. 27 Comparison of assessments giving age scores (expressed as group average) (RDLS CA appears lower because some RDLS administered prior to pregroup assessments.)

The syntactic analysis

As four different therapists were involved in the syntactic analysis, two measures were taken for conformity: cross-checking and adoption of certain conventions of analysis. These measures were necessary in that they revealed some interesting idiosyncrasies of analysis.

The speech sample was ten minutes of free play with toys, after a suitable warm-up period. The original transcript and analysis were made by the child's own therapist, as she was best equipped to make any semantic interpretations. A check of the analysis was made by a different therapist and a final check was made by the author, partly to collect all the problems of analysis. The majority of these were then resolved through discussion.

Our 'conventions of analysis' are problematical themselves, in that hard and fast rules cannot be created however desirable conformity may be. There is no one 'correct' analysis when dealing with something as idiomatic as language and as variable as child language acquisition. We made context and general syntactic maturity our most important yardsticks, just as Crystal *et al.* did in their analysis of Hugh's use of *can't* in *can't draw my buggy* (*GALD*, 153). At first sight there appears to be a negative verb phrase—Neg V Stage IV. However this is unlikely, considering the general syntactic maturity, as Hugh was not using either *can* or contraction. It is more likely that Hugh learnt *can't* as a whole. (In normal use of the profile for therapy, one could easily check this assumption at the child's next visit.) Our conventions, therefore, were introduced not to do away with discerning analysis, but to clarify points on which we were unclear and make our analyses as standard as possible.

No *incomplete* or *ambiguous* utterances were analysed at any point in our investigation. Remedially these often provide extra information, particularly necessary when structured or intelligible utterances are few. Frequently it is the clause structure that is the problem, whilst the structural relationships at phrase and word level may be clear. We rejected problematic utterances for two reasons, firstly because these problem utterances are more time-consuming, and secondly, because the fact that the utterance is incomplete or ambiguous may indicate that the child does not have complete control over the syntax involved. Our aim in the group was just as much to improve and consolidate 'shaky' syntax as to promote new constructions.

Semi-auxiliaries were marked as auxiliaries only if (a) the child was beyond Stage II and using Aux, and (b) the auxiliary was marked and therefore being used differently from a VV Stage II, e.g.

   (i) *they got go playschool* → VV
   (ii) *he('s) got to sit there* → Aux + V

In (ii) *got* is marked by *to* and *got to* seems equivalent to a modal, *must*, which would be marked as Aux.[27]

---

[27] *Got* is analysed above as a catenative, cf. p. 66.

Verb particles and *auxiliaries* were only recorded as such when used with a main verb. In fact, utterances without a main verb, which were felt semantically to contain a V Part were recorded as ambiguous, because without the main verb the intention is syntactically unclear, e.g.

$$
\text{that on} \begin{cases} \text{that television is } \underline{\text{turned on}} \\ \qquad\qquad\qquad\quad \text{V Part} \\ \\ \text{that television is } \underline{\text{on the table}} \\ \qquad\qquad\qquad\quad \text{A} \\ \qquad\qquad\qquad \text{Pr D N} \end{cases}
$$

Although constructions such as *I can* were often less ambiguous, we were reluctant to credit the child with the use of an auxiliary which by very definition should be an auxiliary of something. The child seems to be using *can* as a main verb with no verb phrase structure. In addition an utterance such as *he is* was ambiguous as to whether *is* was an Aux, or acting as the main verb and therefore a Cop.

Some sleepless nights were had over the recognition of *discourse features* (*GALD*, 81). Some children appeared to be using genuine 'empty' items, such as this method of listing toys present:

there's a chair . there's a bed . there's a table

Location was not being described (the chair is *there*, in a prescribed place). Two other children appeared to have words with some kind of comment status—

get daddy some then (where *then* was not time related)
he do it see (where there was no evidence of *see* being used as an imperative *look!* but rather an adult, *he's doing it you see*)

Possibly these children were exhibiting features more appropriate to their chronological age levels than their general syntactic levels. We remained unsure about discourse features in these children and did not attribute discourse-feature status unless a child was at Stage V or beyond.

Unmarked *3s* was not consistently recognized and, as it was felt to be of little remedial significance (rightly or wrongly), *3s* was omitted altogether.

Perhaps it is the infrequency of *subordinate clauses* when working with language-delayed preschool children, and consequent unfamiliarity, that led us to be unhappy in dealing with subordinate clauses. In the group samples, the majority of subordinate clauses were single instances, and therefore, marked under Subord. 1 and then under the appropriate heading, e.g. Clause: C/O (cf. p. 88 above for the 'standard' analysis here). This gave a false impression of high proficiency at Stage V clause level. We therefore made a distinction between unmarked clauses and clauses marked by a subordinator:

me know <u>what those are</u>   → Subord. 1
         s
mummy seen him <u>riding my bike</u>   → Clause: C/O

This convention is unsatisfactory when considering such utterances as:

the man says <u>that they must get up</u>→ Subord. 1
          s

the man says <u>they must get up</u>   → Clause: C/O

This does not necessarily mean that all Subord. 1 entries are marked clauses, because there is no separate category for unmarked adverbial clauses. Both the following would be recorded as Subord. 1:

I saw <u>that he was waiting at the bus stop</u> — Subord. 1
S V s   O   (marked)

I saw him <u>waiting at the bus stop</u>   — Subord. 1
S V O   A   (adverbial ummarked)

It may be necessary to reclassify subordinate clauses, not for ease of analysis, but according to remedial significance. With insufficient information on clausal development in the normal and language-delayed child, we were reluctant to make any changes in analysis and so continued to analyse in terms of marked and unmarked subordinate clauses.

Initially pronouns were recorded in the normal manner, i.e. making no discrimination as to type and expressing them as a total figure. Subsequently it was felt more relevant to our remedial considerations to record in more detail pronoun error types (see below).

The profiles

Concerning the range of syntactic ability, we observed the following from the profiles. The majority of children were at Stage III. Those who had more mature structures appearing further down the chart still had the bulk of their utterances within Stage III. Four children had utterances at Stage IV and three children had one or two dependent clauses each. One child, RH, had the bulk of his utterances at Stage II with a few structures at Stage III clause level; but there was little development at phrase level and consequently no expanded utterances. Another child, FO, was at Stage II apart from three X + V : VP and two Pron (ambiguous use of *me*). We did consider omitting RH and FO as they were so far behind the group syntactic level.[28] They were included on the grounds that they would benefit from help in other areas. As will be seen later we were rewarded for keeping them by the information we gained from their progress.

Our separate pronoun count can be seen in Table 2. It shows the *number of children* using personal pronouns and not the number of pronouns used. Eight children used some form of 1st person pronoun (four using *me* and two using both

[28] It is interesting to note, in relation to other areas, that RH and FO were the only two children whose ITPA manual expression scores were significantly below normal. The converse was not true, i.e. those with the most mature syntax did not achieve the highest manual expression score. However, the numbers involved are too small for serious conclusion.

I and *me* in subject position). Pronoun errors were mainly in replacing a subject pronoun with an object pronoun (a normal pattern of development, cf. *GALD*, 72).

Table 2   Numbers of children using Prons in the pregroup sample ($N=11$)

Personal Pron	*I*: 4	*you*: 2	*he*: 6	*she*: 2	*we*: 1	*they*: 3
Error	6		1			1
Correct O Pron	*me*: 2		*him*: 2	*her*: 1	*us*: —	*them*: —
Other: 10			*it*: 8			

Remedial decisions

Our decisions for remediation were not based solely on filling in the gaps and progressing down the chart. (This was partly because when a profile is calculated from a number of children, there is a wider spread of structures present than for one individual, and consequently there are fewer gaps.) Our main concern regarding syntax was to 'make more normal'. This involves attention to the distribution of structures in addition to presence or absence. We took as our normal distribution the normal $3\frac{1}{2}$-year-old in *GALD* (106) and made a comparison with the group's profile. To make them more comparable (the number of utterances varied so widely), each syntactic structure was expressed as a percentage of the individual's major sentence total. On comparison our children were lagging behind the normal $3\frac{1}{2}$-year-old in the following:

Stage III	SVO
	D Adj N
	Pr DN
	Aux
	pl
	ed
Stage IV	XY + A: AP
	SVOA
	AAXY
	Pr D Adj N
	cX
	XcX
	n't
	'cop
	'aux

The biggest discrepancies were for:

XY + A : AP
SVOA —used by 4/11 children
Aux   —used by 5/11 children
pl.   —used by 6/11 children
Pr DN
n't   —used by 3/11 children

In the above lists a common feature relates to the use of adverbials and expanded adverbials (Pr DN, Pr D Adj N). It was decided to work on Pr DN as a preliminary to using it in XY + A : AP structures. By this added attention to adverbials, particularly in VOA, we hoped we could bring about an increase in the use of SVOA.

From experience, children who have problems in acquiring Aux (and usually Cop) seem to have great difficulty, particularly if they have already ventured well into Stage IV without it. It was felt important to try and establish Aux (and Cop) before 'aux and 'cop, because although the latter may be more common, it is difficult to focus on the contracted forms, particularly where there are any phonological restrictions. It was decided to promote the most stressed form, i.e. the negative, or denial of the negative. This would also deal with the lack of *n't*.

Plurals and some personal pronouns were included in the remedial plan, very much on the grounds that developmentally they should have been acquired earlier. Our rather detailed analysis of pronouns (Table 2) was to guide us as to which pronouns needed encouragement and which pronouns were being overworked. Pronoun use can be indicative of limited vocabulary and we did not want to encourage this (cf. also the example on p. 14):

P   *that on there/*
     this one like that/
     got more that/ —
     that do that/
T   *that does what/*
P   *that/*

This type of child often gains a high pronoun total which may disguise a lack of personal pronouns. There was an additional reason for checking the use of personal pronouns. Pronouns are very very suitable for the introduction of new clause structures. This is particularly so with personal pronouns because they require no phrase structure (*the boy → he/him, some big boys → they/them*, etc.), and they are monosyllabic, making less demands in terms of articulation and utterance length. Few of our children had established a system of personal pronouns, so the following basic system was included in remediation: *I, you, he, she* and *it*.

Organization of the group

The children attended the Unit for three mornings a week for five weeks (fifteen $2\frac{3}{4}$ hour sessions). Of the 14 children, the 11 reported here attended approximately 75 per cent of the sessions. The morning was divided roughly into seven periods and a mid-morning break of about fifteen minutes' unstructured play outside. Activities were ordered so that a less physically active task requiring quiet and concentration was followed by a physically active task. Three of the four therapists were present and sometimes a student. There was an overall plan of therapy for the five weeks, but as we did not know how much time would need to be spent on a structure, the detailed planning was made at the end of each session, by the four therapists, for the following session.

Remediation

A description of remedial activities carried out over the five weeks would be too lengthy, so only the daily activities are described here, followed by a few notes on useful and popular tasks.

Daily activities were encouraged to establish a routine as this is often the quickest way to settle preschoolers and get down to work. Daily features involving syntax were a story and scrapbooks. Each week a story was planned to incorporate the topical syntactic structure on a repetitive basis. These stories consisted of a series of pictures with an utterance for each picture. On day 1 of the week, a therapist told the story completely, establishing the model. On day 2 she began to leave some of the target utterances unfinished:

T   *and the little boy is looking ...*
Ps   *in the shed/*
T   *but the dog isn't hiding ...*
Ps   *in the shed/*   etc.

On day 3 the children were encouraged to tell as much of the story as possible, prompted by the pictures. Surprisingly, after a few trials we found that three presentations of the story were not necessary. Two presentations were sufficient, either on two different days or one presentation immediately followed by another—providing that the story was well constructed, syntactically related to other remedial tasks, and pertinent to the experience of the children, e.g. falling off a bicycle and receiving a plaster produces instant involvement and concern. (Such identifiable predicaments seem to compel a response from the child, however limited. Initially FO's contribution was to say *yes* or *no*, with varying degrees of solemnity; but within two weeks his responses had conformed to target utterances.)

The scrapbook task was towards the end of each session, and served both to focus on one aspect of the morning's work and to keep parents in touch with what had been taught. Each picture had an utterance which was said by T, and an underlined utterance which was P's target response. This also helped gain consistency for stimulus questions and target responses.

Four different methods were used:

1 the forced alternative question, e.g.:
    Is it—the ball is in the hat
    or—the ball is behind the hat?
    The ball is in the hat

2 the unfinished sentence, e.g.:
  Here is a duck. Here are lots of . . .
  Ducks
3 the sequence sentence, e.g. (picture of three fat men and one thin man):
  Is he thin? He isn't. He isn't. He isn't (pointing to each in turn)
  He is (pointing to thin man)
  In this example the C is dropped in order to draw attention to the Cop and avoid the child's reply *he fat*.
4 the direct question with indirect models, e.g. (picture of boy climbing with girl looking on):
  He can climb. She can't climb. Can you climb? *I can (climb)*
  The child was allowed to drop the main verb if there was no other way of maintaining the Aux. The indirect models (i.e. with other pronouns) are to project an SV set, indicating a *yes/no* answer is not required.

Syntax games were divided into two types. Firstly, those where T gave a stimulus utterance to produce a target response from one or all of the children, and secondly where the stimulus utterance was also a target utterance, i.e. one of the children took over T's role as game leader and gave the stimulus utterance previously modelled for him. An Example was the *Is it black?* game. T had four large coloured bags in front of her (black, white, red and yellow, chosen on a developmental basis (cf. Cruse 1977). In turn a child selected an object from a box containing objects of the four colours, and placed it out of sight of T but in view of the group. T would pick up the black bag and say of the hidden object *is it black?* aiming for the target utterance *yes it is* or *no it isn't*. None of the children were using VS questions, but we hoped it would be possible, as there were repeated models and we had made the question finite (i.e. the presence of the coloured bags would enable the child to concentrate on the syntax rather than wondering what he should ask). In the event, over half the children managed a VS question, but few managed to produce the utterance without the support of a highly structured situation.

Syntax activity notes

Week 1	Pr DN → Pr D Adj N	e.g. 'musical prepositions'—when music stops children told by child leader *go Pr DN*. Children must state where they are before music recommences.
Week 2	SV (and VS) Pron *I, it* Aux, *can* Cop -n't	e.g. *I can/can't* games *is it black?* game

Week 3	SV Pron *he, she* Aux *is* Neg V pl. -n't	e.g. (*a*) *is he V-ing?* game—boy puppet on same principle as *is it black?* game, but T leader only. Target *he is V-ing/he isn't V-ing.* (*b*) *is he/she V-ing?*—extension of (*a*) with boy and girl puppets. Target *he is V-ing/she isn't V-ing.*
Week 4	V$_{(imp)}$OA (SVOA) Pron *he, she* Pr DN Aux *is* pl.	e.g. *stop/go* game—children run round room until child leader shouts *stop* and gives V$_{(imp)}$OA prompted by a picture, for children to enact. Once command carried out, new leader shouts *go* for game to recommence
Week 5	VOA SVA SVOA pron *I, you, he, she, it* Aux *is, can* Neg V n't	e.g. SVA 'obstacle race'—child commands second child to cross room by overcoming obstacle (*crawl under the chair*). Others asked to describe event. e.g. SVOA house wall frieze—T/child commands other to add to house picture (*stick a chimney on that house*). T asks for description of event.

'After'

Three to four weeks after the group had finished, the children were re-tested in certain areas. LARSP samples were taken and analysed as previously. The results were compared in Figs. 28 and 29 for Stages III and IV.

In Fig 28 Pr N from Stage II is included, because of the work on Pr DN as an expanded adverbial. There is a greater increase in the use of Pr N than in the use of Pr DN (and no real increase in Pr D Adj N at Stage II). Possibly this relates to the use of D. The majority of children appeared to be using DN, but on closer inspection many instances were possessive pronouns, frequently *my*. The context in which Pr DN was being encouraged required a definite article, which had not been established. The increase in Pr N may also be partly accounted for by the number of 'pronominal' children with poor vocabulary. Possibly, having been encouraged to replace their vague Prons and *here* and *there*, they made a straight substitute:

> *in that* → *in box*
> *under there* → *under table*

not recognizing that nouns act differently.

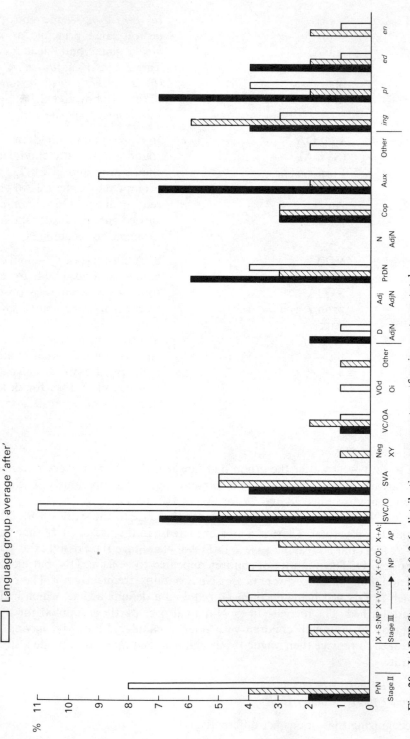

Fig. 28 LARSP Stage III 2;0–2;6: distribution as percentage of major sentence total

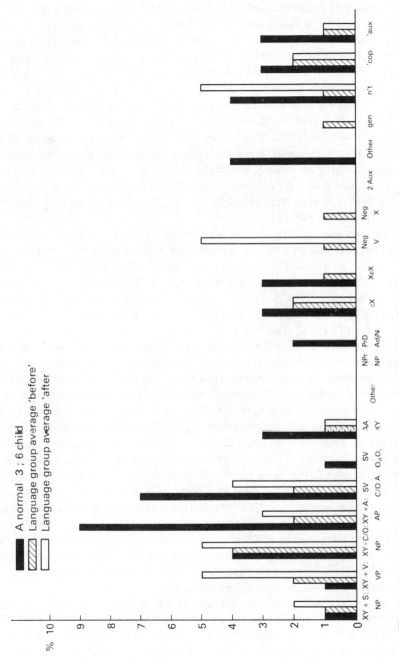

Fig. 29 LARSP Stage IV 2;6–3;0: distribution as percentage of major sentence total

It was initially surprising to see the great increase in SVO structures, but this may have resulted from vocabulary work on verbs which often presented them in this form, and from failed attempts at SVOA. The latter appears unlikely, as language delayed children more often drop S, providing V is secure, where there is length or novelty of vocabulary problems. Also, semantically the aim would have been different, but our approach may have cemented SVO syntactically, and focused on adverbials resulting in SVOA→SVO/AX as two utterances.

There is no increase, despite remediation, in SVA and VOA. Possibly the reduction in VOA is explained by the increase in SVOA. Regarding SVA, the increase in AX (not shown here) and X + A : AP, may indicate that for some children the burden of their new expanded adverbials restricted the number of clausal elements to two only. Looking at Table 3, which shows the number of children using certain structures 'before-and-after', it can be seen that the majority of the children were using SVA before, and all were able to use them 'after'. Four children gained SVOA without its previous use.

The group's use of XY + A : AP appears to be far from the norm. It would be easy to suggest that our normal 3½-year-old was not entirely normal in respect of XY + A : AP. Inspection of the nine instances of XY + A : AP tended to confirm this suggestion: there were only four SVA and one VOA, and no other instances of two clausal elements + A. It could be said that the group were following the normal adult trend of producing more XY + O : NP than XY + A : AP and in this respect were more consistent and normal than the 'normal' 3½-year-old!

The average use of Cop remains the same (both full and contracted forms), although Table 3 confirms that five more children were using it than previously. There is a dramatic increase in Aux (full form, which was how it was presented and encouraged remedially). There were also many instances of auxiliaries as main verbs, *he is* or *she can't*, which were not recorded as Aux (see conventions of analysis.) Again this reflects their presentation, and possibly more emphasis should have been placed on a progression towards Aux + V. In this case perhaps there should be more encouragement of the full form before such wide use of an elliptical form (see comments on ellipsis, *GALD*, 96). Nevertheless there was an increase in the use of VP incorporating Aux. This is a little disguised by the very popular use of V Part, which accounts for the majority of VPs appearing in the pre-group samples.

There is an increase in Neg V and some reduction in the use of Neg XY, reflecting the movement of the negative element from outside the utterance, to a position within the VP. (Neg V was only recorded if the VP was preceded by S, and Aux was followed by V or Cop was followed by C.)

The picture regarding the group's use of VP is a little confusing in relation to the normal child. It looks as though the increase in Neg V, X + V : VP and XY + V : VP has been promoted out of proportion. This reflects the unsuitability of our 'norm'—a group of children would have been preferable. (Sampling problems are more likely to occur with only one child, i.e. there is a lowering of the likelihood of occurrence of certain structures.) In the normal profile there are no Neg X or Neg XY at clause level, and no Neg V and Neg X at phrase level, but

Table 3 A 'before-and-after' comparison of use of structures that received remedial emphasis

☐ Structure used before and after   ▨ Structure used after only

● Structure used before and not after   ○ Structure not used at all

	SL	EL	RL	AC	FO	RH	BR	RG	PW	DW	PH
Age range	3 ; 2										5 ; 1
increase in major sentence total	+17	+7	+13	+10	+31	+21	+34	+18	+29	−11	+34
X + V : VP					▨						
X + A : AP					▨	▨					
SVA						▨					
VOA	○			▨	○	▨	▨	●			
PrN	▨	▨			▨	▨				●	
PrDN	○			●	▨	▨				○	
Cop				▨		○	▨			▨	▨
Aux	○	▨	▨		○	▨	▨				
pl.	○				▨	▨	▨		○		
XY + V : VP		▨	▨		▨	○					
XY + A : AP			▨	▨	○	○					
SVOA	▨		○		○	○	▨				▨
Neg V	▨		○		▨	▨	▨	▨			
n't	○	▨	○		▨	▨	▨	▨	▨		

four instances of *n't*. Also the normal child appears to have some difficulty in combining VP with other clausal elements (use of Aux, 'aux and V Parts, but no X + V: VP and only one XY + V: VP). It was concluded that the normal profile was more atypical than the group profile; but it had served its purpose.

The number of children using pronouns before-and-after is shown below. The results for the 1st person Pron are a little confusing because some children used both the correct and the incorrect forms at the same time. *I* was never used incorrectly, but there were frequent substitutions, usually *me* (and sometimes *my*; perhaps an ingenious blend of *I* and *me*). Eight children used some form of 1st person Pron before, and ten afterwards. During therapy we had encouraged the correct use of the subject Pron, but there was no active discouragement of the developmentally normal use of an object Pron in its place. Gender problems account for more of the *he* and *she* errors than object Pron substitution. For two children, phonological limitations may have caused the lack of differentiation, but for others there appeared to be problems of identification, possibly exacerbated by the cultural swing towards 'unisex' appearance. Also, there were only two girls in the total of eleven samples, which may have biased conversational topics (on the supposition that male children are more likely to identify with, and talk about, things male). This female minority certainly influenced our group work, where children were required to describe another child's actions.

Table 4   Numbers of children using Prons before-and-after ($N=11$)

Personal Pron	I: $4\rightarrow9$	you: $2\rightarrow5$	he: $6\rightarrow8$	she: $2\rightarrow3$	we: $1\rightarrow4$	$they$: $3\rightarrow6$
Error	$6\rightarrow6$		$1\rightarrow4$	$0\rightarrow1$		$1\rightarrow2$
Correct O Pron	me: $2\rightarrow7$		him: $2\rightarrow3$	her: $1\rightarrow1$	us: —	$them$: $0\rightarrow2$
Other: $10\rightarrow11$			it: $8\rightarrow11$			

To return to Table 3, which shows the number of children using remediated structures before and afterwards, there are a few further points to note. All the children, except DW, produced an increase in the number of major utterances for the post-group samples (timing remained the same). One might expect a reduction in the number of utterances if there is an increase in syntactic complexity and utterance length (RG, who has the most mature syntax and uses the longest utterances, produces the fewest). Some increase in the number of utterances is accounted for by a decrease in social minor utterances (from average 27 to average 23) and the increase in spontaneous utterances (from average 36 to 41). We may also be witnessing here the vague intuition expressed before ('he seems to know what he wants to say more'), although it is not easy to prove exactly what is being measured. DW's decrease in major utterances does not invalidate the argument. In the post-group sample he produced the same number of minor utterances, but twenty fewer spontaneous utterances. His own therapist was unable to collect the post-group sample (which should have no effect if one of the benefits of the group is a widening of communicative experience). On looking through the transcript and the accompanying notes, it looks as though the real reason for DW's decrease in major utterances was that his word-finding and word-order problems, which were known to fluctuate, were particularly bad on the day of the post-group sample. The dysrhythmic and disjointed nature of delivery resulted in an increase in the length of time taken to produce an utterance.

The crossed boxes in Table 2 show that a structure was used 'before' and not 'after'. The infrequency of this occurrence, in relation to the designated structures, can be taken as indicative of some reliability in the method of sampling—i.e. if a child could use a structure, he was likely to do so in the ten-minute sampling period.

The last point to be made about Table 3 concerns the progress made by the two children, FO and RH, whom we had considered excluding on the grounds of the severity of their syntactic delay in relation to the syntactic level of the group as a whole. FO and RH had acquired the largest number of new syntactic structures. One might conclude that if our sole aim had been to teach new structures, we could have been very much more ambitious. However, this had not been our aim, because use of certain syntactic structures does not necessarily indicate an increase of effectiveness of communication, or more normal language.

FO and RH used each new structure only once or twice, presumably because they were limited in the use to which their new structures could be put. They were most likely to use their new structures in situations akin to that in which they had been taught. From that point of view they had not made as much progress as the rest of the group. The remainder of the group had not only acquired some new structures, probably nearer their pre-group syntactic levels, but they had also acquired a more normal and confident usage of syntax as reflected in the shifts in the distribution of structures.

Conclusion

We felt that the children in the group had progressed towards more normal syntax. (The syntax can still be seen as more 'normal' despite an unsuitable choice of norm.) The children had also gained new structures, particularly those 'taught'.

Such claims may appear to be of little use without a control or a definition of the child type. It is difficult both ethically and diagnostically to use controls. The children were not homogeneous in their language problems and can perhaps only be loosely described in terms of their common feature—they were all children with language learning problems requiring speech therapy. In that sense, they were all children who would not have made the same sort of progress spontaneously. In fact, the majority of the children already attended a non-remedial group, play-group or nursery, and many of the children had been put forward for the group because of a lack of progress in individual therapy.

The wider issues of whether the benefits of individual and group therapy can be combined, cannot be answered without reference to all the areas of assessment, and so will not be considered here. However, in relation to LARSP we are much nearer the answer to the earlier question—can the measurable aspects and remedial decisions of individual therapy be used within group therapy? Syntax can be taught in a group, but considerable problems remain in identifying the syntax to be taught.

The next step

It is not advocated that LARSP be always used in the way that has been presented here. We would not use LARSP ourselves in this time-consuming manner for normal clinical practice, only for specific projects such as method evaluation. This is not to say that LARSP, as it is at present, is not the best form of evaluating an individual's syntactic progress whilst giving remedial directives. With an individual, there are considerable 'pay-offs' for the time involved, in that a child makes better syntactic progress and therefore in the long run takes less speech-therapy time. For a group of children, the difficulty is in finding time to make a number of analyses at the same time, which urges us to look for a less time-consuming procedure that does not lose us the benefits of LARSP.

It is often the transcription, and not the analysis, that is the most time-consuming. This suggests that some attempt should be made to dispense with transcription and to make a 'live' analysis. It is possible to analyse the stages, if T is very familiar with analysis and P is sufficiently intelligible. T allows mother, student or helper to engage P in conversation, leaving her free to concentrate on marking down utterances as they occur. A taperecording can be made for checking and clarifying or gathering further information such as for Sections A, B, and C and the various totals. Admittedly 'live' analysis is a very difficult task for T if the present LARSP profile is used, because of the great number of structures T must instantly recognize and analyse at three different levels. (It is also about as attractive as three-dimensional chess on a Friday afternoon.)

At the moment such an approach is only really successful with a child using simple language. Conversely it would be possible if the profile were to be simplified. Before such a step is taken more information, in relation to the present profile, is needed on normative data; on the hierarchical relationships in developing syntax; and on indications as to which structures are of most significance remedially. The three are interelated, in that normative data will give some indications of hierarchical relationships, which in turn will give valuable information on remedial significance. Finally one could reduce the profile to remedially significant items only.

More normative data would indicate normally significant items, that is, it would be possible to see by distribution the important remedial goals in 'making more normal'. It may also serve to decrease time spent on remedial decisions. At present, it is difficult to know if a child has really mastered a structure when he uses it only once or twice. FO and RH illustrated this point previously in that, although they had theoretically acquired a number of new structures, it was not felt that they were able to use them normally.

If one accepts the concept of hierarchical development of syntax (*order* is stressed in *GALD*, and is basic to remediation), one assumes certain structures are foundations for the development of further construction. If the key relationships were recognized, it might be possible to reduce the profile and make for easier recognition of a level and readiness for specific forms of remediation. Having identified these relationships, it would then be necessary to recognize which can and which cannot be developed without remediation, that is, we would be evaluating the remedial significance of items. Perhaps it may be possible also to reduce the profile in terms of what may be remediated coincidentally: thus, if the remediation of Neg V always successfully included n't and *do* XY, and use was concurrent, they could all become one entry. It may appear obvious to say that any item which it has not been found necessary to remediate should be omitted, but this cannot be done until experience is confirmed by data.

These are only suggestions, and they need considerable further thought and information; or indeed many of the benefits of LARSP would be dissipated. So far we are only just beginning to recognize the applications and contributions of LARSP; but it is essentially a long-needed practical tool, the effectiveness of which can only be improved through use and evaluation of use.

2.5

A partially-hearing unit

J. E. Williams and D. B. Dennis

The education of severely and profoundly deaf children can only rarely be described as a modified version of normal education. It is more frequently an attempt to provide the child with those prerequisites for learning which the normal five-year-old has acquired before he ever starts school. The education of deaf children is predominantly a question of teaching children their mother tongue—often almost from scratch.

It is questionable, however, whether conventional forms of speech training and language work are adequate for this enormous task. The linguistic attainments of deaf children have proved to be lamentably low and there is increasing criticism of the existing 'oral' approach to deaf education. In the face of this criticism, we would defend the aims of the 'oral' tradition, but would concede that its achievements, and by implication its methodology, leave much to be desired.

We believe that any attempt to improve standards will require a careful appraisal of the rapidly expanding discipline of developmental and applied linguistics and an examination of what we might learn from such related fields as the teaching of dysphasic and mentally handicapped children. Such an examination would reveal that their methodology differs from the language enrichment programmes devised for deprived children and from the 'total immersion' techniques designed for adults learning a foreign language. In the case of the last two groups we can assume that the basic elements of their mother tongue are quite well established, but with dysphasic and mentally handicapped children no such assumption can be made. It is not surprising therefore that in language work with handicapped children there should be a special emphasis on the development of syntax. Indeed, most teachers of the deaf need look no further afield than at their own pupils' spoken and written language in order to see that a substantial proportion of them are lacking not so much in ideas and vocabulary as in the ability to combine words into phrases, phrases into sentences, and to use a wide range of sentence patterns in their appropriate context.

The training of teachers of the deaf has traditionally included the following subjects: child development; language development; curriculum and methods; auditory training; and speech training. In our view, LARSP has direct relevance to the first three and important implications for the last two. What LARSP offers is an explicit, systematic, and comprehensive schedule against which to examine the development of syntax in deaf children. It can be used in the following ways: to assess the spoken or written language of deaf pupils; to examine from a syntactic point of view the appropriateness of materials for reading and language development; to help in the construction of any language development scheme; to plan or review a language teaching schedule for an individual pupil; and to develop a more structured and systematic approach to all forms of language teaching, whether formal or informal, oral or written. During the period 1975–7 teachers of children with impaired hearing in the Cambridge area have used LARSP in each of the ways described above. It is convenient therefore to discuss its use under the three headings of Assessment, Materials and Methodology.

Assessment

Early in 1977 the teachers in Cambridgeshire's Partially Hearing Units were asked to offer the names of those pupils whose language development was causing them the greatest concern. Forty names were submitted out of a total of about 100 pupils. These 40 pupils were visited by an educational psychologist and a sample of their unaided free writing was obtained by asking them to write as much as they could about three large and vivid illustrations from the GOAL language development materials. The samples of free writing were then analysed using the lower section of the LARSP profile. These analyses revealed that 29 pupils had used structures only below the level of Stage V. An examination of their audiograms showed that all but four of these pupils were severely deaf, having an average hearing loss in the better ear of more than 80 dB over the frequency range 500 to 4000 Hz. These 25 severely deaf pupils, aged between 7 and 15, were then further assessed for IQ and Reading Age: the IQ range was from 65 to 125, on the Snijders-Oomen Non-Verbal Test; Reading Age ranged from 6·5 to 8·5 on the Hamp Picture Test.

Using LARSP, a count was made of the number of structures appearing in their sample of free writing at Clause, Phrase and Word levels. The total number of different structures appearing at least once varied from one to 24. Some idea of what these 'scores' indicate can be gained from the observation that a single sentence such as

$$
\begin{array}{ccc}
\underline{\textit{The boys}} & \underline{\textit{are very happy}} & \\
\text{S} & \text{V} & \text{C} \\
\text{D} \quad \text{N}_{\text{pl}} & \text{Cop} \quad \text{Int} \quad \text{X} & \\
\text{XY}+\text{S:NP} & \text{XY}+\text{C:NP} &
\end{array}
$$

would have yielded a 'score' of 7, and one more sentence such as

$$
\begin{array}{ccc}
\underline{\textit{They are not going}} & \underline{\textit{to school}} \\
\text{S} & \text{V} & \text{A} \\
\text{Pron} \quad \text{Aux Neg V} & \text{Pr N} \\
\text{-ing} \\
\text{XY}+\text{V:VP} & \text{XY}+\text{A:AP}
\end{array}
$$

would have added 8 more structures, making a total of 15 for just two sentences.

One of the most attractive features of LARSP is that it provides a detailed and very finely graded assessment for severely deaf pupils' use of language. In this study, for example, it revealed that over half of the 25 pupils had used fewer than 16 different structures in this sample of free writing. This extreme paucity of syntax was not attributable to any great lack of fluency in writing, since the number of sentences written by each pupil varied from 5 to 34 and averaged about 17. A more detailed examination of the 25 profiles revealed, moreover, that, in a total of more than 400 sentences, certain structures were either completely absent or occurred very rarely.

At clause level, for example, we found:

1 only one negative construction, viz. *The baby not can swim*;
2 no exclamatory or imperative forms such as might occur in direct speech, and only one interrogative construction, viz. *The butcher said to the lady do you wanted some ham*;
3 only one indirect object construction, viz. *A big brid give a warm to the baby brids*;

At phrase level we found:

4 no examples of VV;
5 only four instances of V Part, viz. *pull in*, *put in*, *looking round*, *running away*;
6 only two instances of Int X, viz. *very big*, *very soon*;
7 only nine instances of a pronoun, viz. *it* and *she* three times each, *you*, *he* and *her* once each;

At word level we found:

8 only one instance of a past participle (*-en*), viz. *The meat is cooked*;
9 no instance of 3s;
10 only one instance of the genitive, viz. *birds nest*;
11 only one instance of a comparative adjective, viz. *The lake is bigger*;
12 no examples of *-n't*, 'cop, 'aux, *-est*, or *-ly*.

There were on the other hand relatively few 'conventional' grammatical errors of the type one would expect to occur in the course of a normally-hearing child's language development. Those which did occur would be classified by LARSP in the following way:

1 choice of determiner (8 errors), e.g. *a sandwiches, some woman buy ...*, *a money*;
2 inflexion of irregular nouns (5 errors), e.g. *the childrens, some foods, the meats*;
3 choice of preposition (5 errors), e.g. *the cloud is on the sun, the flowers are on the garden, the people are walking at the shop, a boy jumped onto the swimming pool*;
4 wrong tense forms (2 errors), e.g. *the boys are found the fish*; lack of concord (2 errors), e.g. *the two bird is in the nest*; wrong word order (2 errors), e.g. *the tree is on the bird*;

It would appear therefore that conventional teaching procedures have failed to equip these severely handicapped pupils with an appropriate range of syntactic structure, and that what these children most require is not to have their grammatical errors corrected but rather to have their use of syntax expanded, especially in the twelve 'problem areas' listed above. Since, moreover, none of these children can write as fluently as a normal three-year-old can talk, the question arises whether we can afford to allow them to continue to develop language 'naturally' by exposure to traditional methods, or whether, having identified a number of problem areas, we should not seek to remediate these areas by means of more systematic methods, in the hope that what has not been learned 'naturally' may be taught in a more consciously structured way.

In view of the considerable scepticism which exists about systematic and carefully structured teaching methods, it would appear necessary at this point to attempt to dispel some of the illusory misgivings that some teachers of the deaf still have about them. A carefully-structured approach is sometimes thought to imply an emphasis on writing at the expense of talking, an intolerable degree of formality in the classroom, and neglect of the pupils' needs for the convenience of the teacher. These criticisms may possibly have been justified in the past, but it does not follow from this that they are still relevant today. It may well be the case that in the past we lacked both the assessment procedures and the linguistic insight which are the essential prerequisites for a systematic approach to be successfully adopted. Now it should be clear that systematic teaching methods are a logical sequel to systematic assessment procedures. LARSP provides both a systematic assessment procedure and a basis for systematic remediation.

Materials

Having established at what level a pupil is functioning from a syntactic point of view, the teacher is then committed to finding or producing appropriate teaching materials which will lead the pupil through the next stages of his linguistic development without offending either his intelligence or his maturity level. The question of whether or not the pupil's level of syntactic comprehension may exceed his level of syntactic expression is perhaps open to debate. If, however, we are anxious to develop his expressive language along normal lines, then it would appear logical to present him with a variety of linguistic input at a level not grossly exceeding what we can be absolutely sure he understands—that being the level at which he expresses himself. After all, no normally-hearing child who expresses himself like a two-year-old is expected to read or understand language intended for a seven-year-old.

There is unfortunately a dearth of reading material for children with grossly-delayed language development and many teachers feel obliged to produce their own. One of the few publishers of reading books with carefully controlled syntax is the OUP with their Oxford Colour Readers and Oxford Graded Readers; and a commendable attempt is currently being made by the Breakthrough Trust Project to rewrite simple language editions of some standard reading material.

An attempt to teach very elementary sentence patterns through reading is to be found in the Woodford Trust publication *Guidelines*. We find however that this material is rather selective in its choice of structures, and that the order in which they are introduced in no way conforms to the normal developmental schedule suggested by LARSP. Picture material can be an invaluable aid to language development, and an extensive range of picture sets and picture sequences is available from Learning Development Aids (LDA). The advantage of such material is that it can easily be rearranged and used according to a developmental schedule. Picture story material which helps to elicit simple but interesting language is also provided by Nora Wilkinson's books of printed spirit duplicator masters *Pictures and Conversations*.

As far as we are aware, no material has been published in this country which is specifically designed to develop deaf children's use of syntax according to a normal developmental schedule. Such schemes have been attempted, however, for other categories of handicapped children. There is, for example, Lea's (1970) Colour Pattern Scheme for dysphasic children, and a number of projects have been developed for mentally handicapped children at the Manchester Hester Adrian Centre. As far as deaf pupils are concerned, most systematic teaching schemes appear to have originated in the USA, where at the present time there seem to be almost as many language-development programmes as there are Schools for the Deaf. One factor which they have in common, however, is their emphasis upon the teaching of syntactic structure.

Methodology

Most language development schemes for deaf pupils rely largely upon teaching language in its written form. The justification for this is that by so doing they capitalize on the pupil's ability to read—the assumption being that what children have failed to learn by listening to transitory and elliptical speech they can be taught by the use of the more permanent and explicit written form. One disadvantage of using the written form, however, is that teachers frequently require the pupil to respond in full and complete sentences, and to this extent their methodology is likely to conflict with any developmental schedule based on normal child language. This criticism would apply to any system which resembled the Fitzgerald Key. Such a scheme also suffers from the disadvantages of relying on only one overall sentence pattern and requiring pupils to have a full understanding of *wh-*question forms before they can be helped to expand their own utterances. Our reservations about using the John Lea Scheme with deaf pupils are also influenced by what we have learned from LARSP. In this case we would question the value of analysing language into single-word elements which are colour-coded according to their function as parts of speech. When this is done there is no way of identifying consistent patterns of sentence structure without limiting the language to paradigms of rather stereotyped utterances.

What LARSP would appear to suggest is that it is only possible to indicate and identify a linguistically flexible range of sentence structure by an analysis at clause level rather than at phrase level, i.e. SV:SVO:SVC:SVA:SVOA:SVOO: SVOC. Compared with an analysis based on parts of speech, this analysis at clause level provides a much more succinct, practical and flexible guide to the range of sentence structure which severely deaf pupils need to learn. Apart from their use in positive statements, care should also be taken to present them in their negative and interrogative forms and with appropriate expansions at phrase level. A full range of sentence patterns and their expansions can be illustrated by examples of the kind of response to be encouraged at two very different stages of development:

	Basic	*Expanded*
SV	Concorde/is flying	Concorde/is starting to take off
SVO	The plane/makes/lots of smoke	The passengers/have fastened/their safety belts
SVC	The smoke/is/dirty	Concorde/is/a supersonic jet
SVA	Concorde/is/in the sky	A supersonic jet/flies/5 miles up
SVOA	Planes/make/smoke/in the air	A plane like Concorde/can take/passengers/all over the world
SVOO	Can you show/me/the smoke?	Some Americans/did not want to give/Concorde/permission to land
SVOC	Smoke/makes/you/sick	Concorde/may make/Kennedy Airport/very noisy

When the idea of colour-coding is applied to this system of clause analysis, then the result is a limited number of colour sequences which can be used to indicate sentence structure. If, for example, we code:

V	BLUE
any Noun Phrase occurring as S, O, C, or within A	RED
and any other C or A	YELLOW

we produce the following colour sequences:

RED BLUE	Concorde/is flying
RED BLUE RED	The plane/makes/a lot of smoke
	Concorde/is/a jet
	The plane/is/in the sky
RED BLUE YELLOW	Concorde/is/very big
	It/flies/very fast
RED BLUE RED RED	I/can show/you/the smoke
	Planes/make/smoke/in the air
RED BLUE RED YELLOW	Smoke/makes/you/sick

This coding system used in the form of either underlining or colour coded cards and presented in a carefully graded fashion forms the basis of *Graded Syntax*— a language-development scheme devised by the first author of this chapter.

Perhaps the most practical use for LARSP is in the planning or review of a language-teaching schedule for an individual pupil. In illustrating this, however, it is first of all important to know something of the working relationship between the two authors of this chapter. The first author is a Peripatetic Teacher of the Deaf in East Cambridgeshire. Having initiated the use of LARSP with deaf children in the area, he has undertaken a caseload of 20 slower-learning deaf pupils, assessing them with the LARSP Profile and helping and advising six Unit Teachers on appropriate remedial procedures. The second author is a Unit Teacher of the Deaf at a secondary school. Pupils of the Unit (8 profoundly deaf, 4 partially-hearing) integrate in school activities to the best of their ability. Certain pupils integrate for the majority of the timetable; others, owing to greater language problems, have more difficulty in integrating. It is with the latter group of pupils that the authors have concentrated their efforts using LARSP. The first author visits the Unit on one morning, while the second author works to a structured plan throughout the week. Of the less successful pupils, Diane was linguistically the greatest problem until her introduction to a LARSP-based schedule. It was for this reason that we have chosen her as an example of LARSP's effectiveness.

Case study

The four profiles reproduced in this chapter were obtained from samples of free writing by the same pupil in the course of four consecutive school years. This girl was born in 1962, and diagnosed as severely deaf in 1964; she entered a Residential School in 1965. Two years later her family moved into Cambridgeshire and

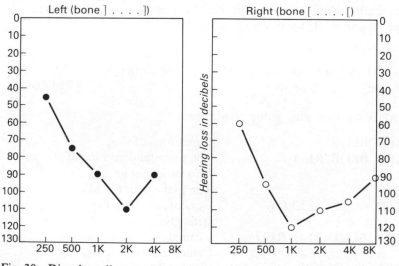

Fig. 30   Diane's audiogram (Nov. 1976)

requested that she be transferred to an Infant Partially-Hearing Unit. They were disturbed that their daughter had begun to use manual signs at home. Progress throughout Infant and Junior School was extremely slow and the first two profiles given below are a fair reflection of her level of language development at the time she started Secondary Education in 1973. Progress continued to be slow until 1975 (see Profile C, below). At this time we began to work with her on a more systematic basis by using the LARSP profile to identify specific areas of syntactic difficulty and by taking what LARSP suggested to be the most appropriate remedial action. An indication of how LARSP can form the basis of a remedial programme is provided by the Outline of Individual Sessions 1975–7. Despite the fact that this is probably the most problematic child in our unit, we are pleased to report that since 1975 her syntactic development has accelerated and is continuing to do so (see Profiles D and E below). This pupil has been accredited with an IQ score of 92 on the Snijders-Ooomen Non Verbal Test (1977). An audiogram made in November 1976 is given as Fig. 30.

Date	Syntactic area	LARSP Chart	Topic
1975			
22/9	Present tense		My day
	Prepositional phrases	Pr N	
		Pr D N	
		Pr Adj N	
29/9	Verb particles	V part	My day
6/10	Irregular past tense	-ed	Yesterday
13/10	Revision		My day
			Yesterday
20/10	Prepositional phrases incorporated in three-element clauses	S V $\overline{\quad}$ A $\overline{\text{Pr D N}}$	
10/11	*is/was*	-ed	The calendar
1976			
12/1	Past tense	-ed	Christmas
19/1	Past tense incorporated in full sentences	S V O A -ed	On Saturday
26/1	Free writing of three-element sentences		Yesterday
2/2	*Who are they?*	S V C	Picture cards
	What are they doing?	S V	
	What are they like?	S V C	
9/2	*When/Where are they going?*	S V A	
	What happened?	S V O (A) -ed	
16/2	Free writing of three- and	S V O (A)	My weekend
23/2	four-element sentences		The dogfight
1/3		S V (O) A	My weekend

Date	Syntactic area	LARSP Chart	Topic
1976			
8/3	Revision		
15/3	Free writing of three-	Stage III	Diane hurts her arm
22/3	element sentences		My teacher
29/3	Improvement and expansion of free writing		
3/5	Ordinal numbers	Adj N	The calendar
17/5	Past tense	-ed	My weekend
24/5	Revision		
14/6	Substitution exercise	$\dfrac{\text{S V} \quad \text{A}}{\text{Pr D N}}$	
	Verbs of movement	pl	
5/7	Revision		Last Christmas
13/9	Free writing of three-	S V A	My trip to Holland
	and four-element sentences	S V O A	
		S V A A	
20/9	*Where are they?*	$\dfrac{\text{S V} \quad \text{A}}{\text{Pr D N}}$	Picture cards
	What do they look like?	$\dfrac{\text{S V} \quad \text{C}}{\text{XcX}}$	
27/9	Free writing	Stage III	Seaside poster
11/10	Revision		
18/10	Present continuous	Aux -ing	Picture cards
	What do they look like?	$\dfrac{\text{S V} \quad \text{C}}{\text{Int X}}$	
1/11	*What are they doing?*	S V O	
		Varieties of	
		Aux -ing	
8/11	Free writing	$\dfrac{\text{S V} \quad \text{A}}{\text{Pr D N}}$	Guy Fawkes Fair
	Use of prepositions		
15/11	Revision		
29/11	Negatives	Neg XY	Contrasting picture cards
		Neg V	
1977			
17/1	Demonstrative and	$\dfrac{\text{S V} \quad \text{O}}{\text{Varieties}}$	
	possessive adjectives	of DN	
24/1	Elliptical responses to	S V	Written conversation
	yes/no questions	Pron	
7/2	Revision		
14/2	Free writing		My boyfriend
28/2	Verbs taking direct and indirect	S V O$_d$ O$_i$	Being kind
	object e.g. *give, read, lend, show,*	S V O$_i$ O$_d$	
	fetch, say		
14/3	Revision	-ed	Christmas presents
21/3	Full responses to *yes/no* questions		Written conversation

Date	Syntactic area	LARSP Chart	Topic
1977			
28/3	Revision		
2/5	Negative elliptical responses to questions	Neg XY Neg V	Incongruous questions
9/5	Full negative responses to questions		Written conversation
23/5	Revision		
30/5	Future tense *going to*	VV	Making plans
20/6	Expansion of the subject noun phrase or the complement	S V C NN D Adj N	My relatives Who's who

Profiles A and B

A retrospective profile analysis was made of Diane's written work, obtained in November 1973. She was asked to look at a series of unrelated pictures on a card and to describe them in writing. In each case we have transcribed the writing as accurately as possible, and then provided a gloss (which in our interpretation of the picture is appropriate and corresponds most closely to what we think Denise was trying to express.) Each item was written on a separate line, and this provides our main evidence of sentence identification (punctuation being somewhat inconsistent). This range of data illustrates a further problem, very typical of written language of the deaf, namely that more than half the sentences are technically deviant or problematic. In sentences (2) and (5) below there is a double determiner; in (3) and (20), auxiliary verb is present at the expense of the main verb; there is verb/noun confusion in (7), (12) and (18); there is word-order deviance in (9) and (13); there is a deviant verb sequence in (11); there are problems of interpretation in (4) and (6). This proportion of 'unanalysed' material is the main reason for the very thin profile A (Fig. 31, p. 227). However, in cases of this kind, we have found it useful to produce a second, 'normalized' profile, where those parts of the sentences that seem to be being accurately used are profiled in the normal way, the deviances classified in the Stage VI Error box, and any 'obvious' irrelevance discounted (e.g. *in* in (13)). We appreciate the dangers involved in any such rationalization, but have found that the fuller profile which emerges can be helpful, in that it points up more clearly the contrast between P's areas of structural strength and weakness. Profile B (incorporating the analyses labelled B below) shows this fuller picture, which is in several respects typical of profiles obtained from the deaf: the over-use of certain sentence types at the expense of others is clearly seen in the relatively high figures for Stage III/IV transitional structure, and for 3s, compared with the several gaps earlier; the expansion of subject NPs at the expense of post-verbal NPs is also visible; and the cluster of errors at Stage VI, with no Stage IV–V development, further illustrates the unbalanced nature of the language learning which has taken place so far.

1
      The   dog   in the basket   (= 'the dog is in the basket')
A,B   S   A
            D   N Pr D   N
            XY + S:NP XY + A:AP

2
      The   car   is   a the   webr   (= 'the car is by the windmill')
B   S   V   A   A   Deviant
            D   N Cop D D N
                   3s
          XY + S:NP   XY + A:AP
                        —Det (DDN)
                        —Prep (omission)

3
      The boy is frsch   (= 'the boy is holding a flag')
B   [clause analysis unclear]   A   Deviant
            D N   [VP analysis unclear]
              3s

4
      The   man   is   on the fish   (= 'the man is fishing')
B   S   V   A   A   Problematic (Ambiguous)
            D   N Cop Pr D N
                  3s
          XY + S:NP   XY + A:AP
                        —Prep (or V)

5
      The   man   is   a the goesr   (= 'the man is a grocer')
B   S   V   C   A   Deviant
            D   N Cop D D   N
                  3s
          XY + S:NP   XY + C:NP
                        —Det

6
      The man is work wall   (= 'the man is working ?on a wall')
B   [clause analysis unclear—   A Problematic (Ambiguous)
      whether SVO or SVA]
         D   N Aux v
              3s
         XY + S:NP XY + V:VP
                —Tense   (-ing)

7
      The Lady is ear Tereraiy (= 'the lady is listening to the telephone')
B   [clause analysis unclear—   A   Deviant
      is *ear* verb or noun?]
         D   N [VP analysis unclear]
               3s
        XY + S:NP

8
          The Lady is in the car (= 'the lady is by the car')
A,B   <u>S</u>   <u>V</u>   <u>A</u>

          D N Cop Pr D N
                   3s

          XY + S:NP   XY + A:AP

9
          The lady mansare   (= 'the ladies are with the men')
B   [clause analysis unclear]   A   Deviant

          D N   Cop

          XY + S:NP
                —Word order
                —N irreg
                —Det
                —Concord

10
          The bady see the bary   (= 'the baby sees the bag')
A,B   <u>S</u>   <u>V</u>   <u>O</u>

          D N   D N

          XY + S:NP   XY + O:NP
                —Concord

11
          Two boy is are the singing   (= 'two boys are singing')
B   <u>S</u>   <u>V</u>   A   Deviant

          Adj N Aux Aux D v
               3s   -ing

          XY + S:NP   XY + V:VP
                —Tense (2 Aux)
                —Det (or possibly —Word order:
                'the two boys')
                —Concord

12
        Two is in the eating   (= 'two men are eating')
B   Deviant (i.e. no clear analysis
       at any level)   A   Deviant

13
          The lady [in] is cleaning the worwr   (= 'the lady is
B   <u>S</u>   <u>V</u>   <u>O</u>   cleaning the

          D N   Aux   v   D N   window')
                    3s   -ing   A Deviant

          XY + S:NP   XY + V:VP   XY + O:NP
             —Prep

14   *The man   are going fis*   (='the men are going fast'
A,B   S   V   A   [picture of racing cars])
      D   N   Aux   v
                        -ing

XY+S:NP XY+V:VP
          —Concord (or possibly
              N irreg)

15   *The lady   is swimming*
A,B   S   V
      D   N   Aux   v
                  3s   -ing

X+S:NP   X+V:VP

16   *The man   is playing the balbr*   (='the man is playing
A,B   S   V   O   the drum')
      D   N   Aux   v   D   N
                  3s   -ing

XY+S:NP   XY+V:VP   XY+O:NP

17   *Two peuple are riding   thehores*   (='two people are rid-
A,B   S   V   O   ing the horses' [two
      Adj   N   Aux   v   D   N   horses in the picture])
                    -ing   ?pl

XY+S:NP XY+V:VP XY+O:NP

18   *The man firen the sleep*   (='the man has fallen asleep')
B   [clause analysis unclear]   A   Deviant
      D   N   [VP analysis unclear]

19   *The lady man are the Spanish*   (='the lady and man are Span-
A,B   S   V   C   ish')
      D   N   N Cop D   N
XY+S:NP   XY+C:NP
—Conjunction   —Det

20   *queen is the cohw*   (='the queen is wearing the crown')
B   [clause analysis unclear—   A   Deviant
      'is'=Aux? or 'has'?]
             D   N
      3s

A	Unanalysed		Problematic	
	1 Unintelligible	2 Symbolic Noise	3 Deviant **9**	1 Incomplete	2 Ambiguous **2**

B Responses

				Normal Response							Abnormal		
					Elliptical Major				Full		Struc-		Prob-
Stimulus Type			Totals	Repet-itions	1	2	3	4	Major	Minor	tural	Ø	lems
	Questions												
	Others												

C	Spontaneous (WRITING) 20		Others	

		Minor			*Social*		*Stereotypes*		*Problems*	

Sentence Type

Stage I (0;9-1;6)

Major				Sentence Structure				
Excl.	Comm.	Quest.			*Statement*			
	'V'	'Q'	'V'	'N'	Other		Problems	
		Conn.		Clause			Phrase	Word

Stage II (1;6-2;0)

	V X	Q X		SV **/**	V C/O	DN **8**	VV	-ing **4**
				S C/O	A X **/**	Adj N **2**	V part	pl **? /**
				Neg X	Other	NN	Int X	
						PrN	Other	-ed

Stage III (2;0-2;6)

	V X Y		X + S:NP **2**	X + V:VP **/**	X + C/O:NP	X + A:AP **/**	
		Q X Y	SVC/O **4**	VC/OA	D Adj N	Cop **2**	-en
	let X Y	VS	SVA **2**	VO$_d$O$_i$	Adj Adj N	Aux **4**	
			Neg X Y	Other	Pr DN	Pron	3s **3**
	do X Y				N Adj N	Other (**Ͻ NN**) **/**	gen

Stage IV (2;6-3;0)

		XY + S:NP **6**	XY + V:VP **4**	XY + C/O:NP **3**	XY + A:AP **/**	
	S	QVS	SVC/OA	A A X Y	N Pr NP	Neg V	n't
		QXYZ	SVO$_d$O$_i$	Other	Pr D Adj N	Neg X	'cop
					cX	2 Aux **/**	'aux
					XcX	Other	

Stage V (3;0-3;6)

			and	Coord. **/**	/ ·	Postmod. **/** clause	/ +	-est
	how	tag	c	Subord. **/**	/ ·			-er
			s	Clause: S		Postmod. **/** · phrase		
	what		Other	Clause: C/O				-ly
				Comparative				

	(+)			(−)		
NP	VP		Clause	NP	VP	Clause

Stage VI (3;6-4;6)

Initiator	Complex		Passive	Pron	Adj seq	Modal	Concord **2**
Coord			Complement	Det **2**	N irreg **/**	Tense	A position
						V irreg	W order
Other				Other	**2** Aux **/**	Conjunction **/**	

Stage VII (4;6+)

Discourse			Syntactic Comprehension	
A Connectivity	*it*			
Comment Clause	*there*		*Style*	
Emphatic Order	Other			

Total No. Sentences **20**	Mean No. Sentences Per Turn /	Mean Sentence Length **5.3**

© D. Crystal, P. Fletcher, M. Garman, 1975 University of Reading

Fig. 31   Diane at 11;0 (Profile A)

D.L. (NOV. '73) 11; 0   B (NORMALISED)

A	Unanalysed					Problematic		
	1 Unintelligible		2 Symbolic Noise		3 Deviant /	1 Incomplete		2 Ambiguous

B Responses

Stimulus Type		Totals	Repet-itions	Elliptical Major				Full Major	Minor	Struc-tural	Ø	Prob-lems
				1	2	3	4					
	Questions											
	Others											

C   Spontaneous (WRITING) 20   Others

		Minor			Social		Stereotypes		Problems	

Stage I (0;9–1;6) — Sentence Type

Major				Sentence Structure				
Excl.	Comm.	Quest.			Statement			
	'V'	'Q'	'V'	'N'	Other	Problems		

Stage II (1;6–2;0)

	Conn.	Clause		Phrase		Word
V X		SV **2**	V C/O	DN **21**	VV	-ing **6**
Q X		S C/O	A X **/**	Adj N **2**	V part	pl **? /**
		Neg X	Other	NN	Int X	-ed
				PrN	Other	

Stage III (2;0–2;6)

V X Y		X · S:NP **2**	X · V:VP **/**	X · C/O:NP	X + A:AP **/**	-en
Q X Y		SVC/O **6**	VC/OA	D Adj N	Cop **6**	3s **//**
let X Y	VS	SVA **4**	VO_dO_i	Adj Adj N	Aux **6**	gen
		Neg X Y	Other	Pr DN **3**	Pron	
do X Y				N Adj N	Other **/**	

Stage IV (2;6–3;0)

		XY · S:NP **14**	XY · V:VP **6**	XY · C/O:NP **6**	XY · A:AP **3**	n't
S	QVS	SVC/OA	AAXY	N Pr NP	Neg V	'cop
	QXYZ	SVO_dO_i	Other	Pr D Adj N	Neg X	'aux
				cX	2 Aux **/**	
				XcX	Other	

Stage V (3;0–3;6)

		and	Coord. **/**	/ ·	Postmod. **/** clause	/ ·	-est
how	tag	c	Subord. **/**	/ ·			-er
		s	Clause: S		Postmod. **/** · phrase		-ly
what		Other	Clause: C/O				
			Comparative				

		(+)				(−)		
	NP	VP		Clause	NP		VP	Clause
Initiator	Complex		Passive	Pron	Adj seq	Modal	Concord **4**	
Coord			Complement	Det **4**	N irreg **/**	Tense	A position	
						V irreg	W order **/**	
Other				Other **2**	Aux **/** Conjunction **/**	Prep **3**		

Stage VII (4;6 +)

Discourse			Syntactic Comprehension	
A Connectivity	it			
Comment Clause	there		Style	
Emphatic Order	Other			

Total No. Sentences	**20**	Mean No. Sentences Per Turn	/	Mean Sentence Length	**5.3**

Fig. 32   Diane at 11;0 ('normalized' profile) (Profile B)

Profiles C, D and E

Profile C (Fig. 33) reflects Diane's written usage in June 1975. The full transcript is given on p. 297; grammatical analysis and profiling details are given on p. 324. The character of the data may be illustrated by the following extract:

> *On Friday I went to home at twelty to four*
> *I drink a cup of tea*
> *Kim is play me*
> *David is a read*
> *I say's about at school*
> *I watch the television*
> *I go to bed at 9 o'clock*

The main contrasts between Profiles B and C reflect the improvement due to the structured work which had been done in the intervening period. Some of the structures absent in B had been selected for teaching, but only in an impressionistic way. As a result, these selected areas show progress, but this progress seems not to have affected the overall language system. Profile C displays just as 'random' an appearance as Profile B. There are now pronouns, where none existed before, mainly in Subject position, and this accounts for the more normal distribution of figures along the Stage III transitional line. AAXY is now used, albeit in a rather stereotyped way. The absence of 3s is presumably fortuitous, given the 'first person' orientation of the writing. But in most other respects (bearing in mind there are nearly twice as many sentences in C), there is little difference between the profiles, and indeed there are some negative signs, especially in the Tense Error figure.

Profile D (Fig. 34) reflects Diane's written usage in May 1976. The full transcript is given on p. 298; grammatical analysis and profiling details are given on p. 329. The character of the data may be illustrated from the opening of the essay, as follows:

> *On Friday I went home at twenty to four*
> *I watched the television*
> *My dog was sleeping*
> *I went to upstairs*
> *I put on the wall*
> *I drank a cup of coffee*
> *I went to bed and I went to sleep*

It is evident that the work on 3- and 4-element clause structures, with particular attention to V (especially in the past tense form), has produced a fuller profile. SVC/OA structures are found for the first time, as are coordinations (both *XcX* and Stage V) and *-ed*. In many respects, Profile D is a conflation of the strengths found in B and C. On the other hand, several of the weaknesses of C carry over also, especially the lack of adjectives, little complex NP structure, poor early word structure, and (for the number of sentences used) a relative lack of integration

D.L. (JUNE '75) 13;6   C

A	Unanalysed					Problematic	
	1 Unintelligible		2 Symbolic Noise		3 Deviant 4	1 Incomplete	2 Ambiguous

B Responses

				Normal Response						Abnormal			
					Elliptical Major				Full		Struc-		Prob-
Stimulus Type		Totals	Repet-itions	1	2	3	4	Major	Minor	tural	Ø	lems
	Questions												
	Others												

C Spontaneous (WRITING) 37   3 *   Others   * not immediate

	Minor				Social		Stereotypes		Problems	

Stage I (0;9–1;6) — Sentence Type

Major					Sentence Structure				
Excl.	Comm.	Quest.					Statement		
	·V·	·Q·	·V·	·N·		Other		Problems	

Stage II (1;6–2;0)

			Conn.		Clause			Phrase		Word
	VX	QX		SV 3		V C/O		DN 12	VV	-ing 3
				S C/O		AX		Adj N	V part 3	pl
				Neg X		Other		NN	Int X	
								PrN 14	Other	-ed

Stage III (2;0–2;6)

			X · S:NP 2	X · V:VP 3		X · C/O:NP	X · A:AP	
	VXY		SVC/O 13	VC/OA	D Adj N 2	Cop	-en
	QXY		SVA 8	VOdOi	Adj Adj N	Aux 7	3s
	let XY	VS	Neg XY	Other	Pr DN 2	Pron 26	gen
	do XY				N Adj N	Other 6	

Stage IV (2;6–3;0)

			XY · S:NP 2	XY · V:VP 5	XY · C/O:NP	XY · A:AP 7	
	·S	QVS	SVC/OA	AAXY 7	N Pr NP	Neg V	n't
		QXYZ	SVOdOi	Other 1	Pr D Adj N	Neg X	·cop
					cX	2 Aux	·aux
					XcX	Other 4	

Stage V (3;0–3;6)

	how	tag	and	Coord. 1	1 ·	Postmod. 1 clause	1 ·	-est
			c	Subord. 1	1 ·			-er
			s	Clause: S		Postmod. 1 · phrase		-ly
	what		Other	Clause: C/O				
				Comparative			Other 1 →	

	(+)				(−)		
NP	VP	Clause		NP		VP	Clause

Stage VI (3;6–4;6)

Initiator	Complex	Passive		Pron	Adj seq	Modal	Concord 1
Coord		Complement		Det 5	N irreg	Tense 2	A position
						V irreg	W order
Other				Other Prep 6 ing 4 pl 3 Part 1			

Stage VII (4;6+)

Discourse		Syntactic Comprehension	
A Connectivity	it		
Comment Clause	there	Style	
Emphatic Order	Other		

Total No. Sentences 37	Mean No. Sentences Per Turn /	Mean Sentence Length 5·2

Fig. 33 Diane at 13;6 (Profile C)

D.L. (MAY '76)   14;5   D

A	**Unanalysed**					**Problematic**			
	1 Unintelligible		2 Symbolic Noise		3 Deviant *I*	1 Incomplete		2 Ambiguous **4**	

B Responses

Stimulus Type		Totals	Repet-itions	Elliptical Major 1	2	3	4	Full Major	Minor	Struc-tural	∅	Prob-lems
	Questions											
	Others											

Normal Response — Elliptical Major / Full Major / Minor / Struc-tural / ∅ — Abnormal — Prob-lems

C	**Spontaneous** 42 (WRITING) **5**	Others		

	Minor			*Social*	*Stereotypes*	*Problems*

Stage I (0;9–1;6) Sentence Type

Major	*Excl.*	*Comm.*	*Quest.*	*Statement*
		·V·	·Q·	·V· ·N· Other Problems
			Conn.	Clause	Phrase	Word

Stage II (1;6–2;0)

Comm.	Quest.	Conn.	Clause		Phrase		Word
V X	Q X		SV **3**	V C/O	DN **22**	VV	-ing **2**
			S C/O	A X **I**	Adj N	V part **8**	pl
			Neg X	Other	NN	Int X	
					PrN **9**	Other **I**	

Stage III (2;0–2;6)

			X + S:NP **I**	X + V:VP **3**	X + C/O:NP	X + A:AP	-ed **34**
V X Y	Q X Y		SVC/O **15**	VC/OA	D Adj N	Cop **2**	-en **5**
let X Y	VS		SVA **9**	VO_dO_i	Adj Adj N	Aux **7**	3s **6**
do X Y			Neg X Y	Other	Pr DN **2**	Pron **29**	gen
					N Adj N	Other **7**	

Stage IV (2;6–3;0)

			XY + S:NP **7**	XY + V:VP **8**	XY + C/O:NP **II**	XY + A:AP **9**	n't
	· S	QVS	SVC/OA **5**	AAXY **3**	N Pr NP	Neg V	'cop
		QXYZ	SVO_dO_i	Other **I**	Pr D Adj N	Neg X	'aux
					cX	2 Aux	
					XcX **3**	Other **4**	

Stage V (3;0–3;6)

	how	tag	*and* **3**	Coord. I **3**	I ·	Postmod. I clause	I ·	-est
			c	Subord. I	I			-er
			s	Clause: S		Postmod. I · phrase		
	what		Other	Clause: C/O				-ly
				Comparative				

	(+)			(−)			
	NP	VP	Clause	NP		VP	Clause

Stage VI (3;6–4;6)

NP	VP	Clause	NP		VP	Clause
Initiator	Complex	Passive	Pron	Adj seq	Modal	Concord
Coord		Complement	Det	N irreg	Tense **7**	A position
					V irreg	W order
Other			Other **Prep I**		**Verb 2**	

Stage VII (4;6+)

Discourse		*Syntactic Comprehension*	
A Connectivity	*it*		
Comment Clause	*there*	*Style*	
Emphatic Order	Other		

Total No. Sentences **42**	Mean No. Sentences Per Turn /	Mean Sentence Length **5·9**

© D. Crystal, P. Fletcher, M. Garman, 1975 University of Reading

Fig. 34   Diane at 14;5 (Profile D)

of phrase and clause structure between Stages III and IV. Diane no longer produces such noticeably deviant sentences, but there are still several whose structure is highly problematic. Repeated sentences are relatively high (one eighth), and the language still reads in a stereotyped way. This last point, however, is as much a matter of lexis as grammar: the vocabulary has increased by some 40 per cent over sample C, but the ratio of vocabulary types to tokens is *very* low, and has in fact deteriorated between C and D (3·3 > 3·1), and favourite items (such as *I*) are used in a constant proportion (1/7 of all tokens in both C and D).

Profile E (Fig. 35) reflects Diane's written usage in July 1977, after structural work that has concentrated on Stages III and IV and the transition between them, along with consolidation of Stage II, and regular work on *-ing*, Aux and Neg. A selection of sentences from this work is as follows:

> *We went to the zoo*
> *My father was driving the car*
> *A long way at 1 hour*
> *I saw the monkey*[29]
> *The monkey was funny*
> *My father holding the monkey hand*
> *I saw the wild cat*
> *Wild cat was very old*
> *The fox was run around*
> *The little monkey was gave an banana it hand*
> *My mother saw a bird*

The developments in *-ing*, Cop, Aux and Adj are notable, in the essay as a whole; also Subjects NPs are more in evidence, at the expense of Pronouns (cf. (D) XY + S:NP 7, Pron 29 in 42 sentences; (E) XY + S:NP 20, Pron 38 in 73 sentences, i.e. NPs increase from 16 per cent to 28 per cent, Prons are down from 66 per cent to 52 per cent). Repetitions hardly occur, but there are still 1/10 of the sentences problematic. The stereotyped appearance still exists (especially with AAXY), but its effect is much reduced through the increase in vocabulary, which produces more varied sentences: the vocabulary increase between D and E is 60 per cent, and the type-token ratio has increased to 3.4, both very positive signs (also the proportion of *I*'s is now 1/13, compared with the 1/7 of C and D). A notable development is in the Stage VI Error columns: Tense Errors have not increased, but several new Error categories have emerged, especially Det, Aux and *-ing*. These new error patterns should not be a cause for pessimism, however: on the contrary, new errors can be a sign of progress—of the child attempting to come to terms with the irregularities and boundaries of grammatical generalizations he has been taught. If more grammar is being used, there will naturally be more opportunity for error. What is abnormal about the Stage VI pattern in profile E is that, unlike the normally-developing child, it lacks the backing of a well-established

---

[29] There were many monkeys. The error could be Plural or Det. Given the difficulties with Det elsewhere, this is more likely.

D.L. (JULY '77) E

A	Unanalysed				Problematic		
	1 Unintelligible	2 Symbolic Noise	3 Deviant		1 Incomplete	2 Ambiguous	7

B	Responses										

					Normal Response					Abnormal	
					Elliptical Major				Full		Struc-		Prob-
Stimulus Type		Totals	Repet- itions	1	2	3	4	Major	Minor	tural	Ø	lems
	Questions											
	Others											

C	Spontaneous (WRITING)	73	1		Others	

	Minor			Social	2	Stereotypes		Problems

Sentence Type

Stage I (0;9–1;6)

	Major					Sentence Structure	
	Excl.	Comm.	Quest.			Statement	
		'V'	'Q'	'V'	'N'	Other	Problems
				Conn.	Clause		Phrase		Word

Stage II (1;6–2;0)

VX	QX		SV 8	V C/O	DN 35	VV 1	-ing 14
			S C/O	A X	Adj N 7	V part 8	pl 2
			Neg X	Other	NN	Int X 3	-ed 58
					PrN 20	Other 1	

Stage III (2;0–2;6)

	VXY	QXY	X + S:NP 2	X + V:VP 4	X + C/O:NP	X + A:AP	-en 1
	let XY	VS	SVC/O 21	VC/OA	D Adj N 2	Cop 8	3s 22
	do XY		SVA 15	VO_dO_i	Adj Adj N	Aux 21	gen 2
			Neg XY	Other	Pr DN 12	Pron 38	
					N Adj N	Other 10	

Stage IV (2;6–3;0)

	. S	QVS	XY + S:NP 20	XY + V:VP 16	XY + C/O:NP 18	XY + A:AP 13	n't 1
		QXYZ	SVC/OA 6	AAXY 17	N Pr NP	Neg V 1	'cop 1
			SVO_dO_i	Other	Pr D Adj N	Neg X	'aux
					cX	2 Aux	
					XcX 4	Other 5	

Stage V (3;0–3;6)

	how		and 1	Coord. 1	1 ·	Postmod. 1 clause	1 ·	-est
		tag	c	Subord 1	1 ·			-er
	what		s	Clause: S		Postmod 1 · phrase		-ly
			Other	Clause: C/O				
				Comparative				

Stage VI (3;6–4;6)

	(+)			(−)		
	NP	VP	Clause	NP	VP	Clause
	Initiator	Complex	Passive	Pron 1	Modal	Concord
	Coord		Complement	Det 12	Tense 12	A position
					V irreg 1	W order 1
	Other			Other prep 4 ing 5 gen 1	Aux 5 Lexical V 2	Part 1

Stage VII (4;6+)

	Discourse		Syntactic Comprehension	
	A Connectivity	it		
	Comment Clause	there	Style	
	Emphatic Order	Other		

	Total No. Sentences	73	Mean No. Sentences Per Turn	/	Mean Sentence Length	5.9

© D. Crystal, P. Fletcher, M. Garman, 1975 University of Reading

Fig. 35 Diane at 15;7 (Profile E)

Stage IV and V. Such a wide range of error categories in Stage VI, with no compar-ably-advanced structures elsewhere, is fairly typical, in the written language of deaf children. It should also be noted that several of the Ambiguous sentences could be interpreted as Diane attempting to express Stage V structures, e.g. *I saw big monkey was funny*. The impression, in short, is one of consolidation to beyond Stage III, with several indications of structural potential further down the chart.

Remedial implications

On the basis of this case, and several other studies of severely and profoundly deaf children made since autumn 1976, we have been most impressed by the rele-vance and effectiveness of the LARSP procedure. In our experience it is the first procedure that has enabled the teacher to comprehensively diagnose and *tackle* in a systematic way the syntactic problems experienced by the deaf.

LARSP has helped and motivated a number of profoundly deaf pupils (11 to 14-year-olds) in new and quite positive ways. The completed Profile Chart gives the teacher:

  (i) a clear indication of where to start a pupil's language remediation;
  (ii) a precise formula on which to structure the pupil's future work.

Subsequent profiles enable the teacher to:

  (iii) measure the relevance and efficacy of his remedial methods;
  (iv) pinpoint the structural 'areas' in which the deaf child continues to have difficulty.

We have been using LARSP's syntactic structures as a basis for systematic remediation. We have tried to concentrate in detail on each individual structure within each division (clause level, phrase level, word level etc.) of each Stage. We have tried to make use of all the 'meaningful' syntactic combinations within each Stage before moving on to the next Stage. We have been able to produce many examples of syntax, even for Stage II, which are not 'telegraphic' and which—particularly important to the deaf—do not rely too heavily on prosodic contour. Working steadily, from the simplest syntax through the different chronological Stages (although not, of course, adhering to *age* norms), the pupils seem to have already acquired a better syntactic 'awareness'. We believe that as a result of the thoroughness of the approach, our profoundly deaf pupils are for the first time getting a 'feel' for their mother tongue: a realistic experience from which we 'hearers' benefited in our first years of life.

This has been another interesting development and it has led to what *may* be a new approach in the use of LARSP. The second author deals with deaf children in the older age range, 11–16, some of whom, for varying reasons, have not achieved much linguistic success so far. He therefore has to take into consideration the fact that, although their language corresponds to that of much younger hearing children, they are maturing quickly in other ways. They need 'something to be going on with' while working through the early Stages of LARSP, something they can use immediately whilst building up more complex structures.

Accordingly, it was decided to use normal, mature language—limiting it according to the developmental Stages of LARSP, but without resorting to 'baby talk', i.e. *use adult colloquial expressions conforming to the earliest syntactic patterns*. Admittedly much of such conversation is crudely contrived, but it is a start for older deaf pupils who had not previously been doing well, who had been attempting to stumble through Stage III, IV or V statements and been cruelly embarrassed by their own and other people's lack of comprehension.

Other pupils have taken to similar exercises, to varying degrees, and are making better progress in lipreading and comprehension. They are also progressing more naturally and often independently to more complicated structures. Further, whilst making receptive language less confused, the above method seems to have engendered a growing confidence in expressive language.

It seems that by 'saturating' pupils in the structures of a given Stage, e.g. Stage II, before encouraging any more complex language, the teacher can help them to advance more confidently into the next intermediary Stages (X + S : NP etc.) and then on to language of the next Stage with fewer fundamental errors.

We understand the importance of not adhering too strictly to Stage 'divisions'. However we have found it illuminating to liken the process of using LARSP to that of a tiered water fountain, with Stage I at the top. Provided each Stage is filled, it will naturally 'overflow' into the next Stage. Eventually the whole thing flows and all the Stages are in action. If language structures are thrown in at random, the Stages do not fill in the correct sequence, and the whole thing fails. (We are now convinced that 'high rates of input' and 'total immersion in language' are major contributory factors to the failure of many deaf children in linguistic achievement.)

Here are some of the several hundred adult colloquial sentences devised for working on early syntactic patterns—in this case, Stage II. It is possible to have a dialogue in a certain Stage, which the deaf can more easily understand as a 'starter' and which builds up confidence. (We are here of course referring to those deaf children who have not achieved linguistic success so far.) For instance,

T	Hello Wayne. Mum home?
P	No. Not yet. Gone out.
T	Where to?
P	To town. To Cambridge.
T	What for?
P	Shopping. My birthday, next week. Home soon. For tea.
T	What time?
P	About four.
T	Thank you. Bye.

Stage II

VX	QX
go away	how much?
come here	what colour?
shut up	what time?
watch out	where to?
sit down	how many

SV	VC	VO	AX
dogs bark	being careful	drink (your) milk	clothes off
birds fly	looking pretty	eat eggs	home now
dad smoke(s)	being silly	play golf	running late
people talk	look(s) bad	draw pictures	keys here
love hurt(s)!	feel(s) good	read(ing) books	all out

Neg X	Other
not today	yes please
not there	no thanks
not me	thank you
not likely!	well done
no exit	

DN	VV	Adj N	V part
a boy	going shopping	next door	running away
an apple	keep going	good game	getting off
the weather	going swimming	lovely day	hold on
some people	went fishing	nice weather	come along
my fault	need(s) cleaning	hot food	moving out
this way			
that man!			

NN	Int X	Pr N
breakfast time	too much	at school
boat house	so hot	to school
tomorrow morning	very nice	at home
John Smith	just right	at work
garden tools	too big	to work
		in London
		on Monday ...
		'At school. In Cambridge. On Monday. In July.'

The use and development of some of the above examples can be seen in the following extracts from a profoundly deaf 13-year-old girl with low attainments until 1977.

January 1977

Using 'normal' conversation, she understood only the italicized words:

T   *Hello Judith.*   Isn't it hot today?
                        It is hot today.
P   *Hello.*
T   *Come in* and sit down. (Pointing to the blackboard) I want you to write this work on that piece of paper.
P   —
T   Just do one page but don't use your *book.*

By now she was confused.

Same date
Next, 'Stage II talk' was used, and there was an immediate improvement in rapport. (Full stops represent good pauses.)

T   *Hello Judith. Hot today!*
P   *Hello. Yes, hot. Very hot.*
T   *Come in. Sit down.* (Pointing to the blackboard) *Write this.*
P   *Oh no! How much?*
T   *One page. On paper. No books.*
P   *What colour?*
T   *Use* } *blue.* *Use* } *ink. No pencils. Be careful. Good writing.*
     In   *In*

This is obviously crudely contrived to start with, but the following extracts shows how, six months later, Judith is moving into Stage III·

June 1977

P   *Hello Mr Dennis. How are you?*
T   *Hello Judith. Very well thanks. Come in now. Sit down here.*
     Look at me. Watch my lips. Please write this. (Points to board)
P   *That is hard. In my book?*
T   *No. Not your book. Write on paper.*
P   *What title?*
T   *'Grammar Work'.*
P   *What colour?*

The important point to emphasize here is that comprehension is obviously much improved.

A further example shows the development of a dysphasic, partially deaf boy of 12–13. It is evident that his description of the Wimbledon Final in 1976 was very much in Stage II terms, whereas his syntax in 1977 was much more Stage

III. We have encouraged him this year to build on his original structures and have in both cases italicized the words/endings that we had to help with:

1976	1977
On Saturday	On Saturday afternoon
Saturday *afternoon*	
at home	*sitting* at home
watch*ing* television	watch*ing* the television
watch*ing* tennis	watch*ing* the tennis
	on television on the television
two men	(*I* watch*ed* tennis)
play*ing* tennis	men play*ing* tennis
white shirt*s*	two men play*ing*
white short*s*	play*ing at* Wimbledon
Borg	Wimbledon *in* London
fair hair	no Wombles!
head *band*	Borg *from* Sweden
from Sweden	Connors *from* America
Nastase	Borg
brown hair	*with* fair hair
from Rumania	*a head* band
	Connors
at Wimbledon	*with* brown hair
in London	
hot *weather*	very hot weather
very sun*ny*	very sunny day

Lastly, we give a brief example of how we planned a Stage II conversation between a profoundly deaf girl of 13 and her mother. It is rather staccato to look at, but it is not 'baby talk'. One should not, of course, produce such stimuli at too fast a pace.

(*Upstairs at home*)

M   Hello Judith.
J   Morning Mum. Monday today.
M   Wake up. Get up.
          Get washed.
          Get dressed.
J   All right. Go down.

(*Downstairs*)

M   Come down. Sit here. Be quick. Eat up.
J   Look Mum. My breakfast. No milk.
M   What now? No milk. Sorry. My fault. Poor thing!
     Any sugar? How much?
J   Bye Mum.
M   Kiss (me). Good girl. Goodbye. Be careful.

Most of the pupils have taken to similar exercises to varying degrees and there have been some interesting developments:

(a) *Motivation and confidence*. By giving pupils something they can recognize *quickly*, learn and use intelligibly, they seem more willing to speak and to work at the other more arduous and crucial aspects of language remediation.

(b) *Self-correction*. After persistent use of Stage II structures, pupils began to pounce more quickly on their own mistakes and sustain a higher level of correct structures. For example,

   (i) *My Mum. At work*. The pupils' meaning could be easily understood without the verb, but once made aware of *is*, they rarely forget to use it. They somehow 'feel' that *My Mum is at work* is more acceptable, and seem to sense that to use the original is a retrograde step.

   (ii) After repeated work with accurate (but to 'hearers', exceptional) Stage II Pr N phrases, e.g. *at home, at school, at work, in Cambridge, on Monday*, pupils later on are usually better able to deal with more common Stage III Pr DN structure, e.g. *at the shops, to the post-office*. Could it be that exceptions, as well as the 'normal' rules are best learned as soon as they fit in acceptably with LARSP's developmental schedule?

(c) It is important to plan carefully the means of interrelating oral and written (and any other) modes of expression.

The development of colloquial language based on LARSP depends on the constant interaction of listening (with suitable amplification), lipreading, speaking, reading and writing. We can illustrate this by describing the way in which a daily lesson was arranged for Wayne's 'Wimbledon' example above. The divisions of INTRODUCTION, GRAMMAR, SPEECH, VOCABULARY and TESTING are typical of the overall weekly pattern used with all the pupils in our Unit.

Lesson A

The subject ('Wimbledon 1976') is *introduced* using books, sequenced pictures, newspaper cuttings, videotape, etc. P is encouraged to talk about the subject to the best of his ability. T writes the comments on the board/overhead projector as P speaks. In this way T can check P's meaning and 'refine' language to the Stage which he is encouraging. T transfers finished product to his (T's) record book. Rubs board. P now attempts own 'essay' on subject.

Lesson B

T and P look at *grammar* of lesson A. (Studying 'essay' and record book.) Such a lesson usually has two main sections:

(i) Word level approximating to Stage II (*-ing*, pl, *-ed*). See *watching, playing* and *men, shirts, shorts* etc. Discussion of other examples of these inflections.

(ii) Phrase and Clause levels of Stage II, e.g.

at home	on Saturday	watching television
at Wimbledon	on Saturday	playing tennis
at school	on Monday	reading books

T and P discuss paradigmatic relationships, attempting to widen P's experience and use of structures within Stage II. (The pupil is also delighted to notice the possibility of combining phrases and clauses syntagmatically. This is one of the ploys to encourage, very gradually, progression from one Stage to another.)

Lesson C

Now that P is confident with content and structure, he is more willing to concentrate on articulation improvement. Thus a *speech* lesson, 'brushing up' Wayne's Stage II structures, is an indispensable sequel. Intelligibility will be the ultimate test of any improvement in language. All speech work is supported by the written word.

Lesson D

Once words have been introduced in an appropriate context, the time has come to relate recent *vocabulary* to existing vocabulary, using the simplest form of definition and categorization, e.g.

afternoon	after lunch/before tea	time
home	my house	place (or building)

A list of the above, based on 'Wimbledon 1976', was copied by Wayne and taken home to discuss and learn with his parents.

Lesson E

T *tests* P's ability to lipread, say, write, and define language from lessons A, B, C and D. Homework is set which tests written use of this language and enables parents to 'keep up' with P's progress.

By means of this sequence of lessons, specific examples of language are developed at the morphological, syntactic, phonological and lexical level through the medium of listening, lipreading, speaking, reading and writing, all at the appropriate developmental stage.

In attempting to work to this plan, three specific points are worth separate mention.

(i) The importance of *not* using a question structure of a Stage above that in which the pupil is capable of answering. Question structures are often the last part of a Stage that 'sinks in'.

(ii) The importance of not being too impatient to move on from a given

Stage. It is often because the hearing-impaired pupil has been hurried misguidedly through the 'baby' stages that he has developed poor, inaccurate or stereotyped syntax. Each development must be carefully monitored and recorded. Only in this way can the teacher 'catch' the classic deaf errors of omission, intrusion, direction and substitution at an early stage, before they become too integral a part of the pupil's language.

(iii) A lot of very basic work has to be done in Stage II, if only as a check on what the pupil can or cannot do. Testing at this Stage is fairly straightforward as the teacher is dealing only with two-element structures: e.g. in a written test based on direction, the pupil would have little challenge! However, as we move into Stage III, we can start to 'piece' some exercises together in a structured way. Any failure in an exercise can immediately be analysed and further work suitably planned *to meet the needs of each specific error*. We suggest, therefore, that Stage III is the place to begin 'Structured Exercises' and that the most logical starting point is the three-element phrase structure (D Adj N, Pr D N etc.), intermediary expansions of SV, VC, VO (X + S : NP etc.) and then on to clause structures SVC/O etc.

We have found LARSP to be an excellent guide to the teaching of syntax to hearing-impaired children. It provides the teacher with structural 'know-how' and gives the pupil motivation, confidence and a certain capacity for self-correction. For the hearing-impaired of average intelligence it offers a method of working systematically (and visually) through the Stages that we gained purely through hearing and talking. In LARSP's thoroughness lies a possible scheme of presenting carefully-structured language in spoken, written and visual form, which could help repair the linguistic havoc wreaked by hearing impairment. However, there have as yet been few attempts to apply the procedure to the devising of properly-structured reading schemes, story-telling sessions, or guidelines for superimposing lexical and phonological procedures. There is evidently a great deal still to be done.

Part 3

LARSP in research and teaching

3.1

A grammatical analysis of the speech of partially-hearing children

John M. Bamford and John Bench

This chapter describes the use of the LARSP profile to assess the grammatical knowledge of a large sample of partially-hearing children.[30] This was done as part of a research project to design and standardize a sentence test for speech audiometry with partially-hearing children (Bench and Bamford 1978), and as such our use of the LARSP profile is rather different from its more usual before-and-after remedial use. The study to be described is a research study, rather than a clinical report, in which the LARSP profile provides a crucial scheme for the assessment of the grammatical advancement of partially-hearing children as a preliminary to designing a test of their ability to perceive speech. Hence, in what follows, the reader should bear in mind that our adaptation, use and analysis of LARSP is specific to a particular set of test design requirements.

Audiologists sometimes have to use one of the so-called speech audiometric tests to measure the hearing for speech of their patients. Such tests consist of balanced lists of linguistic items, usually words or sentences, which are played to the listener from a taperecorder, one item at a time, and which he has to repeat back to the tester. Functions (called speech audiograms) are derived relating the percentage reported correctly, in terms of phonemes or words, to the relative intensity of the speech signal.

Since this kind of speech test is primarily a test of hearing and not a test of linguistic ability, it is necessary for the test to be within the linguistic competence of the listener. Graham (1968), for example, working with educationally subnormal children and using sentences containing familiar vocabulary, found that sentence repetition is related to both sentence length and grammatical structure. For speech audiometric tests using sentences as the test items, the words used should be common words which are known to be within the listener's vocabulary, the length

[30] We would like to thank all those education departments, teachers, schools and children who have been involved with this research for their help and cooperation. Most of the work described was funded by the UK Medical Research Council under Project Grant No. G.975/245/N. We are greatly indebted to Ase Kowal for her help and effort as a full-time member of the project team, to Carolyn Webb for analysing the transcripts onto LARSP profiles, and to Lutgen Mentz for his invaluable statistical and computational advice.

of each sentence should be well within the listener's capabilities, and the grammar used should be familiar to the listener. In addition to these structural criteria the sentences should, of course, be semantically 'reasonable'.

There is no sentence test of hearing available in the UK which satisfies all these requirements, particularly in respect of partially-hearing children, whose language ability may be retarded. Hence, the primary aim of our research project was to design and standardize such a test, suitable for use with (at least) partially-hearing children aged between 8 and 15 years, the age range where the need is, for various reasons, particularly acute.

The first phase in the development of a new audiometric sentence test is to obtain information about the linguistic abilities of those listeners for whom the test is to be designed. This information can then be used to provide the linguistic guidelines (permissible vocabulary, grammar, and sentence lengths) for construction of the test sentences. It is well known that the restricted auditory input of partially-hearing children retards aspects of their linguistic abilities with reference to the language of normally-hearing children (e.g. Owrid 1960, Brannon & Murry 1966, Hine 1970). However, precisely what these aspects are, and to what extent they are not only different in degree (i.e. retarded) but also different in kind from the language of the normally-hearing child remains largely unanswered by the data available in the literature.

It was necessary, therefore, for us to discover the required linguistic information, and we did this by analysing the spoken language of a sample of partially-hearing children of the appropriate age range. Our argument was that if the test sentences contain only those words and those grammatical structures used by the children themselves, then they ought to be within the linguistic ability of the proposed listeners. Lackner (1968), for example, studied a small group of mentally-retarded children and a small group of normal children and showed that each group was able to repeat back those sentences constructed from vocabulary items and syntactic types found in its own spoken repertoire.

This chapter, then, is concerned mainly with the problem of collecting and analysing information about the grammatical knowledge of a sample of partially-hearing children with the use of the LARSP profile. The subjects, the procedure and the results are presented and discussed, and some reference is made to the use of the data to construct the sentences for the speech test. Some further analyses of the data which aim to isolate *group* trends in the profiles are also described. No reference is made here to the separate problem of collecting a pool of suitable vocabulary items for use in the sentences (Bench and Bamford 1978), nor to the standardization of the new test, which is ongoing at the time of writing.

Subjects

The subjects were 263 hearing-impaired children (140 males, 123 females), aged between 8 and 15 years inclusive (mean: 11 years 8 months), with a mean nonverbal IQ (WISC performance scales) of 103·4 (standard deviation: 16·6), and a pure-tone hearing loss of not less than 40 dB ISO in the better ear (averaged threshold at 500, 1000 and 2000 Hz). The mean hearing loss was 73·3 dB (standard deviation: 15·6). In order to obtain the fullest range of subjects possible on the dimensions of age, nonverbal IQ and hearing loss, a deliberate policy of quota sampling was adopted (within the limits of residential schools and partially-hearing units in Berkshire and surrounding Counties).

Procedure

We had decided at an early stage in the project to limit the sentence items in the final speech test to statements, avoiding commands and questions (both of which can cause problems where the task is to repeat back rather than to obey or to answer) and exclamations. Information on the grammatical ability of the children with which to guide subsequent sentence construction was required, therefore, only for statements. As a consequence, we were able to use picture description to elicit speech samples from the children, without worrying that such a method elicits mainly statements, with only a small number of exclamations, commands and questions. However, when the grammatical data are examined in their own right, this bias must be remembered.

The children were seen on an individual basis during school hours at their school. Each subject was tested for about an hour and a quarter, divided if necessary into two or more sessions to avoid fatigue. During this time, and for up to 25 minutes, the child described and talked about a set of coloured pictures which were shown to him one at a time in random order. The pictures were unrelated to each other, and depicted people in familiar scenes: a family on a picnic, some boys playing football, a mother and children in the kitchen, and so on. This procedure was conducted in an informal manner in order to elicit more 'natural' utterances. Generally questions (which tend to elicit elliptical replies) were avoided, and unspecific prompts were given, such as *Tell me what's happening here* and *Tell me some more*. Occasionally, however, it was expedient to encourage a hesitant subject by asking him a direct question (e.g. *Who is in the car?*), to which the reply would often be elliptical (e.g. *Daddy, mummy and the dog*.). The interview was taperecorded. The poor articulation and intonation of some of the more severely impaired was not a serious problem, since by actually seeing the child and his articulatory movements, by knowing the picture material to which he was responding, and with the aid of repetition by the interviewer if necessary, the interviewer could record the child's utterances correctly as the interview proceeded. Any doubtful utterances, either at the interviewing stage or at the later transcription stage (see below) were dropped, but these were very infrequent.

The remainder of the testing time was taken up with assessing the child's puretone hearing, and nonverbal IQ, using the WISC performance scales. Also, when available, certain background information about the subjects was noted, including age at onset and age at diagnosis of hearing impairment. These variables are thought to have important consequences for language development, and their effects are being analysed at present.

The taperecording of each subject's picture description was later transcribed by one of four paid transcribers, who were given copies of the pictures and detailed instructions. Transcription was alphabetic rather than phonetic. The task was to some extent interpretive and hence errors could intrude, but not to any significant degree. For example, the presence or absence of elisions such as *there's* is difficult to determine and must to some extent be a source of transcriber variance. As a check, some of the tapes were re-transcribed by another member of our team. The number of discrepancies between the two transcriptions was extremely small. *GALD* (chapter 4) argues strongly that adequate prosodic cues should be noted in the transcription, on the grounds that trying to do without them leads to a high proportion of ambiguous utterances, and indeed makes the delineation of utterances into sentences (the starting point of the grammatical analysis) extremely difficult. Certainly a transcription with neither prosodic information nor punctuation will suffer from these defects. However, given the poor intonation of some of our subjects and their picture-description task (rather than the patient-therapist *interactive* discourse with which *GALD* is largely concerned), we would argue that punctuational cues are as effective as prosodic cues. A punctuated transcription will still contain *some* ambiguities, of course, as will a transcription with prosodic information, but we are satisfied that, in this study at least, these ambiguities constitute a small proportion of the data—indeed, the total number of elicited sentences deemed to be ambiguous was very small (see Results below). It was decided, therefore, not to train the transcribers in a new skill, but to allow them to use commas and full stops (and exclamation marks and question marks where necessary) to mark the major pauses and natural breaks in the recorded speech. In fact, after considerable discussion, it was decided not to mention punctuation of the transcriptions at all in the instructions to transcribers, with the result that they fell naturally into the accepted system.

Each transcription was then analysed on to a slightly modified version of the LARSP profile. The modifications made to the original and the reasons for them are as follows. Transcribers had been instructed to leave out any unintelligible utterances and symbolic noises, and, as we noted earlier, the task was such as seldom to elicit Responses. (Since they constituted such a very small proportion of the utterances, what Responses there were have simply been treated as if they were Spontaneous utterances.) Incomplete utterances were not analysed. Thus there remained at the top of the profile only the Deviant and Ambiguous sections, before the main body of the profile which is concerned entirely with Spontaneous utterances. Within this section, we thought that for the present project an indication of the use of the *to* form of the infinitive (Inf), of the future tense (fut), of preposition-pronoun structures such as *in it* (Pr Pron) and of adverbial elements in the form of a clause (Clause: A) would be useful.[31] Consequently, these structures

---

[31] Certain ambiguities in *GALD* have led to confusion as to where precisely some Stage V clause-level entries are to be marked (compare, for example, 47–8 with 75–7). To deal with this confusion we adopted the following system: subordinate clauses were defined as those dependent clauses (with or without a subordinating device) which formed part of a main clause and which could be deleted still leaving a grammatically acceptable sentence in terms of 'normal' adult grammar. Such clauses would be marked under Subord 1 or Subord 1 + and then subclassified as Clause:S, Clause:C/O,

were added in what seemed to be the most appropriate places on the profile, although Inf and fut might well have been better placed at the phrase level. Fut was indicated by the use of the auxiliaries *will* and *shall*, or by other verb constructions which implied cognitive awareness of futurity (e.g. *is going to ...*). Such occurrences were marked both at Aux and at fut. Because of the relatively heavy emphasis on quantitative trends in the present project, we further decided to drop three of the Stage 7 sections which offer the analyser an opportunity to comment in a qualitative fashion on the Style, the Syntactic Comprehension and the Discourse of the subject. Finally, at the foot of our profile, we simply provided a space for the analyser to record the number of words in each sentence, from which the mean sentence length could be calculated later. For this particular exercise, Deviant, Ambiguous and Stage I 'sentences' were excluded.

The number of sentences to be analysed on to the profile for each subject was left to the discretion of the analyser, given that there should be enough to provide a stable profile picture. In a very few cases the elicited language sample was so short that all the sentences were analysed. In most cases, however, the analyser transferred something in the region of 40 or 50 major sentences on to the profile. As a check on the reliability of the analysis, and upon the homogeneity of the transcripts, different parts of the transcripts of nine randomly-selected subjects were analysed on to two different profiles by the same analyser working 'blind'. The two profiles were compared, and correlation coefficients (Spearmans rho) were calculated for each subject's profile entries grouped into a number of higher-order categories (e.g. Stage II clauses, Stage IV Phrases, etc.). The coefficients were satisfactorily high, ranging from $+0.89$ to $+0.96$, and were all significant beyond the 0.01 per cent level.

Results

The following is an extract from the transcription of an 11-year-old boy of average nonverbal IQ and with a pure-tone hearing loss in the better ear of 90 dB.

> *Mummy carry bag. Man. The mummy carry bag. Car. House. Doggie. Light. Daddy look. Mummy. Boy. Daddy. Boy. Throw. Happy. Weed. The dog. Bread. The dog play the ball. The man throw the ball. The boy read the book. The mummy look at the boy. Bottle. Everybody food and bread. The dog eat food. The boy throw the ball. The mummy. The daddy look the boy. The boy sleep. The boy throw. Mummy. Ball. Mummy hold bag. The boy pull. The boy stop. The girls are look. Ambulance. Ladder. Very cold. The boy hold. Pull. The dog look at the boy. Slide. Snow.*

Clause:A, or Postmod clause. Thus the dependent clause in *She is sleeping because she is tired* is marked both as subordinate (it can be deleted to leave an acceptable sentence), and as Clause:A. The dependent clause in *Having a headache is terrible*, however, is marked only at Clause:S, since its deletion leaves an incomplete sentence. In this scheme, therefore, there is some double-marking in Stage V. In the *GALD* scheme there is none, since apparently Subord. should be reserved for adverbial clauses alone, all other dependent clauses (whether or not they can be deleted) being marked at Clause:S, or Clause: C/O, or Postmod (see pp. 87–9 above). The amount of duplication in the present scheme is not large, however, and the results would remain essentially unchanged if the analysis were to exclude all the duplications in Stage V.

S. 02

A	**Unanalysed**								**Problematic**			
	1 Unintelligible		2 Symbolic Noise		3 Deviant				1 Incomplete		2 Ambiguous	1

B Responses

Stimulus Type	Totals	Repet- itions	Normal Response						Abnormal			Prob- lems
			Elliptical Major				Full Major	Minor	Struc- tural	Ø		
			1	2	3	4						
Questions												
Others												

C Spontaneous — Others

	Minor			*Social*		*Stereotypes*		*Problems*	

Stage I (0;9–1;6) Sentence Type

Major			Sentence Structure				
Excl.	Comm.	Quest.	*Statement*				
	·V·	·Q·	·V· 9	·N· 36	Other 4	Problems	

Stage II (1;6–2;0)

	Conn.	Clause		Phrase		Word
VX	QX	SV 15	VC/O 1	DN 47	VV	inf.
		S C/O 3	A X	Adj N	V part 3	-ing 2
		Neg X	Other	NN 1	Int X 2	pl 4
				PrN 1	Other	-ed 3

Stage III (2;0–2;6)

VXY	QXY	X · S:NP 14	X · V:VP 5	X · C/O:NP 1	X · A:AP	-en
let XY	VS	SVC/O 16	VC/OA	D Adj N	Cop	fut.
		SVA 5	VO_dO_i	Adj Adj N	Aux 4	3s
do XY		Neg XY	Other	Pr DN 2	Pr Pron	
				N Adj N	Other	gen

Stage IV (2;6–3;0)

	XY · S:NP 17	XY · V:VP 2	XY · C/O:NP 8	XY · A:AP 3	
·S	QVS	SVC/OA	AAXY	N Pr NP	Neg V	n't
	QXYZ	SVO_dO_i	Other	Pr D Adj N	Neg X	·cop
				cX	2 Aux	·aux
				XcX 2	Other	

Stage V (3;0–3;6)

		and 1	Coord. 1 1	1 ·	Postmod. 1 clause	1 ·	-est
how	tag	c	Subord. 1	1 ·			-er
		s	Clause: S	:A	Postmod. 1 · phrase		
what	Other		Clause: C/O				-ly
			Comparative				

	(+)			(−)		
NP	VP	Clause	NP		VP	Clause
Initiator	Complex	Passive	Pron	Adj seq	Modal	Concord
Coord	Complement	Det	N irreg	Tense	A position	
				V irreg	W order	

Stage VI (3;6–4;6)

Other			Other	

Stage VII (4;6+)

Discourse		*Syntactic Comprehension*
A Connectivity	it 2	
Comment Clause	there	*Style* * excluding Stage I
Emphatic Order	Other	

Total No. Sentences * 41	Mean No. Sentences Per Turn	Mean Sentence Length * 3·95 (MAX. = 6)

© D. Crystal, P. Fletcher, M. Garman, 1975 University of Reading

Fig. 36 LARSP profile for an 11-year-old boy with a severe hearing impairment, and an average nonverbal IQ score

Fig. 36 shows the completed profile for the same subject. Although the essential interest of our project is in trends for groups of subjects, rather than in individual profiles, nonetheless it should be noted that Fig. 36 is an illustration of a profile clearly less advanced than one would expect from an 11-year-old: number of words per sentence is low; recursions and Stage IV structures are rare; pronouns, auxiliary verbs and many phrase structures are simply not present; nor are many of the more advanced word endings; even the simple -*ing* ending is hardly ever used; and there are as many Stage I entries as there are in all the other Stages (at the clause level) combined. Note, however, the lack of Deviant and Ambiguous sentences.

The use of the data for sentence construction

For the purposes of drawing up the grammatical guidelines for the construction of the test sentences which were, after all, intended for partially-hearing children, 22 subjects who proved to have a 'profound' hearing loss (an average pure-tone loss of 96 dB or more in the better ear) were excluded from the following analysis, leaving a sample of 241 children. The profiles of these latter children were treated as follows. Five overall profile measures which were thought to reflect level of grammatical advancement were considered:

1 the Stages which contained the largest and second-largest number of clause entries, excluding the transitional entries (which are not exclusive structures);

2 the number of phrase structures used, irrespective of how often they were used—the maximum score on this measure was 24 (the number of phrase structures in Stages II–IV, excluding cX and XcX, which are not exclusive structures);

3 the number of word structures used, irrespective of how often they were used—the maximum score on this measure was 14;

4 the 'phrase-to-clause ratio'—that is, the total number of phrase entries (excluding cX and XcX) in Stages II, III and IV divided by the total number of clause entries (excluding transitions) in Stages II, III and IV;

5 the mean sentence length.

Frequency distributions of the subjects' scores on each of these measures were drawn, both for the total sample (Figs. 33, 34, 35, 36 and 37) and for subgroups defined according to ranges of age, nonverbal IQ and hearing loss. These subgroup distributions (not shown because too numerous) indicated that, as expected, age, nonverbal IQ and hearing loss all had an effect on the grammatical advancement measures. However, and more importantly from the point of view of the construction of test sentences, it was clear that the overall shapes of the subgroup distributions were similar. Hence we could set a criterion for each *total* distribution such that the criterion included most of the sample (c. 85 per cent), while not being too simple to allow for semantically reasonable sentences to be constructed using the criterion as a guideline. Fig. 38, for example, shows that all but about 15 per cent of the children used 10 or more phrase structures, and the criterion was set at this point to strike a balance between including as much of the distribution

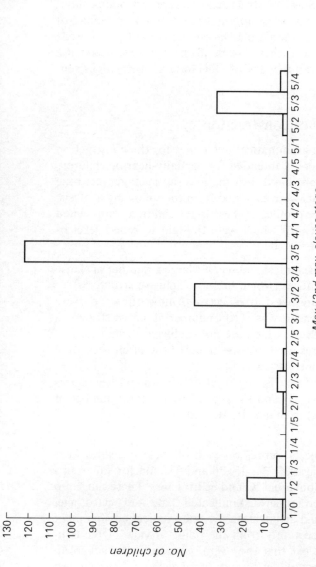

Fig. 37 Frequency distribution of the Stages which contain the largest and second-largest number of entries. Thus 3/2 means that these subjects gave primarily Stage III clauses, followed by Stage II clauses ($N=241$ subjects)

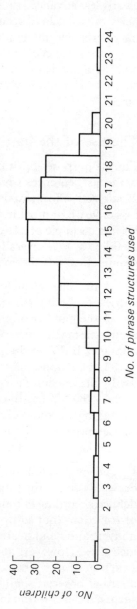

Fig. 38 Frequency distribution of the number of different phrase structures used ($N=241$ subjects)

as possible and keeping the criterion high enough to allow some variety of phrase structures in the test sentences.

On the basis of these arguments, it was decided to use two- and three-element clause structures; to use ten phrase structures; to use seven word-ending structures; to aim to construct sentences with an overall P:C ratio of about 2·0; and to use an average of 5 or 6 words per sentence (other considerations led us to use the

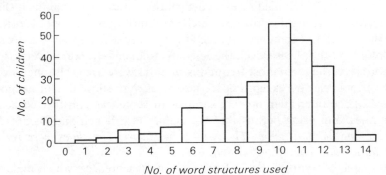

Fig. 39 Frequency distribution of the number of different word structures used (N=241 subjects)

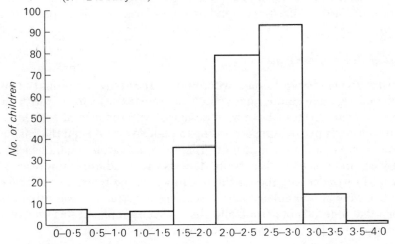

Fig. 40 Frequency distribution of the phrase to clause ratio (N=241 subjects)

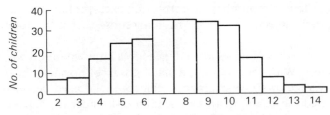

Fig. 41 Frequency distribution of the mean number of words for sentence (N=241 subjects)

number of syllables per sentence as the measure of length, and 7 syllables was set as the limit). The resultant sentences would, it was argued, be grammatically appropriate for all but the grammatically least advanced children, who would probably only be able to report back simple word lists.

In order to decide which *particular* clause, phrase and word-ending structures to use, the grouped profile for all those subjects (N = 208) whose grammatical advancement measures equalled or exceeded all the criteria was examined (Fig. 42). Those structures (within the criteria) which gave the largest number of entries were used in the speech test sentences. Thus, at the clause level, SVC/O, SVA and SV were allowed. At the phrase level, the *ten* most frequent structures were used, and at the word level the *seven* most frequent structures were used (although occasionally, for various reasons, exceptions to these rules were allowed—for example, use was made of the intensifier *very*). Examples of sentences constructed according to these rules, and using permissible vocabulary (see Bench and Bamford 1978) are: *The young boy left home*; *The little baby sleeps*; *The shoes were very dirty*; *The car hit a wall*; *They went on holiday*.

At the time of writing, the 21 lists, each of 16 sentences, which make up the *BKB Sentence Lists for Children* (and the 11 lists, each of 16 sentences, which make up a picture-related test for more 'difficult-to-test' children) have been recorded, and are being standardized and validated on a large sample of partially-hearing children.

Further analyses of the data

This brings the reader up-to-date with events concerning the primary aim of the project, to design and standardize speech audiometric tests for use with partially-hearing children. The tests have been designed, with the help of LARSP, and the standardization is progressing according to plan. We could end the chapter here. However, there is still a great deal of profile and background data which remains unanalysed, and this analysis is being done as the standardization proceeds. The reader might wonder why these analyses, to which the remainder of this chapter is devoted, were not completed *before* sentence construction was attempted. The answer is that time did not permit, and anyway such a sophisticated level of analysis was not required for the purposes of sentence construction.

1 The grouped LARSP profile

Fig. 43 shows the mean number of entries for each profile structure for *all* the hearing-impaired subjects (N = 263), including those with a 'profound' (> 95 dB) hearing loss.

The interpretation of Fig. 43 must depend to a large extent on what a 'normal' profile looks like. With this in mind, a small group of normally-hearing children ($N = 11$), of average or above-average intelligence, and aged between 10½ and 15 years, performed the same picture-description task under the same conditions as the hearing-impaired children. Fig. 44 shows the mean number of entries for each profile structure for these normally-hearing subjects.

Totalled entries, N = 208

A	Unanalysed				Problematic			
	1 Unintelligible	2 Symbolic Noise	3 Deviant		1 Incomplete	2 Ambiguous	**191**	

B	Responses											
						Normal Response					Abnormal	
					Elliptical Major				Full	Minor	Struc-tural	Ø	Prob-lems
	Stimulus Type		Totals	Repet-itions	1	2	3	4	Major				
		Questions											
		Others											

C	Spontaneous			Others	

		Minor			*Social* **192** *Stereotypes* **43** *Problems*			

Stage I (0;9–1;6) — Sentence Type

Minor — *Social* **192** *Stereotypes* **43** *Problems*

Major — Sentence Structure

Excl.	*Comm.*	*Quest.*	*Statement*
	·V·	·Q·	·V· **99** ·N· **812** Other **22** Problems
55	**136**	**11**	

Stage II (1;6–2;0)

Conn.	Clause				Phrase		Word
VX / QX **41** / **18**	SV **1770**	VC/O **743**		DN **11,765**	VV **913**	inf. **1652**
	SC/O **140**	AX **444**		Adj N **876**	V part **2669**	-ing **4753**
	Neg X **20**	Other **1**		NN **130**	Int X **282**	pl **2294**
				PrN **584**	Other **11**	-ed **2882**

Stage III (2;0–2;6)

VXY **7**	QXY **11**	
let XY **1**	VS **16**	
do XY **1**		

X + S:NP **1015**	X + V:VP **1541**	X + C/O:NP **539**	X + A:AP **325**	
SVC/O **5445**	VC/OA **286**	D Adj N **1277**	Cop **1656**	-en **623**
SVA **2047**	VOdOi **24**	Adj Adj N **77**	Aux **4231**	fut. **285**
Neg XY **5**	Other **51**	Pr DN **2979**	Pron **4629**	3s **1822**
		N Adj N	Pr Pron **337**	gen **1177**
			Other **73**	

Stage IV (2;6–3;0)

·S **1**	QVS **22** / QXYZ **15**	

XY + S:NP **3668**	XY + V:VP **3595**	XY + C/O:NP **XY + A:AP 654**	
SVC/OA **1447**	AAXY **366**	N Pr NP **23**	Neg V **340**	n't **299**
SVO₁O₂ **108**	Other **92**	Pr D Adj N **299**	Neg X **51**	'cop **735**
		cX **95**	2 Aux **128**	'aux **1343**
		XcX **1093**	Other **71**	

Stage V (3;0–3;6)

how	tag **4**	
what		

and **3332** / c **288** / s **864** / Other **3**	Coord. 1 **24191** + **527**	Postmod. 1 **271** 1+ **3** clause	-est **74**
	Subord. 1 **892** 1 + **2**		-er **55**
	Clause: S **10** A: **607**	Postmod. 1 + **14** phrase	-ly **172**
	Clause: C/O **757**		
	Comparative **3**		

	(+)			(−)		
NP	VP	Clause	NP	VP	Clause
Initiator **305**	Complex **16**	Passive **2**	Pron **52** Adj seq **5**	Modal **11**	Concord **69**
Coord **30**		Complement **2**	Det **74** N irreg **18**	Tense **117**	A position **1**
				V irreg **18**	W order **40**

Stage VI (3;6–4;6)

Other			Other **2820**		

Discourse	Syntactic Comprehension
A Connectivity **297** it **330**	
Comment Clause **91** there **628**	Style * excluding Stage I
Emphatic Order **3** Other	

Stage VII (4;6+)

Total No. Sentences	Mean No. Sentences Per Turn	Mean Sentence Length * **8·33**

© D Crystal, P. Fletcher, M. Garman, 1975 University of Reading

Fig. 42 The grouped (N=208) excluding those subjects (N=22) with a profound hearing loss, and those subjects (N=33) who failed to reach one or more of the five language-advancement criteria

Mean entries, Hearing-impaired group, N = 263

A

Unanalysed				Problematic		
1 Unintelligible	2 Symbolic Noise	3 Deviant	X	1 Incomplete	2 Ambiguous	1·39

B Responses

Stimulus Type		Totals	Repet-itions	Normal Response							Abnormal			Prob-lems
				Elliptical Major				Full Major	Minor	Struc-tural	∅			
				1	2	3	4							
	Questions													
	Others													

C Spontaneous / Others

Minor — Social 0·92 Stereotypes 0·26 Problems

Major — Sentence Structure

Stage I (0;9–1;6)

Statement

Excl.	Comm.	Quest.	·V·	·N· 12·08	Other 0·37	Problems
0·28	0·61	X / ·V· ·Q·	2·05 Conn.			

Stage II (1;6–2;0)

Clause		Phrase		Word
V X Q X	SV 9·10 VC/O 3·98	DN 42·08	VV 3·56	Int.
0·22 0·10	S C/O 1·00 AX 2·44	Adj N 4·03	V part 11·91	-ing 4·25
	Neg X X Other X	NN 0·66	Int X 1·20	21·05
		PrN 2·70	Other X	pl 9·91

Stage III (2;0–2;6)

Clause		Phrase		Word
V X Y X	X + S:NP 4·72 X + V:VP 7·08 X + C/O:NP 2·53 X + A:AP 1·51			-ed 12·63
X Q X Y	SVC/O 23·35 VC/OA 1·19	D Adj N 5·10	Cop 6·64	-en 2·10
let X Y VS	SVA 8·83 VO$_d$O$_i$ 0·10	Adj Adj N 0·37	Aux 17·27	t. 0·92
X X	Neg X Y X Other 0·24	Pr DN 12·22	Pron 20·87	3s 7·67
do X Y X		N Adj N X	Pr Pron 1·23 Other 0·29	gen 14·17

Stage IV (2;6–3;0)

Clause		Phrase		Word
· S 0·11	X Y + S:NP 15·13 X Y + V:VP 14·80 X Y + C/O:NP X Y + A:AP 6·74			4·72
QVS	SVC/OA 5·87 AAXY 1·44	N Pr NP X	Neg V 1·45	n't 1·20
X Q X Y Z	SVO$_d$O$_i$ Other 0·37	Pr D Adj N 1·18	Neg X 0·22	·cop 3·01
X	0·44	cX 0·48	2 Aux 0·51	·aux 5·37
		XcX 4·57	Other 0·32	-est 0·19

Stage V (3;0–3;6)

Clause		Phrase		Word
how tag	and 13·15	Coord. 19·43 1 · 2·13	Postmod. 1 1·03 1· X	-er 0·22
X X	c 1·17	Subord. 1 2·54 1· X	clause	-ly 0·75
what	s 3·57	Clause: S X A: 2·34	Postmod. 1· X	
	Other X	Clause: C/O 3·21	phrase	
		Comparative X		

Stage VI (3;6–4;6)

(+)			(−)		
NP	VP	Clause	NP	VP	Clause
Initiator 1·14	Complex X	Passive X	Pron 0·22 Adj seq X	Modal X	Concord 0·24
Coord 0·15		Complement	Det 0·29 N irreg	Tense 0·51	A position X
		X	0·10	V irreg X	W order 0·21
Other			Other 11·70		

Stage VII (4;6+)

Discourse	Syntactic Comprehension
A Connectivity 1·22 it 1·37	
Comment Clause 5·37 there 2·45	Style
Emphatic Order X Other	* excluding Stage I

Mean Total No. Sentences * 45·42	Mean No. Sentences Per Turn	Mean Sentence Length * 7·21 (max. 17·37)

© D. Crystal, P. Fletcher, M. Garman, 1975 University of Reading

Fig. 43 The mean number of entries for each profile structure grouped across all subjects (N = 263). Where the mean is less than 0·1 an 'X' is entered. Where an entry was never used, it is left blank.

To further aid the interpretation of Figure 43, we may refer to *GALD*'s profiles for a normally-hearing $3\frac{1}{2}$-year-old and for a normally-hearing adult. In addition, they review the rather limited literature available on the development of grammatical structures, and (113–17) they tentatively discriminate between 11 different patterns or types of profile. Finally, it should be remembered that the profile itself is laid out in such a way as to reflect 'normal' grammatical advancement: that is, a normally-developing child will advance, without obvious imbalance or gaps, on the three levels of clause, phrase and word; by the age of 5 or so it is expected that his language will be fluent and mature, consisting largely of Stage III and IV entries, with some Stage I and II entries, and with a fair proportion of recursiveness, sentence connectivity, and complex sentence patterns.

Armed with these comparators, one can begin to make sense of the grouped profile in Fig. 43. At first glance, both it and the profile in Fig. 44 look reasonably similar and complete, without glaring imbalances or gaps. However, the hearing-impaired children do not constitute a homogeneous group, and it may well be that the grouped profile hides important gaps in the individual profiles. This point will be dealt with later.

Looking at the clause level of analysis, it can be seen that the hearing-impaired group are retarded with reference to the normally-hearing group. They use less of the advanced clause entries, at Stages III and IV, and rather more of the least advanced entries, at Stage I. They exhibit less recursiveness (Stage V) and consequently less coordinating devices (*and* etc.). The figures are compared in Table 5. Expansion entries (e.g. X + S : NP, XY + V : VP) have been kept separate. A chi-squared test on the raw frequencies from which the totalled means in Table 5 were derived (excluding expansions) showed the differences between the two groups to be highly significant ($\chi^2 = 318 \cdot 18$, df $= 5$, $P < 0 \cdot 001$). Notice also that even though both groups give similar numbers of Stage II entries, less of these entries are expanded by the hearing-impaired group than by the normally-hearing group, which is a clear indication of lack of advancement (e.g. *Boy eat*, as opposed to *The boy is eating*). Similarly, the hearing-impaired group expanded a smaller

Table 5 Clause-level analysis: mean number of entries totalled within Stages for the hearing-impaired and the normally-hearing groups

	Group			
Structures	*Hearing-impaired*		*Normally-hearing*	
Stage I entries	14·50		0·36	
Stage II clauses	16·65		16·73	
Two-element expansions		15·84		20·91
Stage III clauses	33·71		39·54	
Three-element expansions		51·04		72·62
Stage IV clauses	8·12		16·00	
Stage V clauses	20·83		31·27	
Connecting devices	17·89		35·08	

Mean entries, Normal hearing group, N = 11

A	**Unanalysed**				**Problematic**		
	1 Unintelligible	2 Symbolic Noise	3 Deviant		1 Incomplete	2 Ambiguous	X

B	**Responses**					Normal Response						Abnormal	
							Elliptical Major				Full	Minor	Struc-tural	Ø	Prob-lems
	Stimulus Type		Totals	Repet-itions	1	2	3	4					
		Questions											
		Others											

C	**Spontaneous**		Others

		Minor			Social	Stereotypes	Problems

Stage I (0;9–1;6)	Sentence Type	**Major**				Sentence Structure	
		Excl.	Comm.	Quest.		Statement	
			·V·	·Q·	0·36 ·V· ·N·	Other	Problems

Stage II (1;6–2;0)

		Conn.	Clause	Phrase	Word
VX	QX		SV 6·91	VC/O 5·73	DN 52·55	VV 6·00	inf. 6·64
			SC/O X	AX 4·09	Adj N 5·73	V part 14·73	-ing 31·18
			Neg X	Other	NN X	Int X 1·55	pl 23·36
					PrN 3·00	Other	

Stage III (2;0–2;6)

				-ed 5·45
VXY		X · S:NP 3·73	X · V:VP 10·00	X · C/O:NP 6·27	X · A:AP 3·09	-en 12·09
	QXY	SVC/O 24·18	VC/OA 1·18	D Adj N 7·91	Cop 12·00	3s 0·73
let XY	VS	SVA 13·18	VO₄O₁ 0·36	Adj Adj N 0·45	Aux 38·73	3s 20·82
do XY		Neg XY	Other 0·64	Pr DN 24·73	Pron 18·91	gen
				N Adj N	Pr Pron 1·82	8·36
					18·18 Other 1·36	n't 1·00

Stage IV (2;6–3;0)

		XY · S:NP 20·18	XY · V:VP 24·54	XY · C/O:NP/XY · A:AP 9·72	'cop 5·91
	S	QVS	SVC/OA 11·09	AAXY 3·09	N Pr NP 1·00	Neg V 1·36	'aux
		QXYZ	SVO₄O₁ 0·18	Other 1·64	Pr D Adj N 2·64	Neg X X	15·36
					cX 0·36	2 Aux 1·45	-est 1·00
					XcX 6·27	Other 1·00	-er 6·64

Stage V (3;0–3;6)

		and 25·27	Coord. 1 11·27 1· 5·64	Postmod. 1 7·45 1· 6·18 clause	-ly 1·52
how	tag	1·18	Subord. 1 7·45 1·		
		S 7·45	Clause: S A: 4·00	Postmod. 1 6·45 phrase	
what		Other 1·18	Clause: C/O 2·71		
			Comparative		

		(+)			(–)		

Stage VI (3;6–4;6)	NP	VP	Clause	NP		VP	Clause
	Initiator 3·45	Complex	Passive 6·36	Pron	Adj seq	Modal	Concord 1·36
	Coord X		Complement 6·27	Det	N irreg 6·27	Tense X	A position
						V irreg	W order
	Other			Other 3·27			

Stage VII (4;6+)	Discourse		Syntactic Comprehension	
	A Connectivity 1·45 ii 2·00			
	Comment Clause 6·27 there 6·72		Style * existing Stage I	
	Emphatic Order Other			

Mean Total No. Sentences * 23·18	Mean No. Sentences Per Turn	Mean Sentence Length * 15·12 (max. +/·30)

© D. Crystal, P. Fletcher, M. Garman, 1975 University of Reading

Fig. 44   The mean number of entries for each profile structure grouped across 11 normally-hearing subjects. Where the mean is less than 0·1 an 'X' is entered. Where an entry was never used, it is left blank.

proportion of their Stage III clauses into Stage IV expansions. Referring back to the expansion entries in Figs. 43 and 44, it can be seen that neither group shows any obvious imbalance in the Stage IV expansions: XY + A : AP is small in both cases, but this is to be expected since the Stage III clauses incorporating an adverbial (A) element are fewer in number; otherwise, subject, verb and object expansions are similar within groups. The same is not true of the Stage III expansions. Here again, X + A : AP is expectedly low, but for both groups the expansion of verb element to verb phrase occurs more frequently than expansion of subject or object to noun phrase. However, in both cases there is a simple explanation: the number of Stage II clauses offering an opportunity for verb expansion is greater than those offering an opportunity for subject or object expansion. In this type of task at least, if two-element clauses are produced, then it is more likely that the 'omitted' element will be subject or object than verb. Considering the relative degrees of subject or object expansion at Stage III by the two groups, it can be seen that the normally-hearing group, despite a (possibly) larger number of Stage II subject elements, have more object expansion than subject expansion. This development of structure in object position rather than in subject position is a regular feature of normal language development. The hearing-impaired group, however, show the opposite trend, having more Stage III subject expansions than object expansions, and this may be important.

At the phrase level of analysis, there are no obvious gaps in the hearing-impaired profile, except perhaps the relative lack of auxiliary verbs (Aux) which are low in comparison with the normally-hearing; there is, however, a somewhat lower level of advancement and a generally depressed level of entries, which partly reflects the lack of clause expansion by the hearing-impaired. In almost every case, the mean number of entries for each phrase structure is less for the hearing-impaired group, despite the fact that both groups gave almost exactly the same number of clauses in toto across Stages I–IV (excluding expansions): 72·83 for the hearing-impaired, 72·63 for the normally-hearing. The surprising exceptions are the pronouns (Pron), usually regarded as a clear indicator of advancement, which are in fact slightly *more* frequent in the partially-hearing profile. The figures for the phrase entries at different Stages are compared in Table 6, and it can be

Table 6 Phrase-level analysis: mean number of entries totalled within Stages for the hearing-impaired and the normally-hearing groups

	Group	
Structures	*Hearing-impaired*	*Normally-hearing*
Stage II phrases	66·14	83·56
Stage III phrases	63·99	105·91
Stage IV phrases	8·73	14·08
Stage V phrases	1·03	8·08
Total	139·89	211·63

seen that the number of entries given by the hearing-impaired group is less than those given by the normally-hearing group at every Stage. Furthermore, as one moves from Stage II to Stage V, less to more advanced, the (percentage) gap between the two groups widens. A chi-squared test on the raw frequencies from which the totalled means in Table 5 were derived showed the differences between the two groups to be highly significant ($\chi^2 = 271 \cdot 69$, df $= 3$, $P < 0 \cdot 001$).

At the word level of analysis, every hearing-impaired entry, except -ed, is markedly smaller. Plurals (pl), third person singular inflections (3s) and contracted auxiliaries ('aux) are particularly depressed. A comparison of the proportion of 'aux (word level) to Aux (phrase level) for each group shows that the smaller number of contracted auxiliaries ('aux) for the hearing-impaired is partly but not wholly due to the lack of auxiliaries (Aux) in general. The total number of mean word entries in Figs. 43 and 44 is 74·10 for the hearing-impaired and 134·36 for the normally-hearing, which is a larger shortfall than at the phrase level. Such a result is not unexpected, since we might suspect that because they are especially difficult to hear, the hearing-impaired face greater problems with these morphological items. It should be noted that by the same token, the error variance due to transcriber error will be greater at this level of analysis than at the previous levels of clause and phrase.

The entries at Stages VI and VII are as expected: the hearing-impaired group show more errors and fewer positive features in Stage VI (especially Initiator), but the numbers are rather small. There was virtually no use of passive clauses by the 263 hearing-impaired children: on a total of only two occasions did they use the passive, as opposed to a total of four occasions by the hearing children (who were only eleven in number). This agrees with previous findings (Tervoort 1970), and is thought to relate to sequencing problems in the hearing-impaired.

Mean sentence length and the mean of the sentence length maxima are considerably smaller for the hearing-impaired group. Note that the former does not include Stage I 'sentences', which if they had been included would have depressed the hearing-impaired figures even more. These sentence length figures are a reflection of the lack of recursiveness and the under-use of phrase and word structures by the hearing-impaired.

It is popularly supposed that much hearing-impaired language is deviant or ambiguous, but such was not the case with this sample of children. This may be partly due to a difficulty of definition (particularly of 'deviant'), but is probably also a genuine reflection of the language of the partially-hearing rather than of the profoundly deaf, since the latter formed only a small proportion of the hearing-impaired group. While on this point, it should be noted that although the inclusion of the 22 profoundly deaf children will have tended to increase the difference between the normally-hearing and the hearing-impaired group means, it cannot be argued that the poorer advancement of the latter is due to the inclusion of this group. For one thing, there were relatively few of them. But also, later analyses have shown (see below) that although pure-tone hearing loss is significantly (negatively) correlated with grammatical advancement, the correlation coefficient is not especially high, and there are many other factors which determine grammatical ability.

The overall pattern of the grouped hearing-impaired profile does not seem to match easily any one of the patterns suggested by *GALD* (chapter 6), although it probably comes nearest to their type 3. The pattern we have in Fig. 43 is one of delay on all fronts overlaid with rather weak phrase structure and even weaker word structure.

Finally, it should be noted that two of our four additions to the profile (Pr Pron and fut) do not seem to be particularly important, although fut was no doubt elicited infrequently because of the nature of the task (picture-description). Inf. and Clause: A, however, look more interesting. For the normally-hearing group Clause: A was used more often than Clause: C/O and Clause: S, which was used not at all by the normally-hearing and rarely by the hearing impaired.

2 Factor analysis of the LARSP profiles

The analysis-by-eye of the profile in Fig. 43, especially when supported by statistical tests of significance for selected language structures, can provide useful indications of some of the important differences between the grammar of the hearing-impaired and that of their normally-hearing peers. However, from the point of view of understanding the effects of hearing loss and other background variables upon grammatical advancement, the grouped profile is of limited value since the group itself consists of a very heterogeneous collection of subjects. We could, of course, present profiles grouped according to our 'background' variables—IQ, hearing loss, type of impairment, and so on—but the reader is still left to sort out the effects 'by eye', and, more importantly, such a presentation of the data omits the interactive effects of variables. Thus mere examination of profiles remains, for this type of project, a rather qualitative approach. One of the problems is that the profile contains some hundred or more structures, and it is just not possible to make sense of these for large groups of subjects. Some of the profile *variables* (i.e. structures) will be reliable discriminators between different types of subjects, others will not. We need a method for isolating these important profile variables and for organizing them (including their relationships with the background variables) in a quantitative way. For these reasons, the data were subjected to a factor analysis.

Initially, all the profile variables (for all hearing-impaired subjects) were included in the analysis. As a result of this it was possible to identify those variables with small means and communalities (the communality of a variable is the proportion of its variance which is common to it and to the optimum factor structure; a variable with low communal variance has a large proportion of error variance or variance unique to itself). These variables were then discarded, leaving a total of 56 'important' profile variables.

The clinician or practitioner who is used to assessing individual profiles in a qualitative manner may find this procedure for excluding certain variables somewhat disturbing, since he may be used to attaching a certain amount of weight to the more advanced, rarer entries. It is unfortunately true, however, that those variables with small means also had small communalities, indicating that they could not be regarded as reliable discriminators between subjects (cf. *GALD*, 105).

The remaining 56 profile variables were again subjected to a factor analysis. This analysis was performed on the covariance matrix rather than the correlation matrix, since it was felt that the natural scaling would be more meaningful than assuming that all variables had equal weight. The remarkable result was that one factor (F_1) accounted for 54 per cent of the total variance, while the next most important factor (F_2) accounted for only 9 per cent of the total variance. Using a standard method (the Scree Test) it was clear that, of the 10 factors extracted in the analysis, only the first was of any significance. To put it another way, our analysis shows that the data can be reduced from well over 100 hundred profile variables to one derived variable (F_1) and yet still account for over half of the total variance. The factor loadings of each of the 56 'important' variables on to F_1, and the communality between each variable and F_1 are shown in Table 7.

Table 7 The loadings of the restricted set of 56 profile variables on to Factor 1, and the communalities between each variable and Factor 1

Variable Number	Variable Name	Loading of Variable on to Factor 1	Communality of Variable with Factor 1
1	Ambiguous	−1·04	20
2	Stage 1 Statement 'V'	−2·84	43
3	Stage 1 Statement 'N'	−18·93	50
4	SV	−1·26	08
5	SC/O	−0·94	32
6	VC/O	−0·47	02
7	X+S:NP	0·21	00
8	X+V:VP	1·19	10
9	X+C/O:NP	0·07	00
10	X+A:AP	0·08	00
11	SVC/O	6·39	43
12	SVA	2·83	41
13	XY+S:NP	4·71	32
14	XY+V:VP	6·89	68
15	XY+C/O:NP	4·53	40
16	XY+A:AP	2·49	45
17	SVC/OA	3·36	61
18	AAXY	1·04	38
19	and	7·80	51
20	s	2·56	51
21	coord. 1	4·74	36
22	coord. 1+	1·64	33
23	subord. 1	2·52	51

Variable Number	Variable Name	Loading of Variable on to Factor 1	Communality of Variable with Factor 1
24	Clause:C/O	1·80	38
25	Clause:A	1·78	45
26	DN	10·03	33
27	Adj N	1·02	07
28	VV	1·44	24
29	V Part	2·54	26
30	D Adj N	2·73	41
31	Pr DN	5·86	62
32	Cop	3·63	43
33	Aux	8·84	61
34	Pron	8·05	37
35	Pr Pron	0·76	21
36	Pr D Adj N	0·86	34
37	XcX	1·79	23
38	Neg V	0·58	11
39	2 Aux	0·31	06
40	Postmod. clause 1	0·80	25
41	Inf.	2·40	40
42	-ing	6·54	44
43	pl.	2·55	14
44	-ed	4·57	21
45	-en	1·17	16
46	3s	3·73	27
47	gen	2·81	49
48	n't	0·41	07
49	cop	1·80	26
50	'aux	3·07	25
51	Initiator	0·58	16
52	it	0·74	20
53	there	1·86	29
54	mean words per sentence	2·65	88
55	maximum words per sentence	6·87	68
56	total number of sentences analysed	2·28	05

Notice that F_1 has both positive and negative loadings. Ambiguous, Stage 1 Statements 'V' and 'N', SV, SC/O, and VC/O have negative loadings, while the remainder are all positive. Thus entries in Stages I and II (clause level) actually count 'against' the subject, while entries at all other levels reflect positive advancement in varying degrees. The factor plays off the occurrence of positively-loaded structures against the occurrence of the negatively-loaded structures. The reader might wonder what is so especially advanced about, for example, the DN structure, which has a high positive loading. DN has a large mean value (Fig. 43), and partly in consequence of this it is a highly reliable discriminator. It discriminates along the dimension of grammatical advancement because, although not highly advanced itself, the 'jump' from using nouns without determiners to using them with determiners is, the analysis shows, a very important and indicative progression for our subjects.

There is, then, only one factor of any importance in determining the results. On reflection this is not surprising: Crystal *et al.* did not pick the hundred-odd variables which go to make up the profile out of a hat containing a wide variety of behavioural skills; they picked their variables from a restricted and specific set of grammatical structures which, according to the literature, reflect grammatical advancement. We would expect the main determiner of a person's performance on the profile to be his grammatical advancement, since that is precisely what the profile was designed to reflect. F_1, then, may be labelled 'Grammatical Advancement Factor'. Examination of the communalities (which are equal to the squares of the correlation coefficients between the variables and F_1) in Table 7 supports this interpretation. Mean and maximum words per sentence, XY + V:VP, SVC/OA, Aux and Pr DN, for example, all correlate highly (> 0.78) with F_1.

It is possible to derive a 'Grammatical Advancement Score' for each subject by calculating a weighted sum of the observed variable values, the weights being proportional to the factor loadings. The scaling of these scores is arbitrary and, following precedent, they have been scaled to have zero mean and unit variance. The scores so derived range from $+1.88$ (most advanced) to -2.12 (least advanced). The correlations between these scores and various background variables were calculated, and these correlation coefficients are presented in Table 8.

Table 8 The correlations (Pearson's r) between certain 'background' variables and Grammatical Advancement Scores

Background Variable	Correlation Coefficient	Number of subjects for whom data available	Significance level
Pure-tone hearing loss (Ave. at 500, 1000, 2000 Hz)	-0.42	263	< 0.001
Nonverbal IQ	0.24	263	< 0.001
Age	0.36	263	< 0.001
Age at onset of hearing impairment	0.17	188	< 0.05

While it comes as no surprise that Grammatical Advancement is affected by hearing loss, age, nonverbal IQ, and age at onset of impairment, it is of considerable interest to be able to specify the magnitude of the relationships, and to realize that although the correlations are significant, there is some degree of unexplained variability. If all the background variables from Table 8 are included, the multiple correlation coefficient between these and Grammatical Advancement is 0·66. Clearly, there are other background variables which are of importance in determining Grammatical Advancement. These will include such factors as the time between onset of the impairment and its diagnosis, the type of impairment, educational background and parental occupation, and attempts are currently being made to analyse their effects.

At the time of writing, the analysis of the data has not been taken beyond Table 8, and this chapter will be concluded with a few words about the intended analyses. It is certainly useful and important to be able to quantify the relationships which are known to exist between Grammatical Advancement and such variables as hearing loss, age at onset of impairment and nonverbal IQ, and to compare their relative and combined effects. We will wish to go beyond this, however, and return to the simplified profile (if we think it useful, we may reduce the set of profile variables even further by discarding those remaining items which exhibit low communality with Factor 1), in order to determine what exactly *is* the grammatical basis of poor F_1 scores. Groups of subjects with similar F_1 scores will be isolated and their profiles analysed for significant trends on particular profile variables such as function words, pronouns, SVO's, etc. An important question will be whether similar F_1 scores reflect similar profile patterns, and if not, whether, within a group of similar F_1 scorers, different measures on the background variables tend to go with different profile patterns. To give a rather simple and speculative example, it might be the case that, within a group of children with F_1 scores of, say, about $-1·00$, those with low IQs and mild hearing losses tend to lack four-element clauses and recursive devices, and tend to use rather short sentences; while those, on the other hand, with high IQs but severe high-frequency hearing loss tend to fall down on the word-endings. Indeed, different patterns of pure-tone hearing loss may tend to produce different profile patterns with similar F_1 scores.

Finally a cautionary note. The analysis presented here, and in particular the factor structure, is the optimum structure for discriminating amongst the hearing-impaired individuals who constituted our sample. The sample is representative of hearing-impaired children, and the factor structure will not necessarily, therefore, be a particularly effective discriminator within a group of normally-hearing children of similar age or within another group of different pathology. For example, there may well be normally-hearing children who vary significantly and reliably on some of the structures found in Stages VI and VII. Such a group would probably give a rather different factor structure and weighting, reflecting the increased importance and reliability of these advanced variables. As always, more normative data is required.

3.2

Sentence-repetition tasks compared with expressive language performance

Julie Brinton

The present investigation was carried out by a speech therapist, with the primary intention of seeing if a sentence imitation task could provide useful information about a child's expressive language ability, in the context of language delay. It is known, from the work of Slobin and Welsh (1971) and others, that imitation tasks can be used as a 'probe' to test hypotheses about syntactic competence in normally-developing children. What is not clear, however, is the extent to which similar tasks might be used in clinical context, as part of a screening or assessment procedure. Use of the LARSP procedure, it was felt, might provide a more precise means than is routinely available for estimating the nature and extent of the correlation between expression and imitation at the grammatical level.

Ten children with delayed language development (the LD group) were selected to form the experimental group. They had expressive language scores (as measured by the Reynell Developmental Language Scales) of one or more standard deviations below the mean. The age range of the group was 3;1–4;10, mean 48·3 months. In all cases their comprehension was equal to, or above their expressive language, and their articulation was not grossly deviant. The language assessment was carried out by the speech therapist in charge of the case, and was done within one month prior to the experiment. All the children came from English-speaking families, were of normal intelligence, and had no hearing-loss. In some cases the children had had their intelligence assessed, and the rest were considered of average intelligence by the Medical Officer of Health and the speech therapist. The children were all boys and were attending for speech therapy at one of four health clinics in southwest London.

The experimental group was matched with 20 normal children—10 of the same chronological age (the CA group), and 10 who matched their language age (the LA group). The CA age-range was 3;0–4;10, mean 48·5 months. The age-range for the LA control group was 2;1–3;5, mean 35·5 months. The children selected to form the control groups were attending day nurseries, a playgroup, or a nursery school. Where possible, the social class of each child was documented so that the closest matching for class was made.

The spontaneous speech of each child was taped for 20 minutes, and the tape

Graham　　　　　　　　　　　　　　　　　　　　　　　　　　A

A	**Unanalysed**			**Problematic**	
	1 Unintelligible	2 Symbolic Noise	3 Deviant	1 Incomplete	2 Ambiguous

B Responses

				Normal Response						Abnormal		
		Totals	Repet-itions	Elliptical Major				Full Major	Minor	Struc-tural	Ø	Prob-lems
Stimulus Type				1	2	3	4					
	Questions			8	3	1			31			
	Others			2								

C Spontaneous 　　　　　　　Others

Minor		Social **4**	Stereotypes	Problems

Stage I (0;9–1;6) — Sentence Type

Major			Sentence Structure		
Excl.	Comm.	Quest.	Statement		
	·V·	·Q·	·V· 1 ·N· 7	Other 5	Problems

		Conn.	Clause		Phrase		Word
Stage II (1;6–2;0)	VX	QX	SV	VC/O 5	DN 6	VV	-ing 3
			S C/O 2	AX 4	Adj N 3	V part 6	pl 3
			Neg X	Other	NN 1	Int X	-ed 3
					PrN 4	Other	
Stage III (2;0–2;6)	VXY	QXY	X + S:NP	X + V:VP	X + C/O:NP	X + A:AP	-en
	let XY	VS	SVC/O	VC/OA 2	D Adj N	Cop	
	do XY		SVA	VOdOi	Adj Adj N 1	Aux	3s
			Neg XY	Other	Pr DN	Pron 5	gen
					N Adj N	Other 1	
Stage IV (2;6–3;0)	S	QVS	XY + S:NP	XY + V:VP	XY + C/O:NP	XY + A:AP	n't
		QXYZ	SVC/OA	AAXY	N Pr NP	Neg V	'cop
			SVOdOi	Other	Pr D Adj N	Neg X	'aux
					cX	2 Aux	
					XcX	Other	
Stage V (3;0–3;6)	how	tag	and / Coord. 1	1 ·	Postmod. 1 clause	1 ·	-est
		c	Subord. 1	1 ·			-er
	what	s	Clause: S		Postmod. 1 · phrase		-ly
		Other	Clause: C/O				
			Comparative				

	(+)			(−)		
	NP	VP	Clause	NP	VP	Clause
Stage VI (3;6–4;6)	Initiator	Complex	Passive	Pron — Adj seq	Modal	Concord
	Coord		Complement	Det — N irreg	Tense	A position
					V irreg	W order
	Other			Other		

	Discourse		Syntactic Comprehension	
Stage VII (4;6+)	A Connectivity	it		
	Comment Clause	there	Style	
	Emphatic Order	Other		

Total No. Sentences	Mean No. Sentences Per Turn	Mean Sentence Length

Fig. 45　LD group: example 1

Peter

A **Unanalysed**

			Problematic	
1 Unintelligible 9	2 Symbolic Noise 6	3 Deviant 1	1 Incomplete 2	2 Ambiguous 1

B **Responses**

Stimulus Type		Totals	Repet-itions	Normal Response						Abnormal			Prob-lems
				Elliptical Major				Full Major	Minor	Struc-tural	Ø		
				1	2	3	4						
	Questions			2	3	3	2	9	21			
	Others				1		1					

C **Spontaneous**   Others

Sentence Type		**Minor**			Social 3		Stereotypes 2		Problems	

Stage I (0;9–1;6)

Major					Sentence Structure				
Excl.	Comm.	Quest.			Statement				
	·V·	·Q·	·V·	·N·	Other		Problems		

Stage II (1;6–2;0)

	Conn.	Clause		Phrase		Word
V X	Q X	SV 4	V C/O 1	DN 11	VV	-ing 22
		S C/O	A X 1	Adj N 3	V part 8	pl 11
		Neg X	Other	NN	Int X	
				PrN 1	Other	

Stage III (2;0–2;6)

						-ed 5
V X Y 2 3	Q X Y	X + S:NP	X + V:VP 1	X + C/O:NP	X + A:AP 1	-en 2
let X Y	QXY VS	SVC/O 14	VC/OA	D Adj N 1	Cop 11	3s 6
		SVA 5	VOdOi	Adj Adj N 1	Aux 12	gen
do X Y		Neg X Y	Other	Pr DN 2	Pron 97	
				N Adj N	Other 1	

Stage IV (2;6–3;0)

						n't 9
S	QVS	XY + S:NP	XY + V:VP 2	XY + C/O:NP 2	XY + A:AP 1	'cop 9
	QXYZ 1	SVC/OA 5	AAXY 2	N Pr NP	Neg V	'aux 7
		SVO₁O₂	Other	Pr D Adj N	Neg X	
				cX	2 Aux 1	
				XcX	Other	

Stage V (3;0–3;6)

	how what	and 7 c 5 s 5 Other 1	Coord. 1 7	1·	Postmod. 1 7 clause	1· 2	-est -er 1 -ly
		tag 3	Subord. 1	1·			
			Clause: S		Postmod. 1 5 phrase		
			Clause: C/O				
			Comparative 3				

Stage VI (3;6–4;6)

(+)			(−)			
NP	VP	Clause	NP		VP	Clause
Initiator	Complex 1	Passive	Pron	Adj seq	Modal 1	Concord
Coord		Complement	Det	N irreg	Tense 1	A position
					V irreg	W order
Other			Other 1			

Stage VII (4;6+)

Discourse		Syntactic Comprehension	
A Connectivity	it		
Comment Clause	there	Style	
Emphatic Order	Other		

Total No. Sentences	Mean No. Sentences Per Turn	Mean Sentence Length

© D. Crystal, P. Fletcher, M. Garman, 1975 University of Reading

Fig. 46   LD group: example 2

transcribed within 24 hours. The children were seen individually, and given four miniature dolls and doll's-house material to play with. They were encouraged to play, and when they were at ease the taperecorder was switched on. Some of the LD group were seen with their speech therapist and/or mother so that the child might be more at ease. The conversation that was taped followed *GALD* procedure, and full profiles were made of each child. Two examples are given in Figs. 45 and 46.

Sentence length was selected as the variable for increasing sentence complexity, in order to investigate imitation performance. Twenty-one sentences were used in a repetition-task—7 of 7-word length, 7 of 9-word length, and 7 of 11-word length. Words were selected which were in frequent use to and by children in the preschool age range, and which should be equally familiar to children from different socioeconomic backgrounds. The sentences were given in a random order, but in the same order for each child (see Table 9). In each case, the sentences were given after the spontaneous speech sample had been taken.

Table 9 Sentences used in the sentence-repetition task

---

1 All the children are in the play-ground now
2 Mummy is wearing a new dress for the party
3 The ball is bouncing up and down
4 The little girl likes playing with her big brother
5 All the pretty flowers are growing in the back garden now
6 The girl and her brother are sleeping
7 The girl is running fast to catch the big red bus
8 The big black cat is climbing up a tree
9 All the children like to play in the lovely white snow
10 There are lots of pretty flowers there
11 Daddy is going to drive the big new car
12 The boy and his little sister go shopping with their mummy
13 The man is putting the book there
14 The little girl is playing with her big doll
15 The little boy is bouncing a red ball there
16 The girl plays with the dolls house
17 Daddy is going out to the garden
18 The girl and the boy like playing on the high swings
19 The little girl is playing with her brother and his friend
20 My mummy and her friend are going to the town today
21 The dog is barking at the cat

Fig. 47 shows the increasing order of complexity for the three groups of sentences. There is very little difference in overall grammatical level, the constituent features being distributed fairly evenly between Stages II and IV, as shown on p. 271.

The instructions given to each child were the same. The children were told they were going to play the 'Smartie game', as follows: 'Now we're going to play a

A	Unanalysed					Problematic		
	1 Unintelligible		2 Symbolic Noise		3 Deviant	1 Incomplete		2 Ambiguous

B   Responses

				Normal Response						Abnormal		
					Elliptical Major				Full		Struc-		Prob-
Stimulus Type		Totals	Repet-itions	1	2	3	4	Major	Minor	tural	Ø	lems
	Questions												
	Others												

C   Spontaneous   Others

	Minor	Social	Stereotypes	Problems

Stage I (0;9–1;6)   Sentence Type

Major				Sentence Structure				
Excl.	Comm.	Quest.			Statement			
	'V'	'Q'	'V'	'N'	Other	Problems		

Stage II (1;6–2;0)

	Conn.		Clause			Phrase		Word
	V X	Q X	SV *1-0-0*	VC/O *0-0-1*	DN *7-0-7*	vv *0-2-3*		-ing *5-6-5*
			S C/O	A X	Adj N	V part *1-2-1*		
			Neg X	Other	NN	Int X		pl *2-1-3*
					PrN	Other *0-0-1*		-ed

Stage III (2;0–2;6)

	V X Y	Q X Y	X + S:NP *1-0-0X* + V:VP *1-0-0X* + C/O:NP *X* + A:AP					
		Q X Y	SVC/O *0-2-0*	VC/OA	D Adj N *0-7-1*	Cop *1-1-0*		-en
	let X Y	VS	SVA *2-1-2*	VO_dO_i	Adj Adj N	Aux *5-5-3*		
			Neg X Y	Other	Pr DN *2-3-1*	Pron		3s *5-6-1*
	do X Y				N Adj N *0-1-0*	Other *2-1-1*		gen *1-0-0*

Stage IV (2;6–3;0)

	S	QVS	X Y + S:NP *4-3-3X Y* + V:VP *4-4-3 X Y* + C/O:NP *X Y* + A:AP					n't
		QVS	SVC/OA *3-3-1*	AA X Y *1-1-3*	N Pr NP *5-3-3*			
		Q X Y Z	SVO_dO_i	Other	Pr D Adj N *0-0-2*	Neg X		'cop
					c X	2 Aux		
					X c X *2-0-3*	Other *0-2-3*		'aux

Stage V (3;0–3;6)

	how	tag	and	Coord. 1	1 +	Postmod. 1 clause	1 +	-est
			c	Subord. 1 *0-0-1* 1 +				-er
			s *0-0-1*	Clause: S		Postmod. 1 phrase		
	what		Other	Clause: C/O				-ly
				Comparative				

(+)			(−)				
NP	VP	Clause	NP		VP		Clause

Stage VI (3;6–4;6)

Initiator *1-1-2*	Complex *0-2-1*	Passive	Pron	Adj seq	Modal		Concord
Coord		Complement	Det	N irreg	Tense		A position
					V irreg		W order
Other			Other				

Stage VII (4;6 +)

Discourse		Syntactic Comprehension	
A Connectivity	it		
Comment Clause	there *1-0-0*	Style	
Emphatic Order	Other		

Total No. Sentences	Mean No. Sentences Per Turn	Mean Sentence Length

Fig. 47   Conflated profile of 7-, 9- and 11-word sentences

	No. of structure tokens		
Level	*7-word*	*9-word*	*11-word*
Stage II	9	4	12
III	14	20	8
IV	19	17	21
V	0	0	2
VI	1	3	3
VII	1	0	0
Word level	13	13	9

game. It is "Say what I say". If I say "The doll is standing up", you must say ..., etc.' Each practice sentence was rewarded with a Smartie. If the child was still uncertain, these sentences were repeated until he knew what to do. The test sentences were administered in the same way, and rewarded with verbal praise or Smarties. If the instructor felt that the child did not hear the sentence, then it was given again. If there was no reason to believe the child had not heard, then the sentence was not repeated, and 'no response' was noted. The child was reminded during the testing to 'say exactly what I say', and was given much verbal encouragement. Care was taken to ensure that the child was attending before the stimulus sentence was given, and the child's name was sometimes called to direct his attention to the task. The sentences were given one after the other, with no breaks, and all the children—even the youngest—could cope with this length of concentration. The task took between three and ten minutes.

The imitations were transcribed and scored for omissions, substitutions, repetitions, and the total number of correct imitations. The total number of possible omissions or substitutions at each level—clause, phrase, and word—was calculated for each sentence. For example, in the sentence

```
The ball   is bouncing  up and down
   S            V             A
───────   ──────────   ──────────
 D  N  Aux   v      X   c   X
        3s     -ing
```

the total number of possible omissions would be 3 at clause level, 7 at phrase level, and 2 at word level (transitional information was excluded). If the child's response was *ball bounce*, one omission error is made at clause level, five at phrase level, and one at word level. If the child did not respond at all, he was scored with the total possible omissions for that sentence.

The same measure was taken for substitutions, as substitutions in responses were all found to be word for word, or phrase for phrase, for example

Stimulus: *The girl plays with the doll's house*
Response: *The girl plays with her baby*
(Errors: 2 substitutions at phrase level, 1 omission at phrase level, 1 omission at word level)

The individual child's total number of errors scored was converted into a percentage of the total possible at each syntactic level for each sentence length.

The number of repeated elements was calculated if repetition was immediate with no change at all (even a change of stress), e.g. *her girl girl big doll* was counted as a repetition of one phrase-level element (cf. stimulus sentence 14, Table 9); *the boy bounce, the boy bounce the ball* was a repetition of one clause (cf. sentence 15, Table 9) etc.

The number of correctly-imitated sentences was calculated for each child at each sentence length.

The data for the sentence-repetition task was examined, and the distribution of the scores for the omission errors permitted a 3-way analysis of variance to be carried out (Winer 1962). The data for substitution errors, although calculated in the same way, did not show a normal distribution, and so this data, and that for repetition errors and sentences repeated correctly were prepared for the Fisher Exact Probability Test (Siegel 1956).

Grouping profiles

It was found by examining the profiles that the children in each group were functioning at different stages, and fell into clear subgroups, as follows:

LD Group: 1 Stage III (3 children), including no commands/questions, and up to 4 different word-endings
2 Stage IV (3 children): most utterances at III or even II, but a few in IV; very restricted development at word level (1 or 2 endings)
3 Stage V (4 children): even spread at IV and one or two different constructions at V or VI; word-endings well developed

CA Group: 1 Stage IV (3 children): even spread with fewer constructions at IV than III; fewer constructions at III than (2) below; between 4 and 7 different word-endings
2 Stage V (3 children): spread across the chart; no comparatives; 2 tags; 7 or 8 word-endings
3 Stage VI (4 children): spread more in the negative box than the positive box; well-established Stage V structures, with more here than in (2) above

LA Group: 1 Stage III (2 children): Stage I well-established; one child had poor phrase level development and 2 different word-endings; the other had better phrasal development and 3 word-endings
2 Stage IV (4 children): (a) 2 children had a few structures overall and only a few at IV; 3 or 4 different word-endings; (b) 2 children had many structures overall, and more at IV than in (a); 6 different word-endings in both cases
3 Stage V (2 children): a few Stage V structures and 5–7 different word-endings

4 Stage VI (2 children): even spread at early stages, well-developed in all areas; 7 different word-endings in each case; great use of auxiliaries and pronouns

These groupings suggest the way that children develop through the stages of the profile. If a child is just entering one stage, most of his utterances are found in the previous stage (see Fig. 45); he remains in the new stage until it is consolidated before being able to produce more complex structures. In some cases it appeared that the phrase-level utterances developed first, followed by clause-level structures. Usually, however, there was a greater variety of structures at clause level that appeared first. The use of pronouns becomes very marked at Stage III or IV. The word-level endings did not show a development from the top of the list to the bottom, but showed two clusters, as illustrated in Fig. 46.

Results and discussion

Substitutions, repetitions and correct imitations showed no significant differences across the three groups, and are not discussed further here. The analysis of variance of the omission errors did however display some points of interest, as shown in Table 10.

Table 10 Omission errors in the repetition task

Source of Variation	SS	df	MS	F
Sentence length	7797·541	2	3898·77	6·562 $P < 0.05$
Group	23197·608	2	11598·80	19·522 $P < 0.01$
Syntactic level	29464·208	2	14732·1	24·522 $P < 0.01$
Sentence length x group	197·748	4	49·44	0·083 ns
Sentence length x syntactic level	4036·948	4	1009·24	1·699 ns
Group x syntactic level	1241·214	4	310·3	0·522 ns
Sentence length x group x syntactic level	438·330	8	54·79	0·092 ns
Within cell	144373·4	243	594·13	
Total	210746·997	269		

The profiles were then rank-ordered against the rank-ordered omission errors obtained from the sentence repetition task. The results of the subsequent analysis by Spearmans rho are given in Table 11.

Analysis of variance of omission errors showed a significant result for the three main effects of groups (language delay, chronological-age controls, and language-

Table 11 Breakdown of group omission errors

Group	Level		
	Clause	Phrase	Word
LD	0·32 ns	0·16 ns	0·64 $P < 0·05$
CA	0·33 ns	−0·25 ns	0·33 ns
LA	0·59 $P < 0·05$	0·60 $P < 0·05$	0·51 ns

age controls), syntactic level (clause, phrase and word), and sentence length (7, 9, 11 words). Syntactic level showed the following order of difficulty: clause level had the least omissions, then phrase level, and word level had the most. When the means were examined across all levels, the most errors were seen at sentence length 9, and when the transcriptions were analysed, a recency effect was noticed at sentence length 11. The results showed a change in strategy, i.e. when the longer sentences were repeated, the last few words of the stimulus sentence were repeated exactly and sometimes followed by some words from earlier in the sentence, e.g.

Stimulus   *The little girl is playing with her brother and his friend*
Response   *Friend, her brother and friend*

The child appears to use the meaning of the whole sentence when repeating 7- and 9-word sentences, and repeats more than the last few words only. However, when the sentence to be recalled is of 11 words, then the child no longer reproduces the meaning of the sentence, but repeats only the last few words that are still in his short-term memory.

The above results show that for the LA control group, the omission errors on sentence-repetition tasks closely resemble their performance on the LARSP profile. This is true at clause and phrase level ($P < 0·05$) for the LA group, but not at word level. This suggests that sentence-repetition tasks may be appropriate to investigate the linguistic ability of the younger age group who are developing language normally (supporting Slobin and Welsh 1971). The chronological-age controls and the LD group, however, do not show this correspondence between expressive language and repetition tasks. It may be that at a certain stage in development, the child's encoding and decoding strategies for imitated and spontaneous speech are similar, but that this changes with age. The language-delayed child may have problems of recall of verbal information, but is able to use language at a higher level than his imitative ability would suggest.

Sociolinguistic factors may explain why these two sets of data are not seen to be more predictive of each other. The task of repeating sentences is a strange one for the child, and sets up its own sociolinguistic constraints which are different from those experienced by the child whilst talking about the toys he is playing with. So it is perhaps not surprising that the performance in one speaking situation should not predict the performance in another, except for the very young child who may not yet be as aware as older children of the different situations.

3.3

Some remarks on the teaching of LARSP

J. H. Connolly

During the last few years, several assessment procedures have been published which provide a fairly comprehensive and systematic analysis of grammatical disabilities. Of these procedures, LARSP is probably the best known to clinicians in Britain, at least, though other schemes have been developed elsewhere, notably by Lee (1966), Engler, Hannah and Longhurst (1973), and Dever and Baumann (1974). However, LARSP has two major advantages over these. Firstly, it employs a mode of description which has been worked out in detail and set out systematically in readily available grammars (Quirk *et al.* 1972, Quirk and Greenbaum 1973). Secondly, it embodies the Syntactic Profile Chart, which not only provides a standard format for the detailed representation of patients' abilities and deficits, but also, being arranged developmentally, facilitates immediate comparison of the range of grammatical patterns used by any individual child patient with the range that is available to a normal child of the same age. Clearly, an assessment procedure of this kind cannot fail to be of great value to clinicians, once they have been trained in its use. Of course, there is more to the assessment of a child with delayed or deviant language, or of an adult with an acquired language disability, than simply the analysis of the patient's grammatical patterns. The assessment needs to include other factors, such as his or her physical and psychological state. But nevertheless, a refined grammatical assessment procedure like LARSP is a vital part of the clinician's armoury, and the effort involved in learning to employ it is well invested.

The efficient administration of LARSP demands both familiarity with the Syntactic Profile Chart and a reasonable degree of skill in grammatical analysis. In order to train clinicians in its use, therefore, courses need to be provided to help them acquire the necessary experience. In the case of student speech therapists, the provision of courses should present no great problem. Such courses can simply be integrated into their training programme. It is pleasing to note that some skill in grammatical analysis is now required of all candidates taking the College of Speech Therapists' Diploma examination, while the subject is also taught in various degree courses which lead to a qualification in Speech Therapy. However, with regard to those qualified therapists whose training has not included much, or even any, formal linguistics, the situation is less straightforward. Various courses on

LARSP have been organized for the benefit of therapists and others interested in the analysis of language disorders, and the authors of LARSP have, in fact, visited some Area Speech Therapy Services to give instruction in its use. Moreover, in more than one Area, the therapists have been given courses by, and collaborated in the clinic with, members of staff of the local speech-therapy training centre, to the mutual benefit of both parties. One hopes that until all practising therapists have had courses in grammatical analysis as part of their initial training (a situation which is not likely to obtain until the next century!), in-service and refresher courses will continue to be provided, and that therapists will continue to be encouraged and given the financial support to attend them. It is, clearly, to the ultimate benefit of patients that therapists should be given the best possible opportunity to learn to use the latest grammatical assessment and remediation procedures.

Assuming that such courses are to be provided, what should they contain? Let us consider courses for student therapists, where the time available is sufficient for a reasonably thorough training to be given in LARSP and in the techniques of grammatical analysis, which constitute an essential prerequisite to its use. In my opinion, such training should be integrated into the students' overall linguistics programme, a view which seems to be shared by others whom I have consulted.[32] The exact placement of LARSP within this general programme depends, however, on the overall time available for the latter. In Leicester, the linguistics programme proper, excluding psycholinguistics, at present extends over the first two years of a three-year training course. It begins with an introduction to the scientific study of language, and of grammar in particular. This lasts for one term, the second and third terms then being devoted to a study of the structure of adult English together with an outline of its development in childhood. It is here that LARSP is introduced, the Syntactic Profile Chart being, in fact, a useful teaching-aid in this context. Practice in grammatical analysis also begins at this stage. The first year linguistics course also includes phonetics and elementary phonology. The second year involves semantics, sociolinguistics, and more advanced aspects of grammatical theory, phonology and language acquisition. It also includes training in phonological analysis and further practice in grammatical analysis. The compression of all this into two years is necessitated by the structure of the College of Speech Therapists' examination system. In departments which do not prepare students for this particular examination, the linguistics programme can be extended over a period of up to four years, and LARSP introduced later than the first year. Thus in Reading and Glasgow (Jordanhill), LARSP is taught in the third of four years. The chief considerations, however, which apply to all the different full-time courses, are firstly that LARSP should not be introduced until

[32] I should like to thank Dr Michael Garman (Reading), Dr Pamela Grunwell (Birmingham), Mr Trevor Hill (Glasgow), and my colleague Mrs Rae Smith, for the information with which they have kindly supplied me on the teaching of LARSP within the courses in which they are or have been involved, and for pointing out the aspects of LARSP which students have, in their experience, found most difficult. They should not, of course, be assumed to share all the opinions which I have expressed here.

students have done sufficient linguistics for them to find it reasonably easy to follow, and secondly that it should not be introduced too late for students to gain adequate practice in using it before they qualify and perhaps find themselves with no-one to ask for advice on, for example, the finer points of grammatical analysis or profiling.

Having placed the introduction of the teaching of LARSP within the overall training programme, we may next consider the internal structure and content of the LARSP course. In Leicester, in fact, the teaching of LARSP takes place mainly within the first-year Structure of English course. This means that students are familiar with at least the theory behind LARSP in time for their first clinical placement, and furthermore, it helps to show the relevance of a course in English grammatical structure to the needs of the clinician. The Structure of English course begins with an outline of clause-rank (or clause-level) structures in adult English statements, questions and commands. Next, the Syntactic Profile Chart is introduced, even though this means a slight digression from the study of English structure as such. The purpose of the Chart is explained, and its arrangement illustrated with reference to the development of clause-rank structures, which development is, of course, thereby covered in outline. Furthermore, an explanation is given of how a suitable sample of a patient's speech may be obtained and transcribed, and how, when the data have been analysed, the Chart can be completed to yield a quantitative profile of the patient's grammatical ability. The categorization of utterances as Unanalysed, Responses and Spontaneous is also dealt with at this stage, as is their classification as Full Major, Elliptical and Minor. The last three terms are, in fact, already familiar from the earlier, introductory course on the study of grammar, but the distinction between Elliptical and Incomplete utterances needs, nevertheless, to be emphasized here. The calculation of sample length in terms of Total Number of Sentences (important for the comparison of successive profiles of the same patient) and of Mean Sentence Length is also described at this point. Thus, as far as the Syntactic Profile Chart is concerned, all that remains outstanding is coverage of structures at ranks other than that of the clause. These are dealt with one rank at a time, following a description of adult grammar at the rank concerned. The Chart is thus made available for use as quickly as possible, the remainder of the Structure of English course then being devoted to more advanced topics, such as the syntax of non-finite constructions. Whenever a particular area of grammar is covered, students are referred to the appropriate sections of Quirk and Greenbaum 1973.

The order of exposition within the Structure of English course is thus as follows:

(i) introduction to adult English clause-rank syntax;
(ii) outline of clause-rank development in children, with reference to the Syntactic Profile Chart, which is introduced at this point;
(iii) introduction to adult phrase-rank syntax;
(iv) outline of phrase-rank development in children. with reference to the

    (v)   introduction to adult word structure;

   (vi)   outline of the development of word structure in children, with reference to the Syntactic Profile Chart;

  (vii)   introduction to connectivity in adult syntax;

 (viii)   outline of the development of connectivity in children, with reference to the Syntactic Profile Chart;

   (ix)   more advanced adult syntax (e.g. nonfinite constructions).

I would not, of course, claim that this is the only way of introducing LARSP or organizing a Structure of English course. It is simply the way that seems best to fit the overall scheme of the particular training course provided by one particular establishment. As long as a course is internally coherent, the details of its design must depend on the general form of the training programme in the institution concerned.

What teaching methods are appropriate for courses in English grammar and in the use of LARSP? Since neither of these subjects is very easy to learn out of books, most people appear to find some form of face-to-face tuition helpful, and this is generally provided partly in the form of lectures and partly in the form of small-group tutorials or seminars. Personally, I teach grammatical theory, adult English syntax and morphology, and grammatical development in childhood, through the medium of lectures. This enables points of difficulty to be given a more detailed explanation than is available in any textbook; and although I view lectures as being supplementary to students' reading, and not a substitute for the latter, I consider that students will benefit more from a grammar like Quirk and Greenbaum (1973) if they are introduced to it gradually through lectures than if they are faced with the forbidding prospect of finding their way round it on their own while still fairly new to the subject. Of course, it is not possible to cover the whole of English grammatical structure in a lecture course. Ultimately, therefore, students must learn to refer to the grammar-book when faced with the analysis of a difficult construction, rather than relying solely on lecture-notes. Sooner or later, in the course of clinical practice, they are sure to encounter problematic constructions, and the more familiar they are with the grammar-book, the more efficiently they will be able to use it as an aid.

During lectures on English grammar, I feel it is a good idea not only to explain grammatical constructions, but also to indicate how to analyse these constructions on paper (or rather, on the blackboard, in the first instance!). The rationale behind this is that although students may be led to understand, for example, the function of the subordinate clause in the sentence *He arrived after she had left*, this does not of itself mean that they can actually set out the analysis of the sentence in terms of clause-rank functional elements in a manner such as the following:

He   arrived after she had left
  S   V   A
           s   S   V

Plainly, students also need practice in performing grammatical analysis themselves. This they obtain during small-group tutorials, where a better opportunity exists than in lectures for individuals to be helped with the particular points which they find difficult. They also acquire further experience through exercises which they perform in their own time, with the aid of a grammar. These exercises, when completed, are discussed at the next tutorial. It has been found prudent to give a number of examples of a given construction in exercises if students are to come to recognize it readily and thus gain fluency in analysis. Similarly, facility in placing structures, once analysed, on the Syntactic Profile Chart comes only with practice, though certain rules of thumb can be given as a guide; for example, two-element structures generally figure at Stage II and three-element structures at Stage III, though there are some exceptions. Fortunately, practice in placing structures on the Chart can easily be combined with practice in actual analysis. The need for a good deal of practice in these areas deserves to be emphasized. It is easy for experienced linguists to underestimate the difficulties which newcomers find in acquiring the skill of practical analysis. Most students have been taught very little of the structure of English in school, let alone practical analysis—a trend which I personally consider most regrettable—and for this reason, it is necessary to guard against proceeding too quickly.

Although the aim of training in grammatical analysis within a speech therapy course is ultimately to equip students to analyse patients' utterances (see further Grunwell 1975, Connolly 1977), it is better to confine initial practice to the analysis of normal adult structures. These are difficult enough in themselves, without the extra problems presented by non-adult data. A useful source of material here is Algeo 1974. Practice in the analysis of grammar at a particular rank can profitably begin as soon as the area concerned has been covered in lectures. In order to equip students to use LARSP, however, it is essential to build up to a stage where they can not only perform analysis at clause rank, phrase rank and word rank, but also perceive the relationship between sentences, and between clauses within the same sentence, categorize sentences as full major, elliptical and minor, and identify sentence types such as statement or question.

This goal must, of course, be attained gradually. In particular, it is advisable to begin with exercises containing no embedded structures whatever, before proceeding step by step towards the analysis of multiply-embedded sentences. Thus, for instance, students should learn to cope with simple sentences like *The dog has upset the bin* (with no embedding) before they progress to sentences like *The dog has upset the box of chocolates* (with a prepositional phrase embedded within the object noun phrase), while a sentence such as *The dog avoided the house of the man who hated animals* should be presented only to reasonably experienced analysts, containing as it does a relative clause within a noun phrase within a prepositional phrase within another noun phrase!

There is, of course, a limit to the extent to which students can be prepared for all the different structures that they might encounter. Consequently, teaching should emphasize the principles of analysis, rather than attempting merely to provide a set of model analyses for particular types of structure, since the structural variety found in English is enormous. Students should, therefore, in my opinion, be taught to recognize elements of structure in terms of criteria; for example, the subject of a clause can be identified through concord, position and realization type (for details, see Quirk and Greenbaum 1973, 170). There is no harm in using semantic criteria, either, as a source of hypotheses, provided that these hypotheses are then checked against the crucial grammatical criteria. For instance, since the subject often represents the entity which performs the process identified by the verbal element, this particular semantic role can be used as a clue to help in the syntactic analysis. Accordingly, in the sentence *The cat chased the mouse, the cat*, representing the performer of the process of 'chasing', may be taken as a candidate for the category of subject, as, indeed, it proves to be when tested against the syntactic criteria mentioned above. Students must, however, be warned against uncritical reliance on such semantic clues; in the sentence *The mouse was chased by the cat*, it is *the mouse* which is the subject, despite the fact that the semantic roles of the two participants are the same here as in the previous example.

It is worth mentioning at this juncture some points which students of grammatical analysis tend to find particularly difficult. With regard to the mechanics of analysis, four such areas of difficulty may be noted:

(i) segmentation (e.g. deciding whether the sentence *He arrived yesterday at three o'clock* should be divided into three or four clause-rank elements);

(ii) multiple class-membership (e.g. realizing that a word like *fast* may on different occasions be categorized as a noun, an adjective, a verb or an adverb, depending on the function it fulfils in the sentence concerned);

(iii) application of appropriate categories to structures of particular ranks (e.g. describing clause-rank patterns in terms of subject, adverbial etc., rather than in terms of noun, adverb etc.);

(iv) embedding (e.g. identifying structures like subordinate clauses, or postmodifying phrases within noun phrases).

Embedding is probably the most difficult of the four. The deeper the embedding, the harder the task of analysis tends to appear, embedded nonfinite clauses being especially difficult. Often students find that, although they can understand the analysis of a sentence when it is demonstrated to them, they are unable to perform such an analysis on their own. Competence in this area improves with practice, of course, but the ability to recognize a particular construction, for example a postmodifying prepositional phrase within a noun phrase, may be fostered by first demonstrating the analysis of a sentence containing the construction and then asking students to produce new sentences containing the same construction. In performing this essentially creative task, they have to draw upon more than a merely passive understanding of the analysis of sentences containing the construction concerned.

In my view, some grounding in the academic skill of grammatical analysis is necessary before the analysis of unedited data in the form of patients' utterances can be attempted. The analysis of clinical data may, therefore, either be introduced in such a way that clause-rank analysis of such data is attempted immediately after clause-rank analysis of adult sentences but before phrase-rank analysis of the latter, and so on, or else its introduction may be delayed until the analysis of simple adult sentences at all ranks has been covered. My own inclination is towards the second of these two strategies, because of the extra difficulties associated with the analysis of clinical data which, if encountered by students before they have gained confidence in normal analysis, might prove disconcerting and even discouraging.

The analysis of clinical data is far more problematic than that of sentences of the normal adult language. Even the grammatical analysis of the actual speech of normal adults can be difficult, as it tends to contain utterances which do not conform to the pattern of grammatical sentences, being perhaps unfinished, or containing repetitions of words and phrases, to mention but two possibilities. In a dysphasic patient's speech, however, these problems are often more acute, and in some cases, the syntax is so deviant that the scope for normal analysis becomes severely limited. The following extract from the speech of a patient quoted by Critchley (1970, 220) is a case in point:

> *I drove him when the straightaway from he guards and place, I forget to talker, what, where the name of the police I told where the place there . . .*

In this sequence, it is not always possible to decide on the syntactic relationship between the different words, so that a full grammatical analysis in terms of normal syntactic categories cannot be given. Nevertheless, some fragments of the utterance can be related to normal syntactic patterns; for example, the first three words suggest the clause-rank analysis subject + verbal element + object.

The application of normal grammatical categories to the analysis of the utterances of young children is also beset with problems. In fact, attempts have been made to establish special types of category for the analysis of child language. None of these, however, has yet gained near-universal acceptance even in principle. For example, Braine's (1963) distributional categories of 'pivot' class and 'X-class' (which has since become known as 'open' class) have been attacked by Brown (1973, 97–110), while his own mode of analysis (see esp. 189–98) has in turn been criticized by Howe (1976, 34–45). The LARSP approach is to make use of the normal adult categories as far as is practical, but to admit explicitly that their application to early speech is tentative and that, for this and other reasons, problematic utterances will arise. Hence, places are provided on the Syntactic Profile Chart where problematic utterances may be entered. When writing down analysed structures prior to entering them on the Chart, it can be useful to employ a symbol such as X, or U (for 'unclassified'), for elements which cannot be assigned unequivocally to a single category. For example, if the child utterance

> *now mummy*

were encountered in a context where *mummy* could not with confidence be analysed as either subject, object or complement, then a representation of the whole structure as AX or AU might help the analyst to see where it should be entered on the Chart.

It is important that students should be made aware of the problematic nature of the analysis of clinical data, and warned that it is unrealistic to expect to be able to analyse every utterance encountered. They should be advised that rather than puzzle over an utterance for an inordinate amount of time, it is better simply to label it as 'problematic', and they may also take advantage of the fact, when completing the Syntactic Profile Chart, that several categories have been conflated—for example, object and complement. On the other hand, it is important not to inculcate a defeatist attitude, and there are various hints that may be given as an aid to coping with some of the difficulties. First, problem cases should be left until the end of the analysis and solved together, so that inconsistency is avoided (cf. *GALD*, 94). Secondly, it is a good idea to aim fairly early on in the analysis of a particular utterance to identify the verbal element(s) since the identification of such elements generally provides the key not only to the number of clauses, but also to the internal analysis of each clause. Thirdly, it sometimes helps, when confronted with an utterance which lacks certain elements that would be present in a corresponding adult sentence, to imagine that adult sentence and analyse this first. For example, the following utterance (quoted from Brown and Fraser 1964; 63) has no verbal element:

   That Daddy car.

But suppose that one were analysing the adult sentence

   That is Daddy's car.

Here, the clause-rank structure is, clearly, subject + verbal element + complement. On this basis, it may be hypothesized (but not deduced) that the appropriate LARSP-type analysis at clause rank for the original child utterance is subject + complement, there being, as has already been stated, no verbal element. It must be emphasized, however, that the analysis of the corresponding adult structure (or structures, if there is a choice) is only a source of *hypotheses* for the analysis of particular child utterances; these hypotheses should then be tested against the actual data.

Competence in grammatical analysis is essential for the successful use of LARSP. This is why so much attention has been devoted to it here, and why it demands a reasonable amount of course time. In Leicester, the Structure of English course, which includes LARSP, and the tutorials in grammatical analysis, together amount to some 40 student-hours, out of approximately 200 occupied by the entire linguistics (theory) programme. (These figures exclude reading and the preparation of written work.) Ideally, I should like to devote even more time to the subject, but this would require a longer course, which is not feasible at present. Within the four-year course at Glasgow (Jordanhill), for example, 50 hours are available for matters relating to LARSP-type assessment.

In addition to competence in grammatical analysis, however, the efficient use of LARSP involves other attainments as well. One has already been mentioned, namely familiarity with the chart. For instance, if one has assigned to the utterance *here mummy* the analysis adverbial + subject, one still has to realize that it is entered on the chart as an example of AX in the Stage II clause-rank structures. Moreover, one must always remember that a given utterance may require entries at several different places on the chart. For example, it will have to be placed in the appropriate box in section B or C at the top of the chart. It may also yield one or more structures at word rank, phrase rank and clause rank, each of which would need to be entered separately. It may, furthermore, contain one or more instances of a particular element/realization pattern, such as $X+S:NP$. Again, it may exhibit embedding or conjoining, which would require appropriate entries on the chart, and it may also display various other grammatical properties for which credit is to be given, such as 'passive'. In addition, it may exhibit errors which require noting, for example in noun or verb morphology. Not surprisingly, students take a little while to become used to all this.

Another prerequisite for using LARSP is the ability to transcribe stress and intonation. Users need to have achieved a level of accomplishment such that they can at least employ with reasonable confidence the broad transcription suggested in *GALD*, 57–8. Clearly, if this particular skill is not to lag behind that of grammatical analysis, it is desirable that the transcription of stress and intonation should be introduced during a phonetics course either before the commencement of training in the use of LARSP or else fairly soon after it has begun. In Leicester, the second of the two options is the only one which is feasible because LARSP itself has to be introduced so early.

Training in LARSP does not, of course, end with the completion of formal instruction. Experience will grow as students use it in clinics, and it is important that they are encouraged to employ it in this context and given help where necessary.

Although the bulk of formal training in LARSP is inevitably concerned with the mechanics of the exercise, obviously due attention should also be paid to its application in clinic, and especially to the way in which it can be used as a guide to the planning of a remedial programme for a particular patient (cf. *GALD*, 99–127). In this respect, users need to be made aware of the sensitivity of LARSP, especially in the way that it provides separate quantitative information for each rank of structure. They should also be warned that it is intended only as an assessment of syntactic and morphological ability and disability; it has no semantic dimension, and still less does it assess lexical, phonological or articulatory performance. It cannot be assumed that a patient with a grammatical disability will necessarily have any other kind of linguistic disability, or vice versa. Of course, a sample of speech obtained for LARSP purposes *may* exhibit nongrammatical disabilities, such as nonfluency or restricted lexical range, and when this happens it is wise to make a separate note of the details.

If, as is clearly desirable, a course of training in LARSP is to include some discussion of the methods of carrying out the treatment indicated by the assessment procedure, then an interdisciplinary approach to the teaching of LARSP is called for. The grammatical analysis and the production of syntactic profiles need to be taught by someone with a good knowledge of linguistics, while methods of executing remedial programmes based on syntactic profiles can be taught in detail only by a person with clinical experience. On the other hand, the close connection between assessment and remediation needs to be stressed. This means that LARSP should, ideally, be taught either by one person who is adequately versed in both areas or by two (or more) people each of whom is competent in one area and has at least a rudimentary knowledge of the other.

It will be seen that a thorough training in LARSP demands a good deal of time and effort. However, the effort invested is repaid in several ways. Firstly, and obviously, a training in LARSP will enable the student to employ this detailed assessment procedure. Secondly, it will almost inevitably provide the student with more than enough grammatical knowledge to make use of other remedial procedures which require knowledge of certain grammatical categories (notably word classes), for instance Lea 1970 or Conn 1971. Thirdly, it is likely to enable the student to recognize particular grammatical structures fairly readily in the speech and writing of patients, and this will allow the latter's progress to be monitored on a day-to-day basis, between formal assessments.

If students who are pursuing courses in LARSP are to be formally assessed in terms of their academic progress, such assessment may in principle be carried out either continuously or by means of an examination. In either case, a thorough assessment would at least involve testing students' skill in analysing clinical data and their knowledge of how a syntactic profile drawn up on the basis of an analysis may be used as a guide to the planning of a remedial programme. Whether or not there is to be a formal assessment, however, it is advisable from time to time during the course to test informally students' ability to perform grammatical analysis. This will tell the person giving the course whether students are coping with material of a particular level of complexity, or whether they need further practice before proceeding to the analysis of more difficult patterns. It will also indicate areas of unforeseen difficulty and enable any misapprehensions to be cleared up. Students cannot but benefit from such a process.

Almost all the discussion so far has related to the extended type of training in LARSP which can be provided in the context of a three- or four-year speech therapy course. Let us now, however, consider in-service training for qualified therapists, where the time available is far more limited. Qualified therapists naturally have the advantage of experience in the assessment of patients and in the planning and execution of treatment. Consequently, courses provided for them can concentrate on LARSP itself and the linguistic background required by those who wish to use it: adult English grammar, its development in childhood, and the techniques of grammatical analysis.

With regard to LARSP itself, therapists' attention needs to be drawn to the greater sensitivity which it possesses compared with other widely-used procedures, and to the fact that it is not based on the principle of scoring. As for the linguistic prerequisites, these are the same as for student therapists, and those qualified clinicians who have not received a fairly extended linguistic training need to be provided with some guidance in this area within the context of a LARSP in-service course. The content of such an in-service course is thus rather similar to that of the full-time courses discussed above, though obviously neither the same depth of coverage nor a comparable amount of practical analysis can be fitted into even an intensive short in-service course as into a normal full-time course. For this reason, refresher or follow-up courses are highly desirable.

In-service courses in LARSP tend to last from three to five days. A typical course will have a structure such as the following:

(i) lectures on the grammatical categories of normal adult English, followed up by a workshop on grammatical analysis;

(ii) lectures on normal language development, followed by a workshop on the grammatical analysis of normal child data;

(iii) introduction to sections B and C on the Syntactic Profile Chart, followed by a workshop relating to these;

(iv) lectures on patterns of grammatical disorder, followed by a workshop relating to these;

(v) case studies of children;

(vi) case studies of adults;

(vii) demonstration/workshop on the analysis of data provided by therapists pursuing the course.

Such a course is then generally followed up in two ways. First, therapists who have attended the course form working groups, meeting perhaps once a week, to discuss problems that have arisen in the use of LARSP. Secondly, one-day follow-up courses are provided, centring round the analysis of material supplied by the therapists who attend.

Among those who attend in-service courses, it is not uncommon to find some considerable variety in the extent of previous experience in grammatical analysis and of familiarity with LARSP. On at least one occasion, the resulting problems have been overcome with some success through setting up a hierarchy of three groups, membership of which is determined according to experience and ability. Each individual decides for himself or herself which group to join. However, free movement between groups is permitted, so that, for example, someone who initially joins the beginners' group and later finds he can cope more than adequately with the work of that group may then, with his confidence increased, transfer to a more advanced group. In this way, the inexperienced are in less danger of being left behind, while the experienced are not held back by discussion of what for them are elementary points.

In general terms, courses on LARSP should be geared to the needs of the particular students who attend them. Often, these courses will include a good deal of both theory and practice, and subject to the overall constraints of time and staffing, they should be designed in such a way as to provide as sound a training in LARSP as possible. If good training results in maximum efficiency in the use of LARSP, then the consequent benefit to patients may be seen as a reward to the efforts of both the therapists who have learnt to employ it and the lecturers who have instructed them.

Part 4

Exercises and solutions

Exercises

Exercise 1

Section A
Which of the following utterances would you place in Section A, and under which category?

1 'man in the gàrden/
2 all 'cat for 'me no mòre hóuse/
3 he 'got a 'nice
4 'what are you dìd/
5 he 'wanted a 'new càr/
6 that be (*2 sỳlls*)/
7 (where's the box?) 'on the tàble/
8 I 'got a '(*1 syll*) in thére/
9 a 'boy is wàlking/—and a girl 'is/
10 I . I think he's còming/
11 'my boat goes 'glug-glug-glug tòo/
12 'I got twò of/
13 she will slèep will/
14 bòy/—in càr/
15 'them got no drìvers/
16 'where you 'got it

Exercise 2

Sections B and C
2a Profile the following T/P interactions in terms of Sections B and C:

1 T 'where's he gòing/
   P to tòwn/
2 T 'that's a bùs/
   P it's a nîce 'bus/
3 T 'look óut/
   P sŏrry/
4 T is 'that nĭce/
   P yès/—
      vèry nice/
5 T 'what were you dòing/
   P 'kicking a bàll/
6 T 'where did you sèe him/
   P 'in the gàrden/—
      'in the gàrden/
7 T 'can you sèe/
   P (*nods head*)
8 T 'put 'that dòwn/
   P ón/
9 T 'what did you sèe/
   P a 'cow 'sitting in a fièld/
10 T 'I've got a hòrse/
    P 'I've got one tòo—
       it's a rèd one/
11 T 'where's the bòx/———
       can you sée it/
12 T 'who's got the hòrse/
    P Sùsie gót it/—
       Sùsie gót it/
13 T you're peĕping/
    P nŏ/
       my èyes are shút/
       my èyes are shút/

14   T   you weren't reády/———
     I'll 'count agàin/
15   T   'when will it stòp/
     P   when 'that 'wheel hits 'that one
         thère/
16   T   'has Steven 'got a căr/
     P   'Steven a càr/—
         'Steven a càr/

17   T   'where's he gòing/
     P   he's 'going to
18   T   'is the 'cow hĭding/
     P   mòo/
19   T   'what's thàt 'called/
     P   er
20   T   'why is 'that hót/
     P   'why is 'that hŏt/

2b   Interpretation of Sections B and C. What are the most significant features of the following B/C profiles?

1

B Responses Stimulus Type	Totals	Repet-itions	Normal Response Elliptical Major 1	2	3	4	Full Major	Minor	Abnormal Struc-tural	Ø	Prob-lems
36 Questions	36	12	7	5	1		9	10	4		
24 Others	24	7	4	1			5	2	12		
C Spontaneous	103	21	44	Others 59							

2

B Responses Stimulus Type	Totals	Repet-itions	Normal Response Elliptical Major 1	2	3	4	Full Major	Minor	Abnormal Struc-tural	Ø	Prob-lems
32 Questions	30		19					11		2	
80 Others	27	10					10	12		53	5
C Spontaneous			Others								

3

B Responses Stimulus Type	Totals	Repet-itions	Normal Response Elliptical Major 1	2	3	4	Full Major	Minor	Abnormal Struc-tural	Ø	Prob-lems
31 Questions	16	1	1				15			15	
27 Others	9	6	5	4						18	
C Spontaneous			Others								

4

B Responses Stimulus Type	Totals	Repet-itions	Normal Response Elliptical Major 1	2	3	4	Full Major	Minor	Abnormal Struc-tural	Ø	Prob-lems
200 Questions	117	2	48					69		51	
21 Others	10	1	2					8			
C Spontaneous			Others								

Exercise 3

Stage I

Classify the following Stage I utterances:

1 yès/
2 dàddy/
3 móre/
4 mĕ/
5 gòne/
6 chàir/
7 mhṁ/
8 whére/
9 'one 'more tìme/
10 sìt/

11 wàsh/
12 rèd/
13 bў̆e/
14 Lòndon/
15 sŏrry/
16 eàting/
17 mùmmy/ (*calling*)
18 blèss you/ (*after a sneeze*)
19 róund/
20 ùgh/

Exercise 4

Stage II

4a Allocate the following sentences to a Stage II label:

1 'big trèe/
2 'kick bàll/
3 'where gò/
4 mỳ 'car/
5 'baby èat/ (*pointing to baby having milk*)
6 'in gàrden/
7 'want sèe/
8 nòt 'go/
9 'go thère/
10 'very bìg/
11 'boy glàsses/ (*picture of boy wearing glasses*)
12 the pùssy/
13 big 'one/
14 (*puts man inside a bus*) 'man bùs/
15 (*pointing to cow*) 'is còw/
16 Dàvid 'gloves/ (*giving David his gloves*)
17 kick bàll/ (*telling daddy*)
18 'he dòctor/ (*referring to appearance of man in a white coat*)
19 ùnder 'chair/

20 'on thère/
21 sèe 'man/
22 'come ìn/
23 hère 'red/
24 'cat jùmping/
25 thàt 'ball/ (*reply to 'which ball?'*)
26 'man whére/
27 'mummy sàd/
28 thàt 'much/
29 'quite nìce/
30 'help jùmp/
31 'daddy nò/
32 'three trèes/
33 'jumping nòw/
34 àllgone 'car/
35 dòlly 'house/
36 yòu 'see/
37 'sit dówn/
38 'jump thère/
39 'two eàch/
40 'on bòx/

4b Analyse and profile the following sentences (excluding transitional information):

1 'where your cár/
2 'jump in pùddle/
3 'what go dò/

4 'where the bóys/
5 'what he dóing/

Exercise 5

Transitional Stages

Identify the transitional expansions in the following sentences, showing where, if at all, you would place them on the Profile Chart:

1 the 'boy càme/
2 àll the 'people are 'coming/
3 he 'saw the 'man in blàck/
4 the 'man is 'kicking the bàll/
5 'put the 'box thère/
6 he will 'have to 'go/
7 mỳ 'mummy thére/
8 'he hìt him/

9   we 'should be gôing/
10 I 'think he's còming/
11 the 'man kicked the 'ball through the window/
12 the 'boys and 'girls came in/
13 'gone in thère/ ·
14 'where's the màn 'gone/
15 'what I 'said was 'only a pàrt of it/

Exercise 6

Hierarchic phrase structure

Analyse and profile the following:

1 big red hat
2 want to go
3 may be walking
4 very nice blue coat
5 boys and girls

6   isn't going
7   wants to keep trying
8   gone down with (flu)
9   (he) has asked to go
10 (I) have been sitting down

Exercise 7

Stage III

Analyse and profile the following sentences involving Stage III structures:

1   'man 'kick bàll/
2   I sàw yóu/
3   a bìg 'house/
4   'not mummy sèe/
5   'sees mỳ man nów/
6   'am thère 'now/
7   'in the gàrden/
8   'give yòu the 'book/
9   'are they còming/
10 he ìs níce/
11 Ì can 'go/
12 on bìg 'car/
13 'that is Smìth/
14 he sèems háppy/

15 'someone 'knows the ànswer/
16 dóes he/
17 'who 'kicked the bàll/
18 'look ûp to/ (=admire)
19 'what is 'happening hère/
20 hìm/
21 'let me gò/
22 'where my dàddy/
23 'you 'go nomòre/
24 dòn't 'hit 'me/
25 'are they 'going to tówn/
26 ànybody/
27 'put 'book thère/

Exercise 8

Stage IV

Analyse and profile the following sentences involving Stage IV structures:

1 'John 'saw Jim thére/
2 'in my 'new càr/
3 'and yòu/
4 he 'looked under the 'table quìckly/
5 the mán in the mòon/
6 the 'four 'black càts/ and the 'three 'red squìrrels/
7 wòn't/
8 'you 'come here quìckly 'now/
9 he mìght not cóme/
10 'I got a bòok for 'you/
11 mén/ wómen/ and chìldren 'came/
12 he 'came and 'saw the mèss/
13 'certainly nòt/
14 'four and 'five and 'six make fiftèen/
15 'under a 'beautiful 'new mòon/
16 hăppily/ they gòt 'there/
17 he's tripped/——and 'fallen òver/
18 the 'people all 'came to 'see the shòw/

Exercise 9

Word level

Analyse the following in terms of word structure, where this exists, noting any ambiguities:

1 walking
2 biggest
3 gone
4 come
5 boys
6 he's (nice)
7 sent
8 no smoking
9 happily
10 goes
11 his
12 won't
13 I'm (walking)
14 tinier
15 is
16 cat's
17 tooked
18 better
19 mices
20 was
21 am
22 people
23 worst
24 London's
25 swimming
26 I had
27 we
28 yours
29 be
30 were

Exercise 10

Stage V

Analyse the structure of the following sentences:

1 the 'man 'saw a hórse/ and the 'lady 'saw a còw/

2 they wàlked to 'town/ when they 'missed the tráin/

3 'I can 'see a 'lady in a cóat/ 'carrying a bàg/
4 you're stàying/ áren't you/
5 it's as 'big as yòu are/
6 'what a prìce that 'is/
7 the 'car you 'bought is 'very nìce/
8 and 'that's not àll/
9 'when I gó/ 'shouldn't concèrn you/
10 thàt's the 'card to sénd him/
11 'come and sèe/
12 còme if you wánt to/ and 'if you've 'got the càr/
13 'I have an 'answer of some mèrit to that quéstion/
14 'how tàll he 'is/
15 'I can 'see the 'lorry that 'made all the nóise/
16 'who's the 'man 'asking the wày/

Exercise 11

Stage VI

11a   Errors. Identify those sentences which contain errors in the LARSP sense, and classify them at Stage VI:

1 we tóoken it òut/
2 the 'sheeps 'look nìce/
3 'him is 'going hòme nów/
4 màn 'going/
5 he 'posted the 'letter from the pìllar-box/
6 he's 'riding on a hòrses/
7 quìckly 'went he 'home/
8 you are wálk on the gràss/
9 'let's us gò nów/
10 I àin't 'going/
11 'he am hàppy/
12 'it did hùrt me/
13 I 'just will 'put the 'paper òn/
14 'that is mòre 'good/
15 'I want bìscuit/
16 hè's the 'man which I sáw/
17 'give it to shè/
18 I 'got a 'pink 'lovely ıce-crèam/
19 I 'didn't 'do nŏthing/
20 thòse 'mans is cóming/
21 you 'must 'do it yèsterday/
22 he 'have be gòing/
23 he 'shouldn't dò it/ cán he/
24 the 'all pèople 'came/
25 'I've got òne as 'well/

11b   Positive features. Classify the following Stage VI developments:

1 he 'shouldn't hăve to 'do it/
2 'I've been 'stung by a wàsp/
3 the tèlly's 'gone 'wrong/
4 'half my 'money was 'on the tàble/
5 he was 'married on Tuèsday/
6 'my 'brother 'Fred is insìde/
7 'all the 'seats are èmpty/
8 'ask him to come ìn/
9 'I got a bíke/ a wátch/ and a jìgsaw/
10 'he's been sèen/
11 I'm gòod at thát/
12 'he himsélf/ 'couldn't be bòthered/
13 he 'did it instèad of mé/
14 'three-quarters of the swèets have been 'eaten/
15 he's 'ready to jùmp/

Exercise 12

Stage VII

Classify any Stage VII features in the following sentences:

1 it was in tòwn I mét him/
2 ǎctually/ I 'wanted a bòok/
3 by the gàte I 'said I'd sée you/
4 there's a 'lovely pìcture over 'there/
5 'I'll be làte/ I'm afráid/
6 he's stìll cóming/

7 it was the dèntist who 'told me/
8 'up you júmp/
9 it's 'better to 'leave it till tomòrrow/
10 of còurse I 'want one/
11 he 'runs 'down the wing/—shóots/...

Exercise 13

Analyse and profile the following sentences (used in the imitation task in 3.2.):

1 All the children are in the playground[33] now.
2 Mummy is wearing a new dress for the party.
3 The ball is bouncing up and down.
4 The little girl likes playing with her big brother.
5 All the pretty flowers are growing in the back garden now.
6 The girl and her brother are sleeping.
7 The girl is running fast to catch the big red bus.
8 The big black cat is climbing up a tree.
9 All the children like to play in the lovely white snow.
10 There are lots of pretty flowers there.
11 Daddy is going to drive the big new car.
12 The boy and his little sister go shopping with their mummy.
13 The man is putting the book there.
14 The little girl is playing with her big doll.
15 The little boy is bouncing a red ball there.
16 The girl plays with the doll's house.
17 Daddy is going out to the garden.
18 The girl and the boy like playing on the high swings.
19 The little girl is playing with her brother and his friend.
20 My mummy and her friend are going to the town today.
21 The dog is barking at the cat.

Exercise 14

Analyse and profile the following sentences (Sam's Profile A, 2.2, p. 161):

1 hòuse/
2 yès/
3 grèen/
4 wálking/
5 (name of cat)
6 rúnning/
7 hôrse/
8 ? wǒman/
9 pì/ (= 'water')
10 hòme/

11 èat/
12 drìnk/
13 stràw/
14 yés/
15 bírd/
16 ? càge/
17 mùm/
18 *Unintelligible*
19 bàby/
20 fìre/

21 Mùmmy/
22 yès/
23 bèdroom/
24 bèd/
25 Gúy/
26 Màtthew/
27 mè/
28 Jǒhn/

[33] Taken as two words in the experiment reported in 3.2.

Exercise 15

Analyse and profile the following sentences (Sam's Profile B, 2.2, p. 162):

1	hóuse/	31	bèan/
2	'red hòuse/	32	èat/
3	wìndow/	33	flòwer/
4	blùe/	34	wàter/
5	trèes/	35	wàsh/
6	sùn/	36	'round plàte/[35]
7	in sùn/	37	drỳ/
8	bèe/	38	the plàte/[36]
9	'on the gràss/	39	bìke/
10	flówer/	40	in gàrden/
11	'red and blùe/	41	gàrden/
12	sùn/	42	nò/
13	stàlk/	43	yès/
14	blùe one/	44	'meat pìe/
15	yès/	45	ròund/
16	mè/	46	*Unintelligible*
17	dìgging/	47	'apple pìe/
18	mùmmy/	48	and Nìcky/
19	'in sèed/	49	'ride bìke/
20	'brown and blàck/	50	yès/
21	the bàg/	51	yès/
22	lìttle/	52	slèep/
23	sèed/	53	mùmmy/
24	flówer/	54	drìnking/
25	gárden/	55	rìding/
26	yèllow/	56	nô/
27	sèed/	57	nò/
28	bèan/	58	còok/
29	nò/	59	hòuse/
30	grèen 'flower/[34]		

Exercise 16

Analyse and profile the following sentences (Sam's Profile C, 2.2, p. 163):

1	plàying/	5	mènd it/
2	'in the òutside/	6	with hànds/
3	Gùy/	7	yès/
4	'making 'Guy bìke/[37]	8	a lètter/

[34] PGSS signed.
[35] The context suggested that *round* = 'around'.
[36] T prompt: 'Dry—'.
[37] Someone is mending Guy's bike.

9   mùmmy/
10 lòve 'from/[38]
11 Màtthew/
12 'fly the àeroplane/
13 dèntist/
14 'mummy 'tooth is bròken/
15 cròss/[39]
16 'mummy 'tooth is òut/
17 'go to Bògnor/
18 àeroplane/
19 rècords/
20 he's rùnning/
21 hèn/
22 twò/
23 hèn/
24 a bìrd/
25 mè 'saw/
26 at hòme/
27 'in the field/
28 dòg/
29 twò/
30 eàting/
31 thànk you/

32 dòg/
33 fàll/
34 drìnking/
35 fùnny/
36 'be fùnny/
37 'it 'is fùnny/
38 'on my hèad/
39 'on my tùmmy/
40 'on my knèe/
41 'on my chàir/
42 sìt/
43 'going on the mòo-cow/
44 the mìlk/
45 is stànding/
46 the 'girl is 'giving the bìrthday 'cake/
47 the 'girl is 'holding the flòwers/
48 the 'mummy is 'making the brèad/
49 'on the tàble/
50 the bìrds/
51 wàter/
52 'on the tàble/
53 mè/
54 Gùy/

Exercise 17

Analyse and profile the following sentences (Diane's Profile C, 2.5, p. 230):

1   On Friday I went to home at twelty to four.
2   My Mummy say Hello.
3   I drink a cup of tea.
4   Kim is play me.
5   David is a read.
6   I say's about at school.
7   I watch the television.
8   I go to bed at 9 o'clock.[40]
9   On Saturday I got up at 10 o'clock.
10 I have a wash.
11 I go down stair.
12 I eat my breakfast.
13 I go to up stair.
14 I was Kim is sleep.
15 My David is eat at breakfast.
16 I went to the sea.
17 My David is swimming.
18 I go to shop.
19 Kim is swimming.
20 My buy is comie.
21 Kim is playing the ball.
22 I went to home at 6 o'clock.
23 I read a book.
24 I go to bed a 9 o'clock.
25 On Sunday I got up a 10 o'clock.

[38] A favourite phrase, regularly used in a letter-writing context.

[39] I.e. 'She was cross'.

[40] O'clock is best analysed as an Adjectival, postmodifying the numeral, which acts as head of the NP: support for this analysis includes its omissibility (at nine) and the impossibility of at o'clock. There are no grounds for taking o' as a separate Prep, in the modern language.

26 I have a wash.
27 I go downstair.
28 I eat my breakfat.
29 I went to the shop.
30 I drink a cup of tea.
31 I read a book.

32 Kim is drink a cup of milk.
33 My David is sleep.
34 I say get up is David.
35 I went to shop.
36 I went to home a 7 o'clock.
37 I went to bed at 9 o'clock.

Exercise 18

Analyse and profile the following sentences (Diane's Profile D, 2.5, p. 231):

1   On Friday I went home at twenty to four.
2   I watched the television.
3   My dog was sleeping.
4   I went to upstairs.
5   I put on the wall.
6   I drank a cup of coffee.
7   I went to bed and I went to sleep.
8   On Saturday morning I got up at 9 o'clock.
9   I put on my clothes.
10 I had washed.
11 I went downstairs.
12 I ate bacon and egg for breakfast.
13 I took my dog for a walk.
14 I read a book.
15 My father was in the garage.
16 My father was working the wood.
17 On Saturday afternoon I watched the television.
18 My mother was made a cake.
19 My dog was cut her foot.
20 I drank a cup of tea.
21 My mother say bye.
22 I went to bed and I went to sleep.
23 On Sunday morning I got up at 9 o'clock.
24 I had washed.
25 I put on my clothes.
26 I downstairs.
27 I ate roast and cheese for breakfast.
28 My dog was for a walk.
29 I drank a cup of tea.
30 I watched on film the television.
31 I wote was in the letter my friend.
32 My father was made the garden.
33 I saw blackbird was in the nest.
34 My friend was marry. (='Mary')
35 I played with my friend.
36 On Sunday afternoon I played with my dog.
37 I watched the television.
38 My mother and father are talking about the house.
39 I had washed.
40 I put on my nightdress.
41 I went to bed and I went to sleep.
42 This morning I got up at 7 o'clock.

Exercise 19

Analyse and profile the following data (Henry's Profile A, 2.1, p. 147) in terms of (a) developmental stages, and (b) Sections B and C:

```
1    T   'what's thàt/                              playing with
     P   wàsh/—                                     doll's house
         bòwl/
     T   'why is it a 'good i'dea to 'have that
5        'next to your còoker/———
         it is a good idéa/ *isn't it/
```

	P	*yeàh/	
	T	whỳ is it/————	
		ḿm/	
10	P	còoker/ thère/—	
	T	'what would you 'do in hère/	*indicates sink*
	P	wàshing	
	T	'wash whàt/	
	P	'wash pòt/	
15	T	yeàh/	
	P	(*1 syll*)	
	T	òh/—	
		'what's happened hère/—	
		'look what's hàppened/—	
20	P	'don't knôw/————	*stereotype*
	T	'what about having 'something to èat off/	
	P	yès/	
		plàte/	
	T	ṁ/	
25		'somewhere to 'put your plàte/	
	P	(*laughs*)	
	T	would this be any 'good in this róom/	
	P	nô/	
	T	whỳ/	
30	P	bèdroom/———	
	T	you mean this be'longs in the 'bedroom/	
	P	yès/	
	T	whỳ docs it/—	
		it doésn't/.	
35		it belóngs in the kìtchen/	
	P	nò/	
	T	'why nòt/	
	P	er	
	T	yès/	
40		we'll 'have it in the kìtchen/ (*unint*)	
	P	(*3 sylls*)——(*2 sylls*)	
	T	(*unint*) nòw/ 'let's put 'that—thère/———	
	P	(*3 sylls*)	
		kéttle/—	
45		and a cōoker/	
	T	'what're you dòing/—	
		òh/—	
		'what's thàt/	
	P	meàt/	
50	T	ís it/—	
		'where wàs it/———	
		'where was the mèat/—	
	P	er	
	T	'where wàs it/	

55   P   in thère/

      ...

      T   does the bùs go a'long your stréet/—
      P   nó/——
           lòrries/
           'lot of 'noisy lòrries/
60   T   ôh/.
           is it a 'big 'main ròad thén/
      P   er
      T   Nòtown/ isn't it/
      P   yèah/
65   [nà:]
           'one lòrry/ bròke/ their tràbs/
      T   'one 'lorry whát/
      P   bròke/ their tràbs/—
      T   'broke their whát/
70   P   tràbs/
      T   òh/—
           'outside your hoùse/
      P   yéah/
      T   'what happened thèn/——
75   P   màn/—twò mans/ mènded it/——   *visual evidence*
      T   'did they 'come straight awăy/—   *suggests self-*
      P   yès/——   *correction*
           'in (a) mòrning/
      T   'what did the drìver do 'all that 'time/——
80   P   'very 'very dăngerous/
      T   whàt/
           lŏrries/
      P   nò/.
           tràbs/
85   T   whỳ are they 'dangerous/—
      P   '[bɪn] bróken/
      T   ôh/

Exercise 20

Analyse and profile the following data in terms of (a) developmental stages, and (b) Sections B and C:

1   T   'what are you 'going to dò in the 'holidays/——
      P   'open my prèsent 'up/. on 'Christmas Dáy/
      T   'open your prèsent/.
           ôh/
5   P   'very exci . ex . excìted/—
      T   yòu *áre/
      P   *erm yès/
           erm—'at 'Christmas Dáy/
      T   (*laughs*) what èlse do you 'do on 'Christmas 'Day/——

10 P Chrìstmas . 'present and dínner/——
    and . 'play with 'my . Chrìstmas présent/—
  T 'what do you 'think you're 'going to gèt/
  P a bìke/
  T do you knòw that you're 'going to *'get a bíke/——
15 P *yès/
  T ôh/——
    'where will you rìde/—
  P don't knòw/——
  T can you 'ride in your gǎrden/ or 'will you have
20   to 'ride on the strèet/—
  P 'on the strèet/—
    not allòwed 'on . 'ride it 'on the gra . er 'ride
    it 'on the gráss/ .
    kìll . the 'grass/
25 T ôh/—
    m̂/—
    'who does the 'garden in yòur house/—
  P mùmmy/ and dáddy/ and mé/ and Màry/ .
    àll 'family/
30 T àll the 'family 'does/—
    oh gòod/
  P m̂/
  T 'what do you gròw in your 'garden/—
  P béans/—
35   cábbages/———
    ānd
    'don't knòw/—
    cábbages/ .
    béans/ .
40 T m̄/——
    'lots of vègetables/
  P yès/
  T m̂/
    'jolly gôod/ .
45   'what does your dàddy 'do/—
    'what 'kind of wòrk/
  P sell/ . càravan . 'things/
  T dôes he/———
    does he 'have to 'go awày . to do thát/ or
50   'does he 'do it at hòme/—
  P erm '[houdz] mán/ séll/—càravan thíngs/
  T m̀/
  P ànybody/
    (2 sylls)—
55   lòt of—— of——— 'mans—'sell cáravan 'things/
  T m̀/
    òh yes/——
    'does he 'sell the cǎravan/—

        P nò/
60   T nó/ —
           whàt/ —
           'just the 'things to gò in the cáravan/
        P yès/
        T I sèe/
           ...
65   P and — 'feel . a snów/   *describing a*
           and . 'cut the 'trees 'down for Chrístmas/——   *picture of*
           and . cárs 'cover snów/——   *a wintry scene*
           and . the . 'two 'mans — 'move a — the — the 'car
           — 'off 'the snów/
70   T ṁ/
           'moving the snòw óff/
        P yès/
        T yès/ .
           have you 'ever been 'stuck in the snów/ .
75   P yès/
        T ṁ/———
        P it's rāinīng/ it's pōurīng/
        T I 'wonder what that bòy's 'doing/
        P whàt/ —
80   'looking 'out 'of the wìndow/ —
        T I 'wonder why hè 'has to 'stay in/——
        P be'cause . the . ràin 'came 'down/———
           'that wāter/

Exercise 21

Bottom line

Calculate the total number of sentences, the mean number of sentences per turn, and the mean sentence length, for the following extracts:

A 1   T thère we are/
           you're 'sitting ón the/
        P chaìr/
        T the chàir/
    5   thàt's 'right/——
           lóok/
        P dòggy/ (*laughs*)
        T a dòggy/
           thère he ís/
10   P dòggy/
        T yès/
        P 'here dòggy/
        T 'that's ríght/
        P hulló/——

15   dòwn/
        T   'that's ríght/
              the 'dog's 'going to 'jump dòwn/
              'where are yòu 'going to 'jump/
        P   (*laughs*)
20   T   you're 'going to 'jump — ùp/
        P   nò/

B   Profile B, p. 149 (Henry)

Solutions

In the following pages, these abbreviations are used, in addition to those found on the Profile Chart or in the transcriptional conventions (cf. *GALD*, Chs. 4, 5):

I   = Stage I, II = Stage II, etc.
C   = Clause column
P   = Phrase column
W   = Word column
O   = Other
Q   = Question column
E   = Exclamatory column
—   = Error box
T   = Transitional Stage
Ellipt. = Elliptical

Solution 1

1 Normal developmental possibility—unproblematic, hence not in A
2 Deviant
3 Incomplete (no nucleus, see p. 30)
4 Normal developmental possibility
5 Normal adult sentence
6 Unintelligible (the syllables have a falling tone, hence not Incomplete)
7 Normal ellipsis
8 Carry out normal analysis (the unintelligibility must be lexical, being only 1 syllable)
9 Ambiguous (how many sentences?)
10 Normal adult sentence (ignore the first *I*)
11 Symbolic Noise (see p. 27)
12 Normal developmental possibility (not Incomplete, because tone-unit complete)
13 Deviant (for discussion, see papers by Kuczaj, Fay and others in *Journal of Child Language*, 5.1)
14 Ambiguous (one sentence or two: cf. p. 32)
15 Normal developmental possibility (and in some adult dialects)
16 Incomplete (no nucleus)

Solution 2

2a

1	Q stimulus	Ellipt. Major 1
2	Other	Full Major
3	Other	Minor
4	Q	Minor—Spontaneous Ellipt. 1
5	Q	Ellipt. Major 2
6	Q	Ellipt. Major 1 + Repetition
7	Q	Zero
8	Other	Structural Abnormality
9	Q	Ellipt. Major 3
10	Other	Full Major—Spontaneous Other
11	Q	Zero
12	Q	Full Major—Repetition
13	Other	Minor—Spontaneous Ellipt. 1—Spontaneous Ellipt. 1—Repetition
14	Other	Zero
15	Q	Ellipt. Major 4
16	Q	Ellipt. Major 2— Repetition
17	Q	Not analysed (Section A)
18	Q	Structural Abnormality
19	Other	Zero
20	Q	Full Major

2b

1   Considerable spontaneity and repetition together (? hyperactive child); high Spont. Ellipt. 1 suggests not as fully in control of syntax as the Spontaneous total might indicate; rather 'random' look of other columns—everything is being used, but perhaps not very systematically.

2   More Other stimuli than Q, i.e. it is more like normal conversation. P however does not like Other stimuli: note the high Zero figure, and the use of Minor (presumably as an 'easy' response); the Full Major sentences probably account for most of the Repetitions. Q stimuli help P more, as suggested by the 1-element elliptical responses.

3   More than half the responses are Zeros; no Spontaneous; Full Major rather than elliptical; Repetitions increase as Elliptical does. Suggests a severely sub-normal P, using taught full sentences, and perhaps some echolalia in other contexts, where clear structural cues absent.

4   This is Hugh's first profile (*GALD*, 131): compare your interpretation with that given in *GALD*, 130. The discrepancy in total is because a lot of Hugh was Unintell. at that time.

Solution 3

1	Minor, Social	11	Major, Problem (N or V?)
2	'N'	12	Other
3	Other	13	Minor, Social
4	Other	14	'N'
5	'V' Statement	15	Minor, Social
6	'N'	16	'V' Statement
7	Minor, Social	17	Minor, Social (see p. 62 on Vocatives)
8	'Q'	18	Minor, Stereotype
9	Minor, Stereotype	19	Major, Problem (Adj? Prep? N? V? Adv?)
10	'V' Comm	20	Minor, Social (*not* Exclamatory; see p. 90)

Solution 4

4a

1	Adj N	21	V C/O
2	V C/O	22	V part
3	QX	23	AX
4	DN	24	SV
5	SV	25	DN
6	Pr N	26	QX
7	VV	27	S C/O
8	Neg X	28	Other (Phrase)
9	AX	29	Int X
10	Int X	30	VV
11	S C/O	31	Neg X
12	DN	32	Adj N (+pl. in W)
13	Other (Phrase)	33	AX (+ing in W)
14	AX	34	Other (Clause) (*allgone* = V? C? Adj?)
15	V C/O	35	NN
16	NN	36	SV (+Pron at III)
17	VX	37	V part
18	S C/O	38	VX
19	Pr N	39	Other (Phrase)
20	Other (Phrase)	40	Pr N

4b

1 Q $\underline{\quad C\quad}$ (=QX)
       D N

2 V $\underline{\quad A\quad}$ (=VX)
       Pr N

3 Q $\underline{\quad V\quad}$ (=QX)
       V V

4 Q $\underline{\quad C\quad}$ (=QX)
       D N
            pl

5 Q $\underline{\quad V\quad}$ (=QX)
       Aux v
             ing

Solution 5

1 the boy X+S: NP
2 all the people/ are coming X+S: NP, X+V: VP
3 the man in black XY+O: NP
4 the man/ is kicking/ the ball XY+S: NP, XY+V: VP, XY+O: NP
5 the box XY+O: NP
6 will have to go X+V: VP
7 my mummy X+S: NP
8 No expansions
9 should be going X+V: VP
10 he's coming XY+O: NP
11 the man/ the ball/ through the window   No expansions marked on chart
    (Stage IV structure)
12 the boys and girls/ came in X+S: NP, X+V: VP
13 in there X+A: AP
14 the man/ 's gone XY+S: NP, XY+V: VP
15 what I said/ only a part of it XY+S: NP, XY+C: NP

Solution 6

1 Adj Adj N   III
2 VV   II
3 Aux Aux V   IV (2 Aux)
4 Int Adj Adj N   IV Other
5 XcX   IV
6 Aux Neg V   III (Aux), IV (Neg V)
7 VVV   III Other
8 V part part   III Other
9 Aux VV   III (Aux), II (VV), VI (Complex VP)
10 Aux Aux V part   IV (2 Aux), II (V part), VI (Complex VP)

Solution 7

1 'man 'kick bàll/
     S   V   O

2 I sàw yóu/
   S   V   O
   Pron   Pron
         -ed

3 D Adj N

4 Neg X Y

5 'sees my màn nów/
     V   O   A
           D N
   3s
         XY+O:NP

6 V A A (=Other)

7 Pr D N

8   'give yòu the 'book/
    V O_i O_d
        Pron   D   N
               XY+O:NP

9   'are they cŏming/
    V   S
    Aux Pron
             ing
    X+V:VP

10   he   is   níce/
    S   V   C
    Pron Cop
        3s

11   Ì   can   'go/
    S   V
    Pron Aux   v
        X+V:VP

12   Pr Adj N (Other)

13   'that   is   Smìth/
    S   V   C
    Pron Cop
        3s

14   he   sèems háppy/
    S   V   C
    Pron
         3s
        (*not* Cop)

15   'someone 'knows the ànswer/
    S   V   O
       Pron   D   N
           3s
             XY+O:NP

16   dóes   he/
    V   S
    Aux   Pron
    3s

17   'who 'kicked the bàll/
    Q   V   O   (=QXY)
             D   N
        ed
            XY+O:NP

18   V Part Part (=Other)

19   'what is 'happening hère/
    Q   V   A   (=QXY)
        Aux   v
            ing
        XY+V:VP

20   Pron

21   *let* XY

22   'where my dàddy
    Q   C   (=QX) (see p. 64)
        D   N
         X+C:NP

23   'you 'go nomòre/
    S   V   Neg   (=Neg XY)
    Pron

24   dòn't   'hit 'me/
    do   X   Y
    Neg V   Pron
    X+V:VP

25   'are   they 'going to tówn/
    V   S   A   (=VS, or VS (+X), see p. 77)
       Aux   Pron   Pr Adv
            ing
    XY+V:VP   XY+A:AP

26   Pron   27 V X Y

Solution 8

1 S V O A
   ed

2 Pr D Adj N

3   c   X
      Pron

4 he 'looked under the 'table quìckly/
   S   V   A   A
  Pron   Pr   D   N
       ed   ly

5 NP Pr NP

6 the 'four 'black càts/ and the 'three 'red squìrrels/
          X   c   X
   D Adj Adj N   D Adj Adj   N   (= Other × 2)
             pl   pl

7 Neg V

8   S   V   A A A (= Other)
  Pron   ly

9 he might not còme/
   S   V   IIC
 Pron Aux Neg v   IIIP (Pron)
                       IIIP (Aux)
                       IVP (Neg V)

10 'I got a bòok for 'you/
    S V   O$_d$ O$_i$
  Pron   D N Pr Pron
       ed

11 mén/ wómen/ and chìldren 'came/
              S   V   IIC
   NP   X   c   X   IVP (XcX)
   pl   pl   pl   ed   VI+ (Coord)
         X + S: NP   W (× 4)
                           IIT

12   he 'came and 'saw the mèss/
     S   V   O
          X c X
   Pron   D   N
       ed   ed
      XY+V:VP   XY+O:NP

13   Neg X
        ly

14   'four and 'five and 'six make fiftèen/
            S   V   C
     X c X
           X c X
     XY+S:NP

15   Pr D Adj Adj N (=Other)

16   hăppily/ they gòt 'there/
      A   S   V   A   (=AAXY)
             Pron
       ly   ed

17   he's   trìpped/ —— and 'fallen òver/
     S   V   c   X
   Pron Aux   V   part
     'aux ed   en
     X+V:VP

18   the 'people all 'came to 'see the shòw/
        S   A   V   O   (=SVC/OA)
    D   N   V   V D N
                ed

Solution 9

1	-ing	10	3s
2	-est	11	Ø (only Nouns are gen.)
3	-en	12	n't
4	Ø (i.e. nothing marked in Word column)	13	'aux
5	pl	14	-er
6	'cop	15	3s
7	Ambig. -ed or -en	16	gen
8	Ø (*smoking* is N)	17	-ed (plus V_{irreg} at VI)
9	ly	18	-er
		19	pl (plus N_{irreg} at VI)

20	3s	25	Ambiguous (-ing or N)
21	Ø (*be* only marked in 3rd person)	26	-ed
22	Ø (despite a plural meaning, it is not plural in form)	27	Ø (only plurals of nouns are pl.)
		28	Ø (only nouns are gen.)
23	-est	29	Ø
24	gen	30	-ed

Solution 10

```
the  man  saw   a   hórse / and  the  'lady 'saw   a   còw/      V Conn; VC: Coord 1
       Clause              and       Clause
   S     V    O            S      V     O              IIIC (×2)
   D  N       D   N        D   N        D   N          IIP (×4)
       ed                      ed                      W (×2)
XY+S:NP     XY+O:NP      XY+S:NP     XY+O:NP            IIIT (×4)
```

```
2  they wàlked  to  'town /. when they missed the  tráin/
   S    V       A                    A                    IVC: AAXY
                       s     Subord Clause                V Conn; VC: Subord 1
                             S    V     O                 IIIC
   Pron         Pr   N       Pron      D   N              IIIP (×2); IIP (×2)
        ed                        ed                      W (×2)
        XY+A:AP                   XY+O:NP                 IIIT (×2)
```

```
3  'I  can 'see a 'lady in a cóat/ 'carrying  a  bàg/
   S    V          O                                    IIIC
                   V          O                         IIC; Postmod P 1+
   Pron Aux  v   NP  Pr  NP        D   N                IIIP (×2); IVP; IIP
                              ing                       W
        XY+V:VP  XY+O:NP         X+O:NP                  IIIT (×2); IIT
```

```
4  you're  stàying/ áren't  you/
   S     V          V    S                    VC: Coord 1; IIC; Question III(VS)
                   Neg V                       IVP
   Pron Aux  v    Aux  Pron                    IIIP (×4)
        'aux  ing  n't                         W (×3)
        X+V:VP  X+V:VP                          IIT (×2)
```

5   it's   as 'big as yòu are/
      S V   C
                 Comp   s S   V
    Pron Cop   Pron Cop
        'cop
        3s
                XY+C:NP

IIIC
V Comp; V Conn: s; IIC
IIIP (×4)
W (×2)

IIIT

---

6   'what a price that 'is/
      Q–C   S   V
      Int D N Pron Cop
                    3s
    XY+C:NP

V Exclam: *what*
IIIPO; IIIP (×2)
W
IIIT

---

7   the 'car you 'bought is 'very nice/
            S   V   C
            S   V
      D N Pron   Cop Int   X
                    ed 3s
      XY+S:NP   XY+C:NP

IIIC
IIC; Postmod C 1
IIP (×2); IIIP (×2)
W (×2)
IIIT (×2)

---

8   and 'that's   not àll/
      and S V   C
          Pron Cop Neg X
             'cop
                XY+C:NP

V Conn: *and*; IIIC
IIIP (×2); IVP
W
IIIT

---

9   'where I   gò/ 'shouldn't concèrn you/
            S   V   O
      s   Subord Cl.
          S   V
        Pron   Aux Neg   v   Pron
                  n't
      XY+S:NP   XY+V:VP

IIIC
V Conn: *s*; Clause: S
IIC
IIIP (×3); IVP (Neg V)
W
IIIT (×2)

---

10   thàt's   the 'card to sénd him/
      S V   C
                    V   O
    Pron Cop D N   Pron
         'cop
              XY+C:NP

IIIC
IIC; V Postmod C 1
IIIP (×3); IIP
W
IIIT

11 'come   and   sèe/
    Cl.   *and*   Cl.
    V$_{imp}$ V$_{imp}$

V: Coord 1; Conn: *and*
Command V (× 2)

12 'come if you wànt to/ and 'if you've   'got   the   càr/
    V$_{imp}$ A   A
           s Subord Clause *and* s   Subord Clause

           S   V   S   V   O
           Pron   V Part   Pron   Aux v   D   N
                                        'aux en

    XY+A:AP   X+V:VP   XY+V:VP   XY+O:NP;   XY+A:AP

VXY
V Conn: *and, s* (× 2)
V Subord 1+
IIC; IIIC
IIIP (× 3); IIP (× 2)
W (× 2)
IIT; IIIT (× 4)

13   'I   have an 'answer of some mèrit to that quéstion/
      S   V   O
      Pron   D   N   Pr   D   N   Pr   D   N
                        XY+O:NP

IIIC
VP (Postmod P 1+)
IIP; IIIP (× 3)
IIIT

14 'how tàll   he   'is
    Q–C   S   V
    Int   X   Pron Cop
                      3s
    XY+C:NP

IIIC
IIP; IIIP (× 2)
W
IIIT

15 'I   can   'see the 'lorry that 'made all the nóise/
    S   V   O
                            s   V   O
    Pron   Aux v   D   N   I   D   N
                                  ed
         XY+V:VP   XY+O:NP

IIIC
V Conn: *s*; IIC
IIIP (× 2); IIP; IIIPO; VI+(I)
W
IIIT (× 2)

16 'who's   the 'man 'asking the wày/
    Q   V   C
                        V   O
         Cop   D   N   D   N
         'cop   ing
         XY+C:NP   X+O:NP

QXY
V Postmod cl. 1
IIIP; IIP (× 2)
W (× 2)
IIIT; IIT

Solution 11

Errors

1 V_{irreg}
2 N_{irreg}
3 Pron
4 Ø (normal II)
5 Other: Prep
6 Det
7 W .order
8 Tense
9 Other: Command
10 Ø (a normal non-standard dialect form)
11 V_{irreg}
12 Tense
13 A position
14 Other: Comparative
15 Det
16 Concord
17 Pron
18 Adj seq
19 Ø (a normal non-standard dialect form)
20 N_{irreg}; Concord
21 Modal
22 Tense; Concord
23 Other: Tag Q
24 W order
25 Other: Inton. Tonicity

Positive

1 Complex VP
2 Passive
3 Complement
4 I
5 Passive
6 NP Coord
7 I
8 Complex VP
9 NP Coord
10 Passive
11 Complement
12 NP Coord; Passive
13 Other: Complex Prep
14 I; Passive
15 Complement

Solution 12

1 *it*
2 A Connectivity
3 Emphatic Order
4 *there*
5 Comment Clause
6 A Connectivity
7 *it*
8 Emphatic Order
9 Other (extraposition)
10 A Connectivity
11 Style

Solution 13

1 All the children are in the playground now.

	S		V		A		A	IVC: AAXY
I	D	N	Cop	Pr D	N			IIIP ($\times$2); IIIPO; VI+
		pl						W

2 Mummy is wearing a new dress for the party.
      S   V   O   A   IVC
              Aux   v   D Adj N   Pr D   N   IIIP (×3)
              3s   ing   W (×2)

3 The ball   is bouncing up and down.
      S   V   A   IIIC
    D   N   Aux   v   X c   X   IIP; IIIP; IVP
              3s   ing   W (×2)
   XY+S:NP XY+V:VP XY+A:AP   IIIT (×3)

4 The little girl likes playing with her big brother.
         S   V   O   IIIC
    D Adj N   V   V   Part D Adj   N   IIIP (×2); IIP (VV); IIP (V Part)
               3s   ing   VI+(Complex VP)
    XY+S:NP   XY+V:VP   XY+O:NP   W (×2)
                                            IIIT (×3)

5 All the pretty flowers are growing in the back garden now.
          S   V   A   A   IVC: AAXY
    I D Adj   N   Aux   v   Pr D Adj   N   IVPO; VI+; IIIP; IVP
              pl   ing   W (×2)

6 The girl and her brother are sleeping.
              S   V   IIC
    X   c   X   IVP
    D N   D N   Aux   v   IIP (×2); IIIP
                        ing   W
          X+S:NP   X+V:VP   IIT (×2)

7 The girl is running fast to catch the big red bus.
      S   V   A   A   IVC: AAXY
                  s⁴¹   Subord Cl.   V Conn; VC: Subord 1
                       V   O   IIC
    D N Aux   v   D Adj Adj N IIP; IIIP; IVPO
         3s   ing   W (×2)
                             X+O:NP   IIT

8 The big black cat is climbing up a tree.
          S   V   A   IIIC
    A Adj Adj N Aux   v   Pr D N   IVPO; IIIP (×2)
                 3s   ing   W (×2)
    XY+S:NP   XY+V:VP XY+A:AP   IIIT (×3)

⁴¹ *To*='in order to' and is not the usual infinitive marker, cf. p. 66.

9 All the children like to play in the lovely white snow.

	S		V			A				IIIC
I	D	N	V	V	Pr	D	Adj	Adj	N	IIIPO; VI+ ; IIP; IVPO
		pl								W
	XY+S:NP		XY+V:VP			XY+A:AP				IIIT (×3)

10 There are lots of[42] pretty flowers there.

S	V		C		A	IVC
there Cop	I		Adj	N		VII Discourse; IIIP; IIIPO
	pl			pl		W (×2)

11 Daddy is going to drive the big new car.

S		V			O			IIIC
	Aux	v	v	D	Adj	Adj	N	IIIP; IIP (VV); IVPO
	3s	ing						W (×2)
	XY+V:VP			XY+O:NP				IIIT (×2)

12 The boy and his little sister go shopping with their mummy.

	S			V			A		IIIC
X	c	X							IVP
D	N	D	Adj	N	V	V	Pr	D	N	IIP (×2); IIIP (×2)
						ing				W
	XY+S: NP			XY+V:VP		XY+A:AP			IIIT (×3)

13 The man is putting the book there.

S		V		O		A	IVC
D	N	Aux	v	D	N		IIP (×2); IIIP
		3s	ing				W (×2)

14 The little girl is playing with her big doll.

	S		V			O			IIIC
D	Adj	N	Aux	v	part	D	Adj	N	IIIP (×3); IVP; VI+(Complex VP)
			3s	ing					W (×2)
XY+S:NP			XY+V:VP			XY+O:NP			IIIT (×3)

15 The little boy is bouncing a red ball there.

	S		V		O		A	IVC
D	Adj	N	Aux	v	D	Adj	N	IIIP (×3)
			3s	ing				W (×2)

[42] The internal structure of Initiators is not analysed further on the Chart. *Lots of* is taken as a single element, cf. *GALD*, 53.

16   The   girl   plays with the doll's house.   IIIC
     —S—   —V—   ———O———   IIP ($\times 2$); IIIP
     D   N   V   part D   N   N   W ($\times 2$)
              3s   gen   IIIT ($\times 3$)
     XY+S:NP XY+V:VP   XY+O:NP

17   Daddy   is   going out to the garden.[43]   IVC
     —S—   ——V——   —A—   ———A———   IIIP ($\times 2$)
             Aux   v   Pr D   N   W ($\times 2$)
             3s   ing

18   The girl and the boy like playing on the high swings.   IIIC
     —————————S—————————   ——V——   ——————A——————   IVP
       X   c   X   IIP ($\times 3$); IVP
      D N   D N   V   V   Pr D Adj   N   W ($\times 2$)
                            ing   pl   IIIT ($\times 3$)
         XY+S:NP   XY+V:VP   XY+A:AP

19   The little girl is   playing with her brother and his friend.   IIIC
     ——————S——————   ————V————   ——————————O——————————   IVP
                                         X   c   X   IIP ($\times 3$); IIIP ($\times 2$)
     D Adj N Aux   v   part D   N   D   N   VI+ (Complex VP)
             3s   ing   W ($\times 2$)
     XY+S:NP   XY+V:VP   XY+O:NP   IIIT ($\times 3$)

20   My mummy and her friend are going to the town today.   IVC: AAXY
     ————————S————————   ——V——   ——A——   —A—   IVP
       X   c   X   IIP ($\times 2$); IIIP ($\times 2$)
      D N   D N   Aux   v   Pr D N   W
                          ing

21   The dog   is barking at the cat.   IVC
     —S—   ——V——   ———A———   IIP; IIIP ($\times 2$)
     D   N   Aux   v   Pr D N   W ($\times 2$)
              3s   ing   IIIT ($\times 3$)
     XY+S:NP XY+V:VP XY+A:AP

Solution 14

		Analysis	*Profiling*
1	house	N	I
2	yes	Minor	I: Social
3	green	Adj	I: O
4	walking	V ing	I; W
5	(*name of cat*)	N	I
6	running	V ing	I; W
7	horse	N	I
8	? woman	N	I
9	pi (= '*water*')	N	I
10	home	N	I
11	eat	V	I
12	drink	V	I
13	straw	N	I
14	yes	Minor	I: Social
15	bird	N	I
16	? cage	N	I
17	mum	N	I
18	Unintelligible	—	Section A
19	baby	N	I
20	fire	N	I
21	mummy	N	I
22	yes	Minor	I: Social
23	bedroom	N	I
24	bed	N	I
25	Guy	N	I
26	Matthew	N	I
27	me	Pron	I: O; III P
28	John	N	I

Solution 15

		Analysis	*Profiling*
1	house	N	I
2	red house	Adj N	II P
3	window	N	I
4	blue	Adj	I O
5	trees	N pl	I; W
6	sun	N	I
7	in sun	Pr N	II P

		Analysis	*Profiling*
8	tree	N	I
9	on the grass	Pr D N	III P
10	flower	N	I
11	red and blue	Adj c Adj	IV P: XcX
12	sun	N	I
13	stalk	N	I
14	blue one	Adj Pron (indef.)	II O
15	yes	Minor	I: Social
16	me	Pron	I O; III P
17	digging	V ing	I; W
18	mummy	N	I
19	in seed	Pr N	II P
20	brown and black	Adj c Adj	IV P: XcX
21	the bag	DN	II P
22	little	Adj	I O
23	seed	N	I
24	flower	N	I
25	garden	N	I
26	yellow	Adj	I O
27	seed	N	I
28	bean	N	I
29	no	Minor	I: Social
30	green flower[44]	Adj N	II P
31	bean	N	I
32	eat	V	I
33	flower	N	I
34	water	N	I
35	wash	V	I
36	round plate	Pr N	II P
37	dry	Adj	I O
38	the plate[45]	DN	II P
39	bike	N	I
40	in garden	Pr N	II P
41	garden	N	I
42	no	Minor	I: Social
43	yes	Minor	I: Social
44	meat pie	N[46]	I

[44] As the PGSS follows the morphology and syntax of English, it would be legitimate to assign the same analysis to sign sequences, if used.

[45] T's prompt is irrelevant to the analysis in terms of Stages. It would be noted only in a micro-profile of Section B stimuli.

[46] T felt that Sam used this as a fixed item, hence N; but in view of *apple pie*, one could be justified in assigning NN. In cases of doubt, it is perhaps wisest to *underestimate* P ability.

		Analysis	*Profiling*
45	round	?Adj/Prep	I: Problem
46	Unintelligible	—	Section A
47	apple pie	N^{46}	I
48	and Nicky	c N	IV: cX
49	ride bike	V O	II C
50	yes	Minor	I: Social
51	yes	Minor	I: Social
52	sleep	V	I
53	mummy	N	I
54	drinking	V ing	I; W
55	riding	V ing	I; W
56	no	Minor	I: Social
57	no	Minor	I: Social
58	cook	V	I
59	house	N	I

Solution 16

1   plàying/
    V   I
      ing   W

2   'in the òutside/
    Pr   D   N   IIIP

3   Gùy/
    N   I

4   'making 'Guy bìke/
      V   O   IIC
         N   N   IIP
      ing   W
         X+O:NP   IIT

5   mènd   it/
    V   O   IIC
       Pron   IIIP

6   with hànds/
    Pr   N   IIP
         pl   W

7   yès/
   Minor   I: Social

8   a lètter/
     D   N   IIP

9   mùmmy/
     N   I

10   lòve 'from/
     Stereo.   I: Stereotypes

11   Màtthew/
     N   I

12   'fly the àeroplane/
     V   O   IIC
     ‾‾‾‾‾‾‾‾‾‾‾‾
         D   N   IIP
        X+O:NP   IIT

13   dèntist/
     N   I

14   'mummy 'tooth is   bròken/
          S   V   C[47]   IIIC
     ‾‾‾‾‾‾‾‾‾‾‾‾
       N   N   Cop   IIP; IIIP
                  3s   W
        XY+S:NP   IIIT

15   cròss
     Adj   IO

16   'mummy 'tooth is   òut/
          S   V   C   IIIC
     ‾‾‾‾‾‾‾‾‾‾‾‾
       N   N   Cop   IIP; IIIP
                  3s   W
        XY+S:NP   IIIT

17   'go to Bògnor/
     V   A   IIC: AX
     ‾‾‾‾‾‾‾
       Pr   N   IIP
        X+A:AP   IIT

18   àeroplane/
     N   I

19   rècords/
     N   I
        pl   W

[47] The alternative analysis of SV, with the VP analysed as Aux v, is possible; there is insufficient linguistic data to resolve the issue. But given the apparently parallel 16 below, which is clearly SVC, this analysis seems preferable (cf. also 37).

20 he's rùnning/
   S   V   IIC

     Aux   v   IIIP
     'aux   ing   W (× 3)
     3s

       X + V:VP   IIT

21 hèn/
    N   I

22 twò/
   Adj   IO

23 hèn/
    N   I

24 a bìrd/
   D N   IIP

25 mè 'saw/
    S   V   IIC
   Pron   IIIP
        ed   W
  –Pron   VI –

26 at hòme/
   Pr N   IIP

27 'in the field/
   Pr D N   IIIP

28 dòg/
    N   I

29 twò/
   Adj   IO

30 eàting/
    V   I
    ing   W

31 thànk you/
   Stereo.   I: Stereotypes

32 dòg/
    N   I

33 fàll/
    V   I

34 drinking/
    V   I
       ing   W

35 funny/
    Adj   IO

36 'be funny/
    V   C   IIC

37 'it 'is funny/
    S   V   C   IIIC
    Pron Cop   IIIP ($\times 2$)
         3s   W

38 'on my head/
    Pr D   N   IIIP

39 'on my tummy/
    Pr D   N   IIIP

40 'on my knee/
    Pr D   N   IIIP

41 'on my chair/
    Pr D   N   IIIP

42 sit/
    V   I

43 'going on the moo-cow/
    V   A   IIC: AX
        Pr D   N   IIIP
      ing   W
           X+A:AP   IIT

44 the milk/
    D N   IIP

45 is standing/[48]
    Aux   v   IIIP
    3s   ing   W ($\times 2$)

46 the 'girl is 'giving the birthday-'cake/
        S   V   O   IIIC
    D N Aux   v   D   N   IIP ($\times 2$); IIIP
             3s   ing   W ($\times 2$)
    XY+S:NP XY+V:VP   XY+O:NP   IIIT ($\times 3$)

[48] This is an interesting example of a transitional stage between I and II, technically V:VP. It is not specified separately on the Chart, as it is so uncommon.

```
47   the  'girl  is  'holding  the  flòwers/
          S        V           O              IIIC
     ───────   ──────────  ──────────
     D   N   Aux    v    D    N              IIP (×2); IIIP
             3s    ing        pl             W (×3)
     XY+S:NP  XY+V:VP  XY+O:NP               IIIT (×3)

48   the 'mummy  is  'making  the  brèad/
          S         V           O            IIIC
     ──────────  ──────────  ──────────
     D    N    Aux    v    D    N            IIP (×2); IIIP
              3s    ing                      W (×2)
     XY+S:NP   XY+V:VP   XY+O:NP             IIIT (×3)

49   'on the tàble/
     Pr  D   N                               IIIP

50   the bìrds/
     D   N                                   IIP
           pl                                W

51   wàter/
     N                                       I

52   'on the tàble/
     Pr  D   N                               IIIP

53   me/
     Pron                                    IO; IIIP

54   Gùy/
     N                                       I
```

Solution 17

```
1   On Friday  I   went  to home at twelty to four.
        A       S    V       A        A           IVCO
    ──────────  ──────  ──────────────────
    Pr   N    Pron     Pr  N  Pr  N  Pr  N        IIP (×2); IIIP; IVPO
                 ed                               W
               −Prep                              VI–O

2   My Mummy  say  Hello.
        S       V    O                            IIIC
    ──────────
    D    N                                        IIP
    XY+S:NP                                       IIIT
          −Tense                                  VI–
```

3   I   drink a cup of tea.
    S   V   O   IIIC
    Pron   D N Pr N   IIIP; IVPO
              XY+O:NP   IIIT
           −Tense   VI−

4   Kim   is   play me.
     S   V   A   IIIC
          Aux   v   IIIP
          3s   W
          XY+V:VP   IIIT
          −Tense   −Part   VI−; VI−O (×2)
          −ing

5   David is a read.
    Deviant   Section A

6   I   say's about at school.
    S   V   O⁴⁹   IIIC
    Pron V   part Pr   N   IIP (×2); IIIP
          -s   WO (add to chart)
          XY+V:VP XY+O:NP   IIIT (×2)
          −Tense   VI− (×2)
          −Concord⁵⁰

7   I   watch the television.
    S   V   O   IIIC
    Pron   D   N   IIIP; IIP
                XY+O:NP   IIIT
             −Tense   VI−

8   I   go   to bed at 9 o'clock.
    S   V   A   A   IVC: AAXY
    Pron   Pr N Pr N   Adj   IIIP; IIP; IIIPO
          −Tense   VI−

9   On Saturday I   got up at 10 o'clock.
         A   S   V   A   IVC: AAXY
    Pr   N   Pron V part Pr N   Adj   IIP (×2); IIIP; IIIPO
                     ed   W

⁴⁹ Assuming the interpretation 'talking about being at school'.
⁵⁰ First person verbs do not end in -s in her dialect.

10   I   have   a   wash.

S	V	O	IIIC
Pron		D N	IIIP; IIP
		XY+O:NP	IIIT
	−Tense		VI−

11   I   go   down stair.

S	V	A	IIIC
Pron		Pr N	IIIP; IIP
		XY+A:AP	IIIT
	−Tense	−Plural	VI−; VI−O

12   I   eat   my breakfast.

S	V	O	IIIC
Pron		D N	IIIP; IIP
		XY+O:NP	IIIT
	−Tense		VI−

13   I   go   to   up   stair.

S	V	A	IIIC
Pron		Pr Pr N	IIIP; IIIPO
		XY+A:AP	IIIT
	−Tense −Prep −Plural		VI−; VI−O (×2)

14   I was Kim is sleep.

      Deviant   Section A

    (*was*=*saw*?, coord. structure?

    or relative?)

15   My David is eat at breakfast.

S	V	O	IIIC
D N	Aux v	Pr N	IIP (×2); IIIP
	3s		W
	−Tense	−Prep	VI−; VI−O (×2)
	−ing		

16   I   went   to   the sea.

S	V	A	IIIC
Pron		Pr D N	IIIP (×2)
	ed		W
		XY+A:AP	IIIT

17 My David is swimming.   IIC
         S   V   IIP; IIIP
    ‾‾‾‾‾‾‾‾‾‾   ‾‾‾‾‾‾‾‾‾   W
    D   N   Aux   v   IIT (× 2)
                      ing   VI–
    X + S:NP   X + V:VP
              – Tense

18 Kim is swimming.   IIC
      S   V   IIIP
         ‾‾‾‾‾‾‾‾‾‾‾   W
         Aux   v   IIT
                 ing   VI–
         X + V:VP
         – Tense

19 I   go   to shop.   IIIC
    S   V   A   IIIP; IIP
              ‾‾‾‾‾‾‾‾‾   IIIT
    Pron   Pr   N   VI– (× 2)
              XY + A:AP
         – Tense   – Det

20 My buy is comie.
       Deviant   Section A

21 Kim   is playing thc ball.   IIIC
     S   V   A   IIIP; IIP
          ‾‾‾‾‾‾‾‾‾‾ ‾‾‾‾‾‾‾‾   W (× 2)
          Aux   v   D   N   IIIT (× 2)
          3s   ing   VI–; VI–O
          XY + V:VP XY + O:NP
          – Tense   – Prep

22 I   went to   home at 6 o'clock.   IVC: AAXY
    S   V   A   A   IIIP; IIP; IIIPO
    ‾‾   ‾‾‾‾‾‾‾‾   ‾‾‾‾‾‾‾‾‾‾‾‾‾‾‾   W
    Pron   Pr   N Pr N   Adj   VI–O
         ed
              – Prep

23 I   read   a   book.   IIIC
    S   V   O   IIIP; IIP
    ‾‾   ‾‾‾‾   ‾‾‾‾‾‾‾‾   W
    Pron   D   N   IIIT
         ed[51]
              XY + O:NP

[51] Giving the benefit of the doubt over *read*.

24   I   go   to bed a 9 o'clock.

      S   V   A   A   IVC: AAXY

   Pron   Pr N D N Adj   IIIP; IIP; IIIPO

         −Tense   −Det   VI− (×2)

25 On Sunday I got up a 10 o'clock.

        A   S   V   A   IVC: AAXY

   Pr   N   Pron V part D N   Adj   IIP (×2); IIIP; IIIPO

                   ed   W

                        −Det   VI−

26   I have a wash.

      S   V   O   IIIC

   Pron   D   N   IIIP; IIP

            XY + O:NP   IIIT

         −Tense   VI−

27   I   go   downstair.

      S   V   A   IIIC

   Pron   IIIP

        −Tense −Plural   VI−; VI−O

28   I   eat my breakfat.

      S   V   O   IIIC

   Pron   D   N   IIIP; IIP

            XY + O:NP   IIIT

         −Tense   VI−

29   I   went to the shop.

      S   V   A   IIIC

   Pron   Pr D   N   IIIP (×2)

         ed   W

            XY + A:AP   IIIT

30   I drink a cup of tea.

      S   V   O   IIIC

   Pron   D N Pr N   IIIP; IVPO

           XY + O:NP   IIIT

         −Tense   VI−

31   I read a book.

      S   V   O   IIIC

   Pron   D   N   IIIP; IIP

        ed   W

32 Kim   is   drink a cup of milk.   IIIC
    S   V   O

       Aux   v   D N Pr N   IIIP; IVPO
       3s   W

       XY+V:VP   XY+O:NP   IIIT ($\times 2$)
       −Tense   −ing   VI−; VI−O

33 My David is   sleep.
       S   V   IIC

    D   N   Aux   v   IIP; IIIP
             3s   W

    X+S:NP X+V:VP   IIIT ($\times 2$)
           −Tense −ing   VI−; VI−O

34 I say get up is David.
    Deviant   Section A

35 I   went   to   shop.
   S   V   A   IIIC

   Pron   Pr   N   IIIP; IIP
       ed   W

        XY+A:AP   IIIT
        −Det   VI−

36 I   went   to   home a 7 o'clock.
   S   V   A   A   IVC: AAXY

   Pron   Pr N D N Adj   IIIP; IIP; IIIPO
       ed   W
           −Prep   −Det   VI−O; VI−

37 I   went to bed at 9 o'clock.
   S   V   A   A   IVC: AAXY

   Pron   Pr N Pr N Adj   IIIP; IIP; IIIPO
       ed   W

Solution 18

1 On Friday I went home at twenty to four.
     A   S   V A   A   IVCO

   Pr   N Pron   Pr N Pr N   IIP; IIIP; IVPO
             ed   W

2   I   watched the television.
   S   V   .   O   IIIC
  Pron   D   N   IIIP; IIP
      ed   W
            XY + O:NP   IIIT

3   My dog was sleeping.
     S   V   IIC
   D N Aux   v   IIP; IIIP
      ed 3s   ing   W ($\times 3$)
  X + S:NP   X + V:VP   IIT ($\times 2$)

4   I   went to upstairs.
   S   V   A   IIIC
  Pron   Pr Adv   IIIP; IIPO
      ed   W
        XY + A:AP   IIIT
        − Prep   VI–O

5   I put on the wall.
    Problematic   Section A: Ambiguous
    (unclear whether O omitted,
    or wrong V, or wrong N)

6   I   drank a cup of coffee.
   S   V   O   IIIC
  Pron   D N Pr   N   IIP; IVPO
      ed   W
        XY + O:NP   IIIT

7   I   went   to   bed and I   went   to   sleep.
       Clause   *and*   Clause   52 VC: Coord 1; V Conn: *and*
   S   V   A   S   V   A   IIIC ($\times 2$)
  Pron   Pr   N   Pron   Pr   N   IIP ($\times 2$); IIIP ($\times 2$)
      ed   ed   W ($\times 2$)
      XY + A:AP   XY + A:AP   IIIT ($\times 2$)

8   On Saturday morning I   got up at 9 o'clock.
             A   S   V   A   IVC: AAXY
   Pr Adj   N   Pron V part Pr N   Adj   IIP; IIIP; IIIPO ($\times 2$)
                          ed   W

---

52 The parallelism suggests SVA, but one might want to argue for SV, with *went to sleep* VV.

9   I   put   on   my clothes.
    S   V   O
         V   part D   N
         ed

    XY + V:VP XY + O:NP

IIIC
IIP (× 2); IIIP
W

IIIT (× 2)

10   I   had washed.
     S   V
     Pron Aux   v
          ed   en
          X + V:VP
          − Tense

IIC
IIIP (× 2)
W (× 2)
IIT
VI−

11   I   went downstairs.
     S   V   A
     Pron
          ed

IIIC
IIIP
W

12   I   ate bacon and egg for breakfast.
     S   V   O   A
     Pron   X   c   X Pr   N
          ed

IVC
IIIP; IVP; IIP
W

13   I   took my dog for a walk.
     S   V   O   A
     Pron   D N Pr D N
          ed

IVC
IIP; IIIP (× 2)
W

14   I   read   a   book.
     S   V   O
     Pron   D   N
          ed

    XY + O:NP

IIIC
IIIP; IIP
W
IIIT

15   My father   was   in the garage.
         S   V   A
      D   N   Cop Pr D   N
                 ed, 3s

    XY + S:NP   XY + A:AP

IIIC
IIP; IIIP (× 2)
W (× 2)
IIIT (× 2)

16   My father was working the wood.
             Problematic
     (unclear whether Prep omitted, or
     replacing *the*, or whether special
     sense of *work*)

Section A: Ambiguous

17   On Saturday afternoon   I   watched the television.
           A   S   V   O   IVC
  Pr   Adj   N   Pron   D   N   IIIP (×2); IIP
                                  ed   W

18   My mother   was made   a   cake.
        S   V   O   IIIC
    D   N   Aux   v   D   N   IIP (×2); IIIP
               ed, 3s en   W (×3)
  XY+S:NP XY+V:VP XY+O:NP   IIIT (×3)
           −Tense   VI−

19   My   dog   was   cut   her   foot.
        S   V   O   IIIC
    D   N   Aux   v   D   N   IIP (×2); IIIP
               ed, 3s en   W (×3)
  XY+S:NP XY+V:VP XY+O:NP   IIIT (×3)
           −Tense   VI−

20   I   drank   a cup of tea.
    S   V   O   IIIC
  Pron   D N Pr N   IIIP; IVPO
        ed   W
             XY+O:NP   IIIT

21   My mother   say   bye.
        S   V   O   IIIC
    D   N   IIP
  XY+S:NP   IIIT
           −Tense   VI−

22   I   went   to   bed   and   I   went   to   sleep.
        Clause   and   Clause   VC: Coord 1; V Conn: and
  S   V   A   S   V   A   IIIC (×2)
  Pron   Pr   N   Pron   Pr   N   IIIP (×2); IIP (×2)
      ed   ed   W (×2)
          XY+A:AP   XY+A:AP   IIIT (×2)

23   On Sunday morning   I   got   up   at 9 o'clock.
          A   S   V   A   IVC: AAXY
  Pr   Adj   N   Pron V part Pr N   Adj   IIP; IIIP; IIIPO (×2)
                             ed   W

24   I   had washed.
   S   V
       ‾‾‾‾‾‾‾‾‾‾
   Pron Aux   v
         ed   en
        X + V:VP
       − Tense

IIC
IIIP (× 2)
W (× 2)
IIT
VI–

25   I   put   on   my clothes.
   S   V   O
      ‾‾‾‾‾‾‾‾‾‾ ‾‾‾‾‾‾‾‾‾‾
   Pron V part D   N
        ed
      XY + V:VP XY + O:NP

IIIC
IIIP; IIP (× 2)
W
IIIT (× 2)

26   I   downstairs.
   S   A
   Pron
       − Verb (verbs being well established
               elsewhere, cf. 4, 11 above)

IIC: AX
IIIP
VI–O

27   I   ate roast and cheese for breakfast.
   S V   O   A
        ‾‾‾‾‾‾‾‾‾‾ ‾‾‾‾‾‾‾‾‾‾
   Pron   X   c   X Pr   N
       ed

IVC
IVP; IIIP; IIP
W

28   My dog was for a walk.
        Problematic
   (unclear if omitted V, and if so,
   what kind)

Section A: Ambiguous

29   I   drank a cup of tea.
   S   V   O
        ‾‾‾‾‾‾‾‾‾‾
   Pron   D N Pr N
       ed
        XY + O:NP

IIIC
IIIP; IVPO
W
IIIT

30   I watched on film the television.
        Problematic
   (on = a? or = on a? or omitted Prep?)

Section A: Ambiguous

31   I wote was in the letter my friend.
        Deviant
   (unclear VP, Preps, Word order; no
   apparent normal developmental trend)

Section A

32   My father   was made   the garden.   IIIC
    S   V   O
   D N   Aux v   D N   IIP (× 2); IIIP
           ed, 3s en   W (× 3)
XY + S:NP XY + V:VP XY + O:NP   IIIT (× 3)
         − Tense   VI−; VI–O
         − Verb (= 'digging'?)

33   I saw blackbird was in the nest.
          Problematic   Section A: Ambiguous
(O clause, i.e. *saw that a* ... or
postmod., i.e. *blackbird that was* ...?)

34   My friend   was   marry.   (= 'Mary')   IIIC
    S   V   C
   D N   Cop   IIP; IIIP
         ed, 3s   W (× 2)
XY + S:NP   IIIT

35   I   played with   my friend.   IIIC
  S   V   O
Pron   V part D N   IIIP; IIP (× 2)
       ed   W
        XY + V:VP XY + A:AP   IIIT (× 2)

36   On Sunday afternoon   I   played with my dog.   IVC
         A   S   V   O
Pr Adj   N   Pron V part D N   IIIPO; IIIP; IIP (× 2)
                   ed   W

37   I   watched   the television.   IIIC
  S   V   O
Pron   D N   IIIP; IIP
   ed   W
      XY + O:NP   IIIT

38 My mother and father   are talking about   the house. [53]
         S   V   O   IIIC
   X   c   X   IVP
 D N   Aux v part D N   IIP (× 2); IIIP; VI+ (Complex VP)
                     ing   W
    XY + S:NP   XY + V:VP   XY + O:NP   IIIT (× 3)
                 − Tense   VI−

[53] Presumably not ... *talking/about* ..., which would mean 'talking in various parts of the house'.

39   I   had washed.
     S   V   IIC
     _____
     Pron Aux   v   IIIP (×2)
           ed   en   W (×2)
           X + V:VP   IIT
           − Tense   VI−

40   I   put on   my nightdress.
     S   V   O   IIIC
     _____ _____
     Pron V part D   N   IIIP; IIP (×2)
           ed   W
           XY + V:VP   XY + O:NP   IIIT (×2)

41   I went to bed and I went to sleep.
        Clause   and   Clause   VC: Coord 1; V Conn: *and*
     _____   _____
     S   V   A   S   V   A   IIIC (×2)
     _____   _____
     Pron   Pr N   Pron   Pr   N   IIIP (×2); IIP (×2)
      ed   ed   W (×2)
         XY + A:AP   XY + A:AP   IIIT (×2)

42 This morning I got up at 7 o'clock.
    _____   A   A   IVC: AAXY
       A   S   V   IIP (×2); IIIP; IIIPO
    _____ _____
    D   N   Pron V part Pr N Adj   W
                    ed

Solution 19

Developmental Profile

line
2   wàsh/
    V   I

3   bòwl/[54]
    N   I

7   yèah/
    Minor   I: Social

10 còoker/ thère
    S   A   II: AX

12 wàshing
    V   I
       ing   W

---

[54] Or, given the rising intonation, *wash bowl*, viz. VO (cf. 1.14), or VA ('wash X in the bowl'), or compound N. The above analysis seems to make the fewest assumptions.

14 'wash pòt/
    V   O   IIC

16 Unintelligible   Section A

20 'don't knôw
    Stereo.   I: Stereotypes

22 yès/
    Minor   I: Social

23 plàte/
    N   I

26 No linguistic analysis possible[55]

28 nô/
    Minor   I: Social

30 bèdroom/
    N   I

32 yès/
    Minor   I: Social

36 nò/
    Minor   I: Social

38 Hesitations not linguistically analysed[55]

41 Unintelligible   Section A

43 Unintelligible   Section A

44 kéttle/
    N   I
    and a cōoker/[56]
      c   X   IVP
          ___
        D   N   IIP

49 mèat/
    N   I

53 No analysis

55 in thère/
    Pr Adv   IIO

57 nó/
    Minor   I: Social

[55] One could add an extra section to Section A Unanalysed, if needed.

[56] Given the rising intonation and pause, an analysis of N c N is possible; again, one makes the analysis with the fewest assumptions.

58 lòrries/
   N   I
     pl   W

59 'lot of 'noisy lòrries/
   I   Adj   N   IVPO; VI+ (Initiator)
                  pl   W

62 No analysis

64 yèah/
   Minor   I: Social

65 Unintelligible

66 'one lòrry / bròke/ their tràbs/
      S   V   O   IIIC
  Adj   N   D   N   IIP ($\times 2$)
            ed   pl   W ($\times 2$)
  XY+S:NP   XY+O:NP   IIIT ($\times 2$)
                 –Concord   VI–

68 bròke/ their tràbs/—
   V   O   IIC
        D   N   IIP
  ed   pl   W ($\times 2$)
     X+O:NP   IIT

70 tràbs/
   N   I
     pl   W

73 yéah/
   Minor   I: Social

75 twò 'mans/ mènded it/[57]
      S   V   O   IIIC
  Adj   N   Pron   IIP; IIIP
        pl   ed   W ($\times 2$)
  XY+S:NP   IIIT
   –N$_{irreg}$ VI–

77 yès/
   Minor   I: Social

78 'in (a) mòrning/
  Pr D   N   IIIP

[57] Self-corrections are not analysed.

80	'very 'very dăngerous/	
	Int Int Adj	IIIPO
82	nò/	
	Minor	I: Social
83	tràbs/	
	N	I
	pl	W
86	'[bɪn] bróken/	
	Ambiguous[58]	Section A

Solution 19

Sections B and C

1	T	'what's thàt/	Question
	P	wásh/—	Struct. Abnorm. (one expects N)
		bòwl/	Spont. 1
	T	'why is it a 'good i'dea to 'have that	
5		'next to your còoker/———	Question Ø response
		it ìs a good idéa/ *ìsn't it/	Other (* indicates P speaks at this point)
	P	*yèah/	Minor
	T	whỳ is it/———	Question Ø response
		ḿm/	Other (discount intonation, cf. p. 40)
10	P	còoker/ thère/—	Struct. Abnorm. (*because*-clause expected)
	T	'what would you 'do in hère/	Question
	P	wàshing/	Elliptical 1
	T	'wash whàt/	Question
	P	'wash pòt/	Elliptical 2
15	T	yèah/	Other
	P	(*1 syll*)	Unintelligible
	T	òh/—	No stimulus (insufficient content/pause)
		'what's happened hère/—	No stimulus (insufficient pause)
		'look what's hàppened/—	Other
20	P	'don't knôw/———	Minor (given the analysis of Stereotypes)
	T	'what about having 'something to èat off/	Question
	P	yès/	Minor
		plàte/	Spont. 1
	T	ḿ/	No stimulus

[58] *Bin* does not seem to fit the context; *been* is unlikely, given the overall language level, as it would have to be analysed as Passive (Stage VI).

25		'somewhere to 'put your plàte/	No stimulus
	P	(*laughs*)	No analysis (not language; but cf. p. 25)
	T	would thìs be āny 'good in this róom/	Question
	P	nô/	Minor
	T	whỳ/	Question
30	P	bèdroom/———	Struct. Abnorm. (*because-* clause expected)
	T	you mean 'this belòngs in the 'bedroom	Other
	P	yès/	Minor
	T	whỳ does it/———	Question Ø response
		it dóesn't/ .	No stimulus
35		it belóngs in the kìtchen/	Other
	P	nò/	Minor
	T	'why nòt/	Question
	P	er	Ø response (from a grammatical viewpoint)
	T	yès	No stimulus
40		we'll 'have it in the kìtchen/ (*sylls*)	Other
	P	(*3 sylls*)——(*2 sylls*)	Unintelligible (× 2)
	T	(*sylls*) nòw/ 'let's put 'that — thère/———	Other
	P	(*3 sylls*)	Unintelligible
		kèttle/—	Spont. 1
45		and a cōoker/	Spont. Other (the *and* is structurally distinct from the clausal element to which it connects)
	T	'what're you dōing/—	No stimulus (insufficient pause)
		òh/—	No stimulus (insufficient content/pause)
		'what's thàt/	Question
	P	mèat/	Elliptical 1
50	T	ìs it/—	No stimulus (insufficient pause)
		'where wàs it/———	Question Ø response
		'where was the mèat/—	Question
	P	er	Ø response
	T	'where wàs	Question
55	P	in thère/	Elliptical 1
		… …	
	T	does the ⌐tréet/—	Question
	P	nó/—	Minor
		lòrries/	Spont.1
		'lot of ⌐s/	Spont. 1 (only 1 *clausal* element)
60	T	ôh/	No stimulus (insufficient content/pause)
		is it a 'big 'main ròad thén/	Question

P	er	Ø response
T	Nòtown/ ìsn't it/	Question
P	yèah/	Minor
65	[na:]	Unintelligible
	'one lòrry/ bròke/ their tràbs/	Spont. Other
T	'one 'lorry whát/	Question
P	bròke/ their tràbs/—	Elliptical 2
T	'broke their whàt/	Question
70	P tràbs/	Elliptical 1
T	òh/—	No stimulus
	'outside your hòuse/	Other
P	yéah/	Minor
T	'what happened thèn/——	Question
75	P màn/—twò 'mans/ mènded it/——	Full Major
T	'did they 'come straight awày/—	Question
P	yès/——	Minor
	'in (a) mòrning/	Spont. 1
T	'what did the drìver do 'all that 'time/——	Question
80	P 'very 'very dǎngerous/	Struct. Abnorm.
T	whàt/	No stimulus (insufficient pause)
	lǒrries/	Other (discount intonation, cf. p. 40)
P	nò/	Minor
	tràbs/	Spont. 1
85	T whỳ are they 'dangerous/—	Question
P	'[bɪn] bróken/	Problem
T	òh/	No stimulus

Solution 20D

Developmental Profile

line

2   'open   my   prèsent   'up/ . on 'Christmas Dáy/[59]

	V		O			A		IIIC
	V-	D	N	-part	Pr	N	N	IIP (×2); IIIPO
	XY+V:VP	XY+O:NP				XY+A:AP		IIIT (×3)

5   'very exci—ex . excìted/—
   Int   Adj   IIP (Int X)

7   *erm yès/
    Minor   I: Social

[59] Given the different use of *Christmas* below, it seems reasonable to analyse this as NN, rather than as a single compound N.

8   erm — 'at 'Christmas Dáy/
       Pr   N   N   IIIPO

10   Christmas . 'present and dínner/——
         X   c   X   IVP
      N   N   IIP

11   and 'play with 'my . Christmas présent/—
  and   V   O   V Conn: *and*; IIC
       V   part D   N   N   IIP; IIIPO
      X+V:VP   X+O:NP   IIT (× 2)

13   a bíke/
    D N   IIP

15   *yès/
    Minor   I: Social

18   don't knòw/[60]——
    Stereo.   I: Stereotypes

21   'on the strèet/—
    Pr D   N   IIIP

22   not allōwed   ['on . 'ride it 'on the gra . er]   'ride it
        V   O   IIIC
    Neg   V   . . .   . . .   V Pron IVPO (Neg VV); VI+ (Complex VP)
          en   W
    Passive   VI+
    XY+V:VP   IIIT
    on the gráss/ .[61]
       A
    Pr D   N   IIIP
    XY+A:AP   IIIT

24   kill . the 'grass/
     V   O   IIC
        D   N   IIP
        X+O:NP   IIT

[60] This still seems the stereotyped utterance of Profile A (1.20): Neg is used elsewhere, but until Aux comes into evidence, it would be unwise to credit P with the structures involved.

[61] The syntactic disfluency can be ignored, as it clearly anticipates the following structure. In this dialect, deletion of *to* before *ride* would be possible, and is therefore not a Stage VI Error.

28   mùmmy/ and dáddy/ and mé/ and Màry/.
    X   c   X   IVP
                X   c   X   IVP
                          X   c   X   IVP
                     Pron   IIIP

29   àll 'family/
    I   N   IIPO; VI+ (Initiator)
        – Det   VI–

32   m̀/
    Minor   I: Social

34   béans/—
    N   I
     pl   W

35   cábbages/—
    N   I
       pl   W

36   ānd
    Incomplete   Section A

37   'don't knòw/—
    Stereo.   I: Stereotypes

38   cábbages/.
    N   I
       pl   W

39   béans/.
    N   I
       pl   W

42   yès/
    Minor   I: Social

47   séll/. càravan . 'things/
    V   O   IIC
         N   N   IIP
             pl   W
    X+O:NP   IIT

51   erm '[houdz] mán/ séll/—càravan thíngs/
    Ambiguous (first item = Adj?)   Section A

53   ànybody/
    Pron   IO; IIIP

54   (2̃ *sylls*)—
      Unintelligible   Section A

55   lòt of——of——'mans—'sell cáravan 'things/
                    S   V   O   IIIC
      ‾‾‾‾‾‾‾‾‾‾‾‾‾‾‾‾‾‾‾‾‾‾‾‾‾‾   ‾‾‾‾‾‾‾‾‾‾‾‾‾‾
      D   N   N   N   IIP (× 2)
                           pl   pl   W (× 2)
      — Det   — N$_{irreg}$ VI– (× 2)

59   nò/
      Minor   I: Social

63   yès/
      Minor   I: Social

65   and—'feel . a   snów/—
      and   V   O   V Conn: *and*; IIC
               ‾‾‾‾‾‾‾‾‾‾‾‾
               D   N   IIP
            X + O:NP   IIT
            — Det   VI–

66   and . 'cut   the   'trees   'down for Christmas/——
      and   V   O   A   V Conn: *and*; IIIC
            ‾‾‾‾‾‾‾‾‾‾‾‾‾‾‾‾‾‾‾‾‾‾   ‾‾‾‾‾‾‾‾‾‾‾‾‾‾‾‾
            V-   D   N   -part Pr   N   IIP (× 3)
                           pl   W
         XY + V:VP   XY + O:NP   XY + A:AP   IIIT (× 3)

67   and . cárs/ 'cover snów/——
      and S   V   O   V Conn: *and*; IIIC
             pl   W
           — Word Order[62]   VI–

68   and . the . 'two 'mans—'move a—the—the 'car—
      and   S   V   O   V Conn: *and*; IVC
            ‾‾‾‾‾‾‾‾‾‾‾‾‾‾‾‾   ‾‾‾‾‾‾‾‾‾‾‾‾
            D   Adj   N   D   N   IIIP; IIP
                      pl   W
            — N$_{irreg}$ VI–
      'off 'the snów/
          A
      ‾‾‾‾‾‾‾‾‾‾‾‾
      Pr   D   N   IIIP

72   yès/
      Minor   I: Social

75   yès/
      Minor   I: Social

---

[62] Alternatively, one could see this as an attempt at a passive, but this is less likely, given his linguistic performance elsewhere.

77   it's rāinīng/ it's pōurīng/   I: Stereotypes
         Stereo.

79   whàt/ —   Question I
         Q

80   'looking 'out 'of the wìndow/ —   IIC: AX
         V   A
         ―――――――――――――――――
              Pr   D   N   IIIP
         ing   W
              XY + A:AP   IIIT

82   be'cause . the . ràin 'came 'down/————   V Conn: s; IIC
         s   S   V
         ―――――――――――――――――――――
              D   N   V   part   IIP (×2)
                        ed   W
              X + S:NP   X + V:VP   IIT (×2)

83   'that wāter/   IIC
         S   C

Solution 20

Sections B and C

	T	'what are you 'going to dò in the 'holidays/ ——	Question
	P	'open my prèsent 'up/ . on 'Christmas Dáy/	Ellipt. 3
	T	'open your prèsent/ .	No stimulus
		ôh/	Other
5	P	'very exci . ex . excìted/ —	Ellipt. 1
	T	yòu *áre/	Other
	P	*erm yès/	Minor
		erm — 'at 'Christmas Dáy/	Spont. 1
	T	(*laughs*) what èlse do you 'do on 'Christmas 'Day/ ——	Question
10	P	Chrìstmas . 'present and dínner/ ——	Struct. Abn.
		and . 'play with 'my . Chrìstmas présent/ —	Spont. Other
	T	'what do you 'think you're 'going to gèt/	Question
	P	a bìke/	Ellipt. 1
	T	do you knòw that you're 'going to *'get a bíke/ ——	Question
15	P	*yès/	Minor
	T	ôh/ ——	No stimulus
		'where will you rìde/ —	Question
	P	don't knòw/ ——	Ellipt. 1
	T	can you 'ride in your gǎrden/ or 'will you have	

20		to 'ride on the strèet/—	Question
	P	'on the strèet/—	Ellipt. 1
		not allòwed 'on . 'ride it 'on the gra . er 'ride it 'on the gráss/ .	Spont. Other
		kìll . the 'grass/	Spont. Other
25	T	ôh/—	No stimulus
		m̀/—	No stimulus
		'who does the 'garden in yòur house/—	Question
	P	mùmmy/ and dáddy/ and mé/ and Màry/ .	Ellipt. 1[63]
		àll 'family/	Spont. 1
30	T	àll the 'family 'does/—	No stimulus
		oh gòod/	Other
	P	m̀/	Minor
	T	'what do you gròw in your 'garden/—	Question
	P	bèans/—	Ellipt. 1
35		cábbages/———	Spont. 1
		ānd	Incomplete
		'don't knòw/—	Spont. 1
		cábbages/ .	Spont. 1
		bèans/ .	Spont. 1
40	T	m̄/——	No stimulus
		'lots of vègetables/	Other
	P	yès/	Minor
	T	m̀/	No stimulus
		'jolly gôod/ .	No stimulus
45		'what does your dàddy 'do/—	No stimulus
		'what 'kind of wòrk/	Question
	P	sell/ . càravan . 'things/	Ellipt. 2
	T	dôes he/———	No stimulus
		does he 'have to 'go awày . to do thát/ or	
50		'does he 'do it at hòmc/	Question
	P	erm '[houdz] mán/ séll/—càravan thíngs/	Full major[64]
	T	m̀/	Other
	P	ànybody/	Problem[65]
		(2 sylls)—	Unintelligible
55		lòt of——of——— 'mans—'sell cáravan 'things/	Spont. Other
	T	m̀/	No stimulus
		òh yes/——	No stimulus
		'does he 'sell the căravan/—	Question
	P	nò/	Minor
60	T	nó/—	No stimulus
		whàt/—	No stimulus
		'just the 'things to gò in the cáravan/	Other
	P	yès/	Minor
	T	I sèe/	No stimulus

... ...

[63] Assuming that this is best analysed as one complex Subject.

[64] The ambiguity does not affect its Response status, in terms of elements of clause structure.

[65] It is unclear what this might be an elision of, hence not analysed as Elliptical 1.

65   P   and — 'feel . a snów/ *describing a picture of a*
                                  wintry scene
           and . 'cut the 'trees 'down for Chrístmas/— —   Spont. Other
           and . cárs/ 'cover snów/— —   Spont. Other
           and . the . 'two 'mans — 'move a — the — the 'car Spont. Other
           — 'off 'the snów/
70   T   m̀/   No stimulus
           'moving the snòw óff/   Other
      P   yès/   Minor
      T   yès/ .   No stimulus
           have you 'ever been 'stuck in the snów/ .   Question
75   P   yès/   Minor
      T   m̀/— — —   Other
      P   it's rāinīng/ it's pōurīng/   Problem⁶⁶
      T   I 'wonder what that bòy's 'doing/   Other
      P   whàt/—   Struct. Abn.
80   'looking 'out 'of the window/—   Spont. Other
      T   I 'wonder why hè 'has to 'stay in/— —   Other
      P   be'cause . the . ràin 'came 'down/— — —   Ellipt. 3
           'that wāter/   Spont. Other

Solution 21

A   Tot. Sentences 7   (lines 3, 7, 10, 12, 14, 15, 21)
     Tot. S per Turn 7/6 = 1·16   (T stimuli 2, 6, 9, 11, 13, 20)
     MSL 8 words/7 = 1·14

B   Tot. Sentences 37   (2, 5, 7, 8, 10, 11, 13, 15, 18, 21, 22–3, 24,
                                         28, 29, 32, 34, 35, 37, 38, 39, 42, 47, 53,
                                         55, 59, 63, 65, 66, 67, 68, 72, 75, 77, 79,
                                         80, 82, 83)
     Tot. S per Turn 37/22 = 1·68   (T stimuli 1, 4, 6, 9, 12, 14, 17, 19–20, 27,
                                         31, 33, 41, 46, 49–50, 52, 58, 62, 71, 74,
                                         76, 78, 81)
     MSL 114 words/37 = 3·1   (NB only 2 words counted in 5; hesitation
                                         ignored in 7, 8, etc.; only 'not allowed
                                         . . . ride it on the grass' counted in 22;
                                         minor vocalization is counted, 32; *and*
                                         ignored, 36; 51, 54, ignored; first *of*
                                         ignored, 55; *a–the* ignored in 68)

---

⁶⁶ After a long pause, P produces a stereotyped utterance. It is difficult to be sure whether the response is best classified as Minor or Structural Abnormality—hence Problem.

References

ALGEO, J. 1974: *Exercises in contemporary English*. New York: Harcourt Brace Jovanovich.

AMES, L. B. 1946: The development of the sense of time in the young child. *J. Genet. Psychol.* **68**, 97–125.

ANTINUCCI, F. and MILLER, R. 1976: How children talk about what happened. *J. Ch. Lang.* **3**, 167–90.

BAX, M. C. O. and STEVENSON, P. 1977: Analysis of a developmental language delay. *Proc. Roy. Soc. Med.* **70**, 727–8.

BENCH, J. and BAMFORD, J. M. (eds.) 1978: *Speech-hearing tests and the spoken language of partially-hearing children*. New York and London: Academic Press.

BENEDICT, H. 1979: Early lexical development: comprehension and production. *J. Ch. Lang.* **6 (2)**.

BLANK, M. 1973: *Teaching learning in the preschool: a dialogue approach*. Columbus: Merrill.

— 1974: Cognitive functions of language in the preschool years. *Dev. Psych.* **10**, 229–45.

BLOOM, L. 1970: *Language development: form and function in emerging grammars*. Cambridge, Mass.: MIT Press.

— 1973: *One word at a time*. The Hague: Mouton.

— 1974: Talking, understanding and thinking. In R. L. Schiefelbusch and L. L. Lloyd (eds.), *Language perspectives—acquisition, retardation and intervention*. Baltimore: University Park Press.

BRAINE, M. D. S. 1963: The ontogeny of English phrase structure: the first phase. *Language* **39**, 1–14.

BRANNON, J. B. and MURRAY, T. 1966: The spoken syntax of normal, hard-of-hearing and deaf children. *JSHR* **9**, 604–10.

BRONCKART, J. and SINCLAIR, H. 1973: Time, tense and aspect. *Cognition* **2**, 107–30.

BROWN, R. 1973: *A first language*. Cambridge, Mass.: Harvard University Press.

BROWN, R. and BELLUGI, U. 1965: Three processes in the child's acquisition of syntax. In P. H. Mussen, J. J. Conger and J. Kagan (eds.), *Readings in child development and personality*. 2nd edn, New York: Harper & Row.

BROWN, R. and FRASER, C. 1964: *The acquisition of language*. Chicago: Chicago University Press.

BRUNER, J. 1974: Organization of early skilled action. In M. P. M. Richards (ed.), *The integration of a child into a social world.* Cambridge: Cambridge University Press.

— 1975: The ontogenesis of speech acts. *J. Ch. Lang.* **2**, 1–19.

BUSHNELL, E. W. and ASLIN, R. N. 1977: Inappropriate expansion: a demonstration of a methodology for child language research. *J. Ch. Lang.* **4**, 115–22.

CARTER, A. L. 1975: The transformation of sensorimotor morphemes into words: a case study of the development of 'more' and 'mine'. *J. Ch. Lang.* **2**, 233–50.

CLARK, E. 1973: What's in a word? On the child's acquisition of semantics in his first language. In T. E. Moore (ed.), *Cognitive development and the acquisition of language.* New York: Academic Press.

CLARK, H. H. 1973: Space, time, semantics, and the child. In T. E. Moore (ed.), *Cognitive development and the acquisition of language.* New York: Academic Press.

CLARK, H. H. and CLARK, E. V. 1977: *Psychology and language.* New York: Harcourt Brace Jovanovich.

CLARK, R. 1974: Performing without competence. *J. Ch. Lang.* **1**, 1–10.

CLARK, R., HUTCHESON, S. and VAN BUREN, P. 1974: Comprehension and production in language acquisition. *JL* **10**, 39–54.

CONN, P. 1971: *Language therapy 1: remedial syntax.* London: Invalid Children's Aid Association.

CONNOLLY, J. H. 1977: The selection of a suitable linguistics course for student speech therapists. *Midland Association for Linguistic Studies Journal*, New Series **2**, 99–104.

COOK, V. J. 1976: A note on indirect objects. *J. Ch. Lang.* **3**, 435–7.

CORRIGAN, R. 1978: Language development as related to stage 6 object permanence development. *J. Ch. Lang.* **5**, 173–89.

CRITCHLEY, M. 1970: *Aphasiology and other aspects of language.* London: Edward Arnold.

CROMER, R. F. 1975: An experimental investigation of a putative linguistic universal: marking and the indirect object. *J. Exp. Ch. Psychol.* **20**, 73–80.

CRUSE, D. A. 1977: A note on the learning of colour names. *J. Ch. Lang.* **4**, 305–11.

CRYSTAL, D. 1966: Specification and English tenses. *JL* **2**, 1–34.

— 1975: *The English tone of voice.* London: Edward Arnold.

— 1976: *Child language, learning and linguistics.* London: Edward Arnold.

— 1979: Prosodic development. In P. Fletcher and M. Garman (eds.), *Language acquisition: studies in first language development.* Cambridge: Cambridge University Press.

CRYSTAL, D. and DAVY, D. 1976: *Advanced conversational English.* London: Longman.

CRYSTAL, D. and FLETCHER, P. 1978: Profile analysis of language disability. In C. Fillmore and W. Wang (eds.), *Individual differences in language ability and language behavior.* New York: Academic Press.

CRYSTAL, D., FLETCHER, P. and GARMAN, M. 1976: *The grammatical analysis of language disability: a procedure for assessment and remediation.* Studies in Language Disability and Remediation 1. London: Edward Arnold.

DARLEY, F. L. and WINITZ, H. 1961: Age of first word: review of research. *JSHD* **26**, 272–90.

DERWING, B. 1977: Is the child really a 'little linguist'? In J. Macnamara (ed.), *Language, learning and thought.* New York: Academic Press.

DERWING, B. and BAKER, W. 1979: Recent research on the acquisition of English morphology. In P. Fletcher and M. Garman (eds.), *Language acquisition: studies in first language development.* Cambridge: Cambridge University Press.

DEVER, R. B. and BAUMANN, P. M. 1974: Scale of children's clausal development. In T. M. Longhurst (ed.), *Linguistic analysis of children's speech: readings.* New York: MSS Information Corporation, 280–320.

DONALDSON, M. and BALFOUR, G. 1968: Less is more: a study of language comprehension in children. *B. J. Psych.* **59**, 461–72.

DORE, J., FRANKLIN, M. P., MILLER, R. T. and RAMER, A. L. H. 1976: Transitional phenomena in early language acquisition. *J. Ch. Lang.* **3**, 13–28.

ENGLER, L. F., HANNAH, E. P. and LONGHURST, T. M. 1973: Linguistic analysis of speech samples: a practical guide for clinicians. *JSHD* **38**, 192–204.

ERVIN, S. 1964: Imitation and structural change in children's language. In E. Lenneberg (ed.), *New directions in the study of language.* Cambridge, Mass.: MIT Press.

FAY, D. 1978: Transformations as mental operations: a reply to Kuczaj. *J. Ch. Lang.* **5**, 143–9.

FERGUSON, C. 1976: Learning to pronounce: the earliest stages of phonological development in the child. *Stanford Papers and Reports on Child Language Development* **11**, 1–27.

FLETCHER, P. 1979: The development of the verb phrase. In P. Fletcher and M. Garman (eds.), *Language acquisition: studies in first language development.* Cambridge: Cambridge University Press.

GLEITMAN, L. R., GLEITMAN, H. and SHIPLEY, E. 1972: The emergence of the child as grammarian. *Cognition* **1**, 137–64.

GOLDIN-MEADOW, S., SELIGMAN, M. E. P. and GELMAN, R. 1976: Language in the two-year-old. *Cognition* **4**, 189–202.

GOODGLASS, H., FODOR, I. G. and SCHULHOFF, C. 1967: Prosodic factors in grammar—evidence from aphasia. *JSHR* **10**, 5–20.

GRAHAM, N. C. 1968: Short-term memory and syntactic structure in educationally subnormal children. *Lg. and Sp.* **11**, 209–19.

GRUNWELL, P. 1975: Trends in teaching speech pathology: linguistics. *Bulletin of the College of Speech Therapists* **281**, 5–8.

HABER, L. 1977: A linguistic definition of language delay: evidence from the acquisition of AUX. Paper presented at the Linguistic Society of America Summer Meeting.

HARNER, L. 1976: Children's understanding of linguistic reference to past and future. *J. Psycholing. Res.* **5**, 65–84.

HINE, W. D. 1970: Verbal ability and partial hearing loss. *Teacher of the Deaf* **68**, 450–59.

HOWE, C. J. 1976: The meanings of two-word utterances in the speech of young children. *J. Ch. Lang.* **3**, 29–47.

HUTTENLOCHER, J. 1974: The origins of language comprehension. In R. L. Solso (ed.), *Theories in cognitive psychology.* New York: Erlbaum.

HUXLEY, R. 1970: The development of the correct use of subject personal pronouns in two children. In G. B. Flores d'Arcais and W. J. M. Levelt (eds.), *Advances in psycholinguistics.* Amsterdam: North-Holland, 141–65.

JOOS, M. (ed.) 1958: *Readings in linguistics.* New York: American Council of Learned Societies.

KARMILOFF-SMITH, A. 1979: Language development after five. In P. Fletcher and M. Garman (eds.), *Language acquisition: studies in first language development.* Cambridge: Cambridge University Press.

KLIMA, E. and BELLUGI, U. 1966: Syntactic regularities in the speech of children. In J. Lyons and R. Wales (eds.), *Psycholinguistic papers.* Edinburgh: Edinburgh University Press.

KUCZAJ, S. A. 1976: Arguments against Hurford's 'Aux Copying Rule'. *J. Ch. Lang.* **3**, 423–6.

— 1978: Why do children fail to overgeneralize the progressive inflection? *J. Ch. Lang.* **5**, 167–71.

LACKNER, J. R. 1968: A developmental study of language behaviour in retarded children. *Neuropsychologia* **6**, 301–30.

LEA, J. 1970: *The colour pattern scheme: a method of remedial language teaching.* Oxted, Surrey: Moor House School.

LEE, L. L. 1966: Developmental sentence types: a method for comparing normal and deviant syntactic development. *JSHD* **31**, 311–30.

LEOPOLD, W. 1949: *Speech development of a bilingual child* **4**. Evanston, Ill.: Northwestern University Press.

LIMBER, J. 1973: The genesis of complex sentences. In T. E. Moore (ed.), *Cognitive development and the acquisition of language.* New York: Academic Press, 169–85.

— 1976: Unravelling competence, performance and pragmatics in the speech of young children. *J. Ch. Lang.* **3**, 309–18.

LITOWITZ, B. 1977: Learning how to make definitions. *J. Ch. Lang.* **4**, 289–304.

LLOYD, P. and DONALDSON, M. 1976: On a method of eliciting true/false judgements from young children. *J. Ch. Lang.* **3**, 411–16.

LUST, B. 1977: Conjunction reduction in child language. *J. Ch. Lang.* **4**, 257–87.

MARATSOS, M. P. 1976: *The use of definite and indefinite reference in young children.* London: Cambridge University Press.

MCCARTHY, D. 1954: Language development in children. In L. Carmichael (ed.), *Manual of child psychology.* 2nd edn, New York: Wiley.

MCNEILL, D. 1970: *The acquisition of language: the study of developmental psycholinguistics.* New York: Harper & Row.

NAREMORE, R. C. and DEVER, R. B. 1975: Language performance of educable mentally retarded and normal children at five age levels. *JSHR* **18**, 82–95.

NELSON, K. E. 1973: Structure and strategy in learning to talk. *Monogr. Soc. Res. Ch. Devel.* **38**.

NELSON, K. E., CARSKADDON, G. and BONVILLIAN, J. D. 1973: Syntax acquisition: impact of experimental variation in adult verbal interaction with the child. *Ch. Dev.* **44**, 497–504.

NUSSBAUM, N. and NAREMORE, R. 1975: On the acquisition of present perfect 'have' in normal children. *Lg. and Sp.* **18**, 219–26.

O'CONNOR, J. D. and ARNOLD, G. F. 1973: *Intonation of colloquial English.* 2nd edn, London: Longman.

OWRID, H I 1960: Measuring spoken language in young deaf children. *Teacher of the Deaf* **58**, 24–34, 124–8.

PALMER, F. R. 1974: *The English verb.* 2nd edn, London: Longman.

PIAGET, J. 1962: *Play, dreams and imitation.* Trans. C. Gattegno and F. M. Hodgson. New York: Norton.

QUIRK, R. and GREENBAUM, S. 1973: *A university grammar of English.* London: Longman.

QUIRK, R., GREENBAUM, S., LEECH, G. and SVARTVIK, J. 1972: *A grammar of contemporary English.* London: Longman.

REES, N. (forthcoming): *The production and comprehension of speech.* London: Edward Arnold.

REICH, P. A. 1976: The early acquisition of word meaning. *J. Ch. Lang.* **3**, 117–23.

RICHARDS, M. M. 1979: Adjective ordering in the language of young children: an experimental investigation. *J. Ch. Lang.* **6 (2)**.

RIEKE, J. A., LYNCH, L. L. and SOLTMAN, S. F. 1977: *Teaching strategies for language development.* New York: Grune and Stratton.

ROBINS, R. H. 1971: *General linguistics: an introductory survey.* London: Longman.

RODGON, M. M. 1976: *Single-word usage, cognitive development and the beginnings of combinatorial speech: a study of ten English-speaking children.* Cambridge: Cambridge University Press.

SACHS, J. and DEVIN, J. 1976: Young children's use of age-appropriate speech styles in social interaction and role-playing. *J. Ch. Lang.* **3**, 81–98.

SIEGEL, S. 1956: *Non-parametric statistics for the behavioural sciences*. New York: McGraw-Hill.

SLOBIN, D. I. and WELSH, C. A. 1968: Elicited imitation as a research tool in developmental psycholinguistics. Working Paper 10, Language Behavior Research Laboratory, University of California, Berkeley. Reprinted in C. A. Ferguson and D. I. Slobin (eds.), *Studies of child language development* (New York: Holt, Rinehart & Winston, 1973), 485–97.

SMITH, M. E. 1926: *An investigation of the development of the sentence and the extent of vocabulary in young children*. University of Iowa Studies in Child Welfare **3**.

SNOW, C. 1977: The development of conversation between mothers and babies. *J. Ch. Lang.* **4**, 1–22.

STARK, R. E. 1979: Prespeech segmental feature development. In P. Fletcher and M. Garman (eds.), *Language acquisition: studies in first language development*. Cambridge: Cambridge University Press.

TERVOORT, B. 1970: The understanding of passive sentences by deaf children. In G. B. Flores d'Arcais and W. J. M. Levelt (eds.), *Advances in psycholinguistics*. Amsterdam: North-Holland, 166–73.

TYACK, D. and INGRAM, D. 1977: Children's production and comprehension of questions. *J. Ch. Lang.* **4**, 211–24.

WARDEN, D. A. 1976: The influence of context on children's use of identifying expressions and references. *B. J. Psych.* **67**, 101–12.

WEBER, J. and WEBER, S. 1976: Early acquisition of linguistic designations for time. *Lg. and Sp.* **19**, 276–84.

WINER, B. J. 1962: *Statistical principles in experimental design*. New York: McGraw-Hill.

Index (names)

Index (subjects)

vocabulary development 119–31, 143, 153, 175, 178, 183–5, 196–7, 202, 205, 208, 232, 240, 245–6
vocalization 119–30, 183
vocative 62, 114
V Part 66–7, 73–4, 108, 110, 173, 187, 199, 208, 216, 221, 236
VV 66, 73–4, 108, 165, 187, 216, 236

Wepman 146
WISC 145, 157, 246–7
Woodford Trust 218
word
    first 124–5, 129–31
    order 63, 97, 99, 101, 102, 113, 210, 216, 223, 225

structure 5, 53, 64, 84–7, 110, 156, 158–60, 165–6, 172, 175, 183, 188, 190, 193, 198, 215, 229, 234, 239, 251–4, 257, 261, 271–4, 278–9, 283, 293
types 123, 130, 153, 165, 175–6, 280, 284
writing, analysis of 24, 33, 104, 153, 177–8, 215–16, 218–19, 284

XcX 73, 79–81, 93–4, 98, 108, 229, 251

zero reaction 57–60
zero response 35, 40, 42–4, 50, 51, 305

3s 86, 170, 199, 216, 223, 229, 260